Mathematical Models in Biomedical Science

Mathematical Models in Biomedical Science

Editor: Duncan Chambers

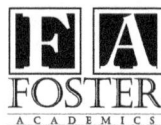

FOSTER
ACADEMICS

www.fosteracademics.com

www.fosteracademics.com

FA FOSTER
ACADEMICS

Cataloging-in-Publication Data

Mathematical models in biomedical science / edited by Duncan Chambers.
       p. cm.
Includes bibliographical references and index.
ISBN 978-1-63242-889-9
1. Medical sciences--Mathematical models. 2. Medical sciences. 3. Biomedical engineering. I. Chambers, Duncan.
R129 .M38 2020
610--dc23

Foster Academics,
118-35 Queens Blvd., Suite 400,
Forest Hills, NY 11375, USA

ISBN 978-1-63242-889-9 (Hardback)

Contents

Permissions

List of Contributors

Index

Preface

This book has been an outcome of determined endeavour from a group of educationists in the field. The primary objective was to involve a broad spectrum of professionals from diverse cultural background involved in the field for developing new researches. The book not only targets students but also scholars pursuing higher research for further enhancement of the theoretical and practical applications of the subject.

The field of biomedical science studies the mechanisms that are at the core of the function and formation of living organisms. It ranges in scope from the study of individual molecules to complex human functions. This contributes to our understanding of how different diseases, traumas and genetic defects alter physiological and behavioral processes. Modern biomedical science works at the cellular, molecular and systems level with the aid of techniques of molecular biology and genome characterization. Such studies have implications on potential medical therapies and clinical studies, and the understanding of disease mechanisms. The integration of mathematics with biomedical sciences has led to many such applications and innovations. Mathematical modeling and analysis, optimization techniques and computational methods, numerical analysis, applied statistics or a combination of these are used for solving problems in this field. Mathematical models and methods also form the basis for the construction of imaging techniques in biomedical science. This has transformed the practice of medicine and furthered the scope of non-invasive diagnosis and surgical planning for guiding surgery, biopsy and radiation therapy. The field of biomedical science and engineering has undergone rapid development over the past few decades. This book elucidates the mathematical concepts and models that have led to advancements in biomedical science. It is an essential guide for both academicians and those who wish to pursue this discipline further.

It was an honour to edit such a profound book and also a challenging task to compile and examine all the relevant data for accuracy and originality. I wish to acknowledge the efforts of the contributors for submitting such brilliant and diverse chapters in the field and for endlessly working for the completion of the book. Last, but not the least; I thank my family for being a constant source of support in all my research endeavours.

Editor

Phase Synchronization Dynamics of Neural Network during Seizures

Hao Liu ⓘ **and Puming Zhang** ⓘ

School of Biomedical Engineering, Shanghai Jiao Tong University, Shanghai 200240, China

Correspondence should be addressed to Puming Zhang; pmzhang@sjtu.edu.cn

Academic Editor: Michele Migliore

Epilepsy has been considered as a network-level disorder characterized by recurrent seizures, which result from network reorganization with evolution of synchronization. In this study, the brain networks were established by calculating phase synchronization based on electrocorticogram (ECoG) signals from eleven refractory epilepsy patients. Results showed that there was a significant increase of synchronization prior to seizure termination and no significant difference of the transitions of network states among the preseizure, seizure, and postseizure periods. Those results indicated that synchronization might participate in termination of seizures, and the network states transitions might not dominate the seizure evolution.

1. Introduction

Epilepsy is a common chronic neurological disease characterized by recurrent epileptic seizures which may cause severe physiological and psychological damage to patients [1]. Tracking the evolution of seizure may be helpful to understand the generation, propagation, and termination mechanism of seizure and to improve the therapy of epilepsy.

Since epilepsy is increasingly considered as a network-level disorder, more and more attention has been paid to dynamic brain network analysis, which has provided new perspectives and insights into the nature of epilepsy [2, 3]. Meanwhile, evidence has shown that seizures result from dynamics of network organization characterized by dynamical evolution of synchronization [4, 5]. Traditional ideas hold that the hypersynchronous activity is the hallmark of epileptiform activity [6]. Recently, a high level of synchronization has been observed prior to the termination of seizures in several studies, which may provide helpful clues to understand the mechanism of seizure termination. Schindler et al. explored status epilepticus electroencephalogram (EEG) signals based on the eigenvalue spectrum of the equal-time correlation matrix, in which EEG signals

were recorded by either intracranial or surface electrodes from patients, and found that synchronization fluctuated at relatively low levels during ongoing epileptiform activity and increased before seizures termination [7]. Then, they established a functional network by computing a cross-correlation matrix based on EEG signals recorded via implanted strips, grids, or depth electrodes from patients undergoing presurgical evaluation for drug-resistant epilepsy and found a global increase of synchronization prior to seizure termination [8]. Furthermore, Evangelista et al. used the nonlinear correlation coefficient to study functional connectivity between the thalamus and selected cortical regions based on stereo-electroencephalogram (SEEG) recorded from patients with drug-resistant mesial temporal lobe epilepsy and found that, at the end of seizure, the global synchronization index and the thalamic synchronization index negatively correlated with seizure duration, which indicated that the thalamocortical synchronization contributed to seizure termination [9]. In addition, Zhang et al. studied on amygdala-kindled seizures in mice and showed that the synchronization measured by mutual information between the thalamus and hippocampus increased prior to the epileptiform discharges' termination [10]. However, by computing Gabor atom density of individual electrode signals from patients with complex partial seizures of both mesial temporal or neocortical onset, Afra et al. found that synchronous seizure termination was a common pattern, which meant most of the ictal activities terminated in all the recording electrodes simultaneously or within 5 s between each other, whereas an asynchronous termination pattern also existed [11]. So, synchronization changes prior to the termination of seizures are debatable and to be further explored.

Several methods, such as coherency [12, 13], mutual information [10, 14], partial-directed coherence [15–17], directed transfer function [18, 19], and phase synchronization [20, 21], have been used to measure the interactions among different areas of the brain to establish a network. Among these methods, phase synchronization measures the interactions between rhythmic signals by detecting the instantaneous phase and is unaffected by the amplitude of signals, which is a useful method to study the synchronization between brain areas, especially when the relationship is too weak to be detected by other measures [14, 22]. Because of the nonlinear property of epileptic brain activities, phase synchronization, as a nonlinear method, has been applied to measure the synchronization between different brain areas [6, 23]. In this study, brain networks would be established by computing phase synchronization between different brain areas.

Studies have applied different indices to characterize brain networks and investigate synchronization dynamics, such as eigenvalue spectrum of the correlation matrix [7], eigenvalue ratio of the Laplacian matrix of the cross-correlation matrix [8], and so on. Evangelista et al. calculated the average of the nonlinear correlation coefficient of all pairs of signals in each time window in regions of interest as a global synchronization index, which was used to measure the thalamocortical synchrony based on SEEG signals [9]. Similarly, in this study, we would calculate the average degree of nodes in each network, which represented the mean phase synchronization of the network, and investigate the dynamics of the average degree prior to seizure termination to investigate the role of synchronization.

Similar network states denote similar brain connectivity patterns. Clustering of the networks over time windows were used to identify a set of distinct network clusters denoting different brain states [24, 25]. Burns et al. investigated the state-space dynamics of patients with partial epileptic seizures based on unsupervised clustering of eigenvector centrality vectors and characterized seizures by a set of network states [24]. Khambhati et al. defined a network state to be the set of all configuration vectors that exhibited a similar pattern of functional connectivity and tracked the dynamic network reconfiguration by clustering time windows (configuration vectors) with similar network geometry via community detection during the seizure generation, propagation, and termination [25]. They found that, during the preseizure epoch, the network demonstrated rapid reconfiguration, but during the seizure epoch, the network showed slower reconfiguration. Liu et al. explored the state transitions of networks of epileptiform discharges in hippocampal slices based on clustering of degree vectors and

identified two network states during the ictal-like discharges which represented tonic and clonic phases, respectively [26]. Since the network states characterized by brain connection patterns represent different stages of the seizure, we would investigate the dynamics of network states during preseizure, seizure, and postseizure periods by using unsupervised clustering of degree vectors to explore the reconfiguration of networks.

The rest of the paper is organized as follows. Section 2 presents the information of data sets and the algorithms for calculating phase synchronization and network states. The results of dynamics of phase synchronization and network states over preseizure, seizure, and postseizure periods are presented in Section 3. Section 4 presents the conclusion of this study.

2. Materials and Methods

2.1. Patient Data Sets. We retrieved ECoG signals recorded from 11 refractory epilepsy patients (Mayo Clinic, Rochester, MN) undergoing implantation of subdural electrodes to localize the seizure onset zone via the International Epilepsy Electrophysiology Portal (IEEG Portal, http://www.ieeg.org), including complex partial seizure and complex partial with secondary generalization seizure. Detailed patient information is given in Table 1. Each of the data sets includes ECoG signals and annotations of seizure time. The ECoG signals were sampled at 500 Hz. We analyzed the largest grid of electrodes in each case to investigate the epileptic network of a local area. The grid sizes are listed in Table 1, which denote the total number and the arrangement of electrodes.

2.2. Data Analysis

2.2.1. Data Preprocessing. We analyzed the preseizure, seizure, and postseizure periods of 22 seizures from 11 patients (2 seizures from each patient). A seizure period denoted the time between seizure onset and termination, and the corresponding preseizure period and postseizure period were defined as the same time intervals of the seizure period before the seizure onset and after the seizure termination, respectively. Since the ECoG signals had high signal-to-noise ratio, we only eliminated the bad channels seriously affected by noise and did not proceed other preprocessing to obtain broadband signals. Then, the theta (4–8 Hz), alpha (8–13 Hz), beta (13–30 Hz), and gamma (30–45 Hz) signals were extracted with finite impulse response filters provided by EEGLAB [27, 28] to ensure zero-phase distortion for further phase synchronization analysis.

2.2.2. Phase Synchronization. The mean phase coherence was calculated to measure the phase synchronization between each pair of ECoG signals. Firstly, for one channel of ECoG signals $x_1(t)$, the Hilbert transform [29] was computed as follows:

TABLE 1: Patient information.

Patient (IEEG portal)	Sex	Age (onset/surgery)	Seizure type	Grid size
Study 006	M	22/25	CP	6×8
Study 010	F	00/13	CP	6×8
Study 011	F	10/34	CP	6×8
Study 014	F	09/33	CP	8×8
Study 016	F	05/36	CPG	4×6
Study 020	M	05/10	CPG	4×6
Study 021	M	Unknown	CPG	6×8
Study 022	F	Unknown	CPG	4×6
Study 023	M	01/16	CP	8×8
Study 026	M	09/09	CP	8×8
Study 037	F	Unknown	CP	8×8

CP, complex partial; CPG, complex partial with secondary generalization. M, male; F, female.

$$H\left[x_1(t)\right] = \frac{1}{\pi} \text{P.V.} \int_{-\infty}^{\infty} \frac{x_1(\tau)}{t - \tau} \, d\tau, \qquad (1)$$

where P.V. means the Cauchy principal value. Then, the instantaneous phase $\phi_1(t)$ of $x_1(t)$ was defined as

$$\phi_1(t) = \arctan \frac{H\left[x_1(t)\right]}{x_1(t)}, \qquad (2)$$

and the mean phase coherence λ between a pair of ECoG signals $x_1(t)$ and $x_2(t)$ was calculated as

$$\lambda = \frac{1}{N} \left| \sum_{t=1}^{N} e^{j\left[\phi_1(t) - \phi_2(t)\right]} \right|. \qquad (3)$$

where $\phi_1(t)$ and $\phi_2(t)$ were the instantaneous phases of the signals $x_1(t)$ and $x_2(t)$, respectively and N was the number of samples in each time window. λ ranges from 0 to 1, and $\lambda = 0$ means no phase synchronization, whereas $\lambda = 1$ indicates the perfect phase synchronization.

To qualify the dynamics of phase synchronization, 1-s moving windows were used with 50% overlap, and the mean phase coherence was calculated for each pair of signals and averaged over all samples in each window (here, the number of samples in each window is $N = 500$). So, a $M \times M$ phase synchronization connectivity matrix (M is the number of electrodes in the grid) was obtained in each time window for each subject. In this way, we would obtain a set of phase synchronization connectivity matrices during preseizure, seizure, and postseizure periods denoting a series of brain networks.

2.2.3. Network Analysis. The network was constructed by the connectivity matrix in each time window, in which the nodes referred to the ECoG channels and the edges were defined as the mean phase coherence value.

In this study, we used the degree to characterize the network. The degree of a node in a network was defined as the sum of the weights of edges which were connected with the given node [2], and the degree vector was formed of the degrees of all nodes in each time window. The mean phase

synchronization of the network was computed as the average value of the degrees of all nodes and was used to measure the phase synchronization of the whole network.

To investigate the transitions of network states, the degree vectors along time were clustered into a set of states by using an agglomerative hierarchical method on Ward's criterion [30]. An agglomerative hierarchical clustering started with each object as a single cluster and then, merged the two nearest clusters repeatedly until only a single cluster remained, and the Ward's criterion was used to measure the proximity (distance) between two clusters through the increase of the sum of the squared error (SSE) resulting from merging the two clusters. The objective function SSE is defined as follows:

$$\text{SSE} = \sum_{i=1}^{K} \sum_{x \in C_i} \text{dist}\left(c_i, x\right)^2, \qquad (4)$$

where K means the number of clusters, C_i is the cluster i, x means an object, c_i is the centroid of the cluster i, and the dist denotes the standard Euclidean distance. Then, the objective function would be minimized to merge the nearest clusters. The optimal number of clusters was determined by the largest second derivative in the distance curve of clustering [26]. Then, we obtained a set of network states and computed the rate of the state change by dividing the number of network state changes by corresponding length of time to investigate the reorganization of brain networks during the preseizure, seizure, and postseizure periods.

2.2.4. Statistical Analysis. The Friedman test with the post hoc Dunn's multiple comparison test was performed to test the difference among multiple groups, with $p < 0.05$ indicating the significant difference.

3. Results and Discussion

3.1. Synchronization Increasing prior to Seizure Termination. For a seizure of patient Study 037 with an 8×8 grid, Figure 1(a) represented the grid and strips' location obtained from the IEEG portal, and the recording data from the grid named "RPG" were analyzed. Figure 1(b) demonstrated 64 channels of ECoG signals recording from the grid RPG, where the left red vertical line denoted the onset time of this seizure and the right red vertical line denoted the termination time. This seizure lasted for 95 s, and we selected the same duration before the onset of seizure as preseizure period and the same duration after the termination of seizure as postseizure period. Then, the seizure period was divided into four periods evenly, named "S1–S4", and preS and postS denoted the periods before the onset and after the termination of seizure with a duration of a quarter of seizure period, respectively. Figure 1(c) shows the phase synchronization connectivity matrix in the 47-48 s time window of broadband signals.

For this patient, the degree vectors, calculated based on broadband signals and formed of the degree of each node during the preseizure, seizure, and postseizure periods, are displayed in Figure 2(b). As shown in Figure 2(c), the mean

(a)

(b)

(c)

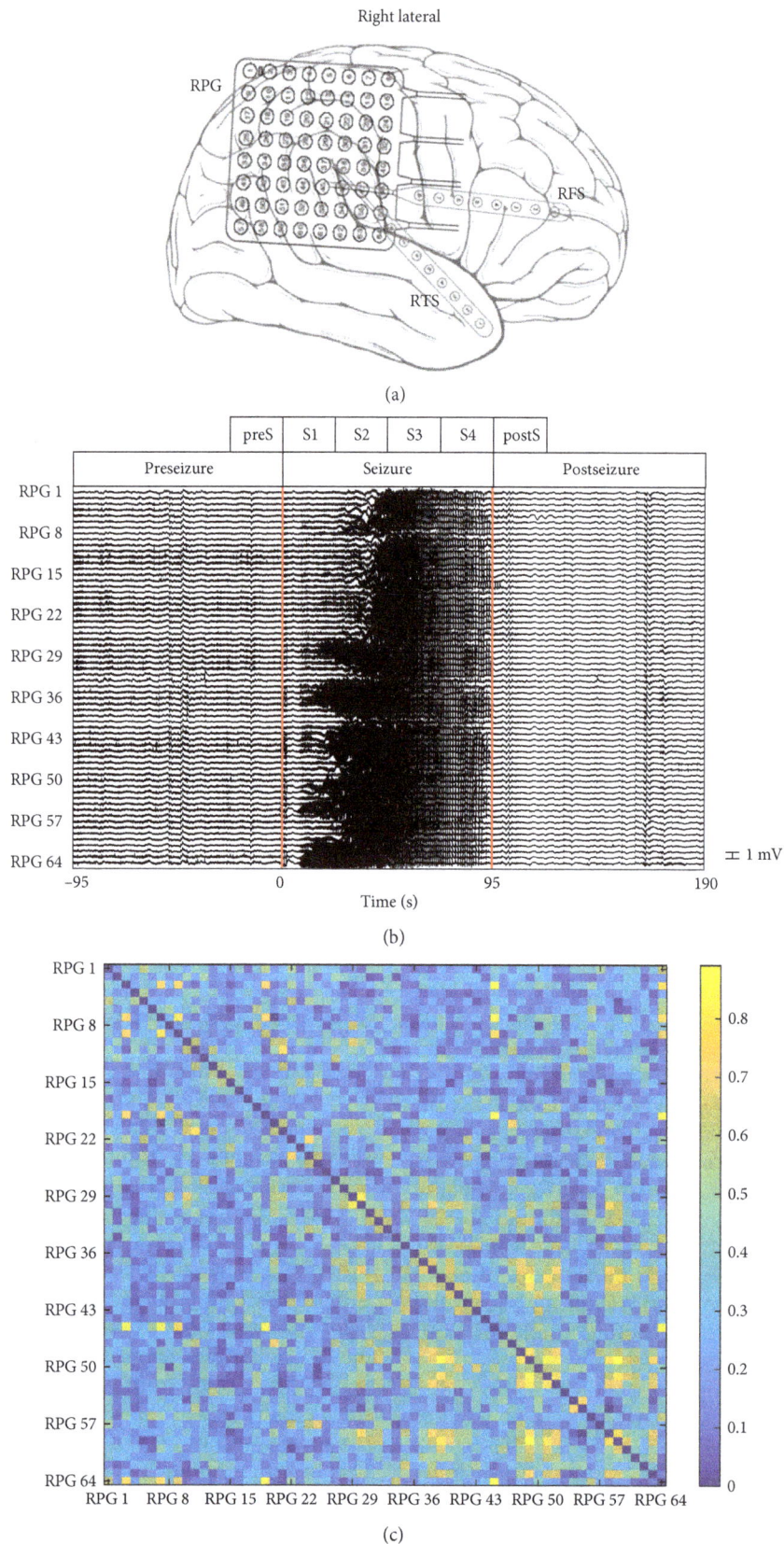

FIGURE 1: ECoG information of Study 037 and one example of the corresponding phase synchronization connectivity matrix. Electrodes positions of the grid RPG are shown in (a) and 64 channels of ECoG signals recorded from the grid are shown in (b). The left red vertical line means the onset time of this seizure and the right red vertical line represents the termination time. The seizure period is divided into four stages evenly, named "S1–S4", and preS and postS represent the period before the onset and after the termination of seizure with a duration of a quarter of the seizure period, respectively. Phase synchronization connectivity matrix in the 47–48 s time window of broadband signals is displayed in (c).

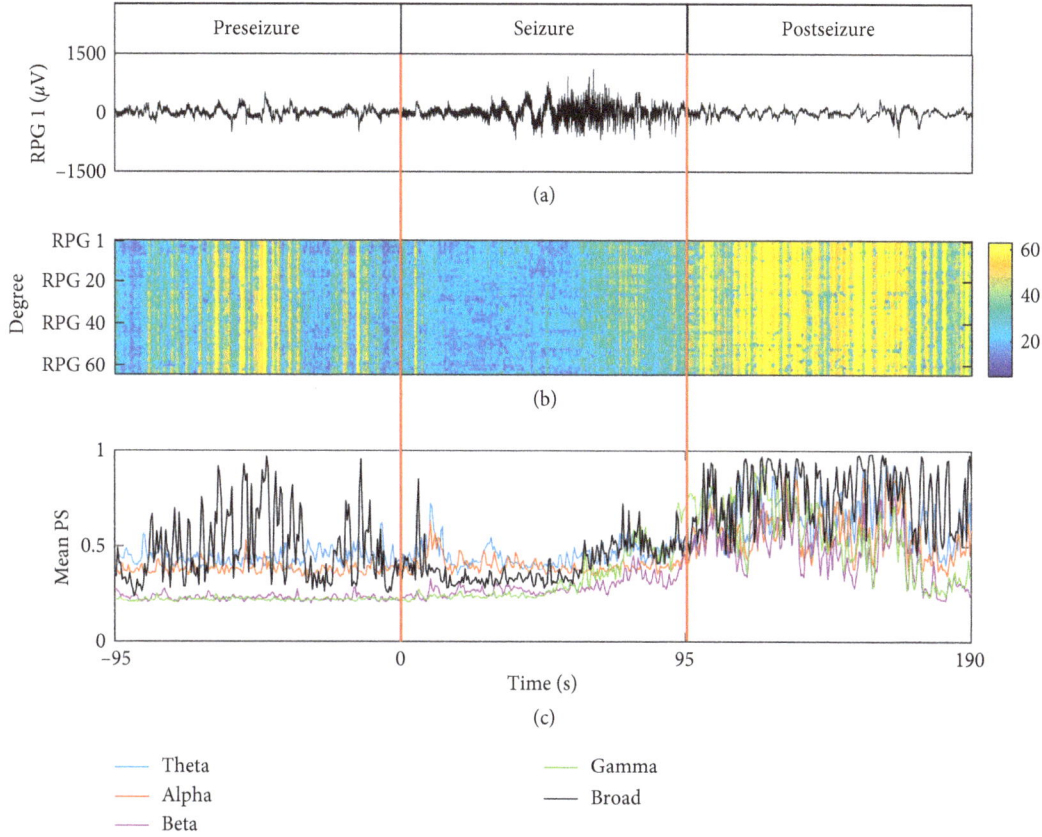

FIGURE 2: Degree vectors and corresponding mean phase synchronization of Study 037. The left red vertical line denotes the onset of this seizure, and the right red vertical line represents the termination of this seizure. (a) shows the #1 channel of the grid signals (RPG1) of the seizure of Study 037. The degree vectors of broadband signals along time are shown in (b), and mean phase synchronization (mean PS) of different frequency components are displayed in (c).

phase synchronization of broadband signals was at a high level in the preseizure period and decreased in the early stage of the seizure period, then it increased significantly in the late stage of the seizure period and remained at the high level in the postseizure period. Moreover, the mean phase synchronization in different frequency bands of Study 037 was different, especially in preseizure periods, in which alpha and theta components showed higher mean phase synchronization than beta and gamma components. However, the mean phase synchronization in all frequency bands increased in the late stage of the seizure period and remained at the high level in the postseizure period.

The statistical analysis results of mean phase synchronization in broadband and different frequency bands across 22 seizures from 11 patients are shown in Figure 3. As shown in Figure 3(a), the mean phase synchronization of broadband signals in S4 was significantly larger than those in preS ($p < 0.01$), S1 ($p < 0.05$), S2 ($p < 0.01$), and S3 ($p < 0.05$). Moreover, the mean phase synchronization of broadband signals in postS was significantly larger than those in S1 ($p < 0.01$), S2 ($p < 0.0001$), and S3 ($p < 0.01$). The mean phase synchronization in the theta band was displayed in Figure 3(b), and the mean phase synchronization in S1, S4, and postS was significantly larger than that in preS. In the alpha band, the mean phase synchronization in S1, S2, S3, S4, and postS was significantly higher than that in preS

(Figure 3(c)). Moreover, the mean phase synchronization in S4 was significantly larger than that in S1, and those in S3, S4, and postS were higher than those in preS in the beta band (Figure 3(d)). As shown in Figure 3(e), the mean phase synchronization in S2, S3, S4, and postS was significantly higher than that in preS in the gamma band. There was no statistical difference between the other pairs. The results demonstrated that the mean synchronization of the network had a significant increase prior to seizure termination and remained at a high level after seizure termination, especially in alpha, beta, and gamma bands.

Several research studies explored synchronization based on broadband signals [7–9], and Li et al. explored the dynamics of phase synchronization of different frequency components and found that the phase synchronization increased before the seizure termination across almost all frequencies [21]. Our study also displayed similar results, which meant multiple brain areas with multiple frequency components may be involved in seizure termination.

Our results confirmed that the phase synchronization increased at the late stage of seizure compared with the early periods and remained high after seizure. In recent years, several studies have reported that a high level of synchronization was observed prior to the termination of seizures in vitro and in vivo models and human seizures [7–10, 21, 31].

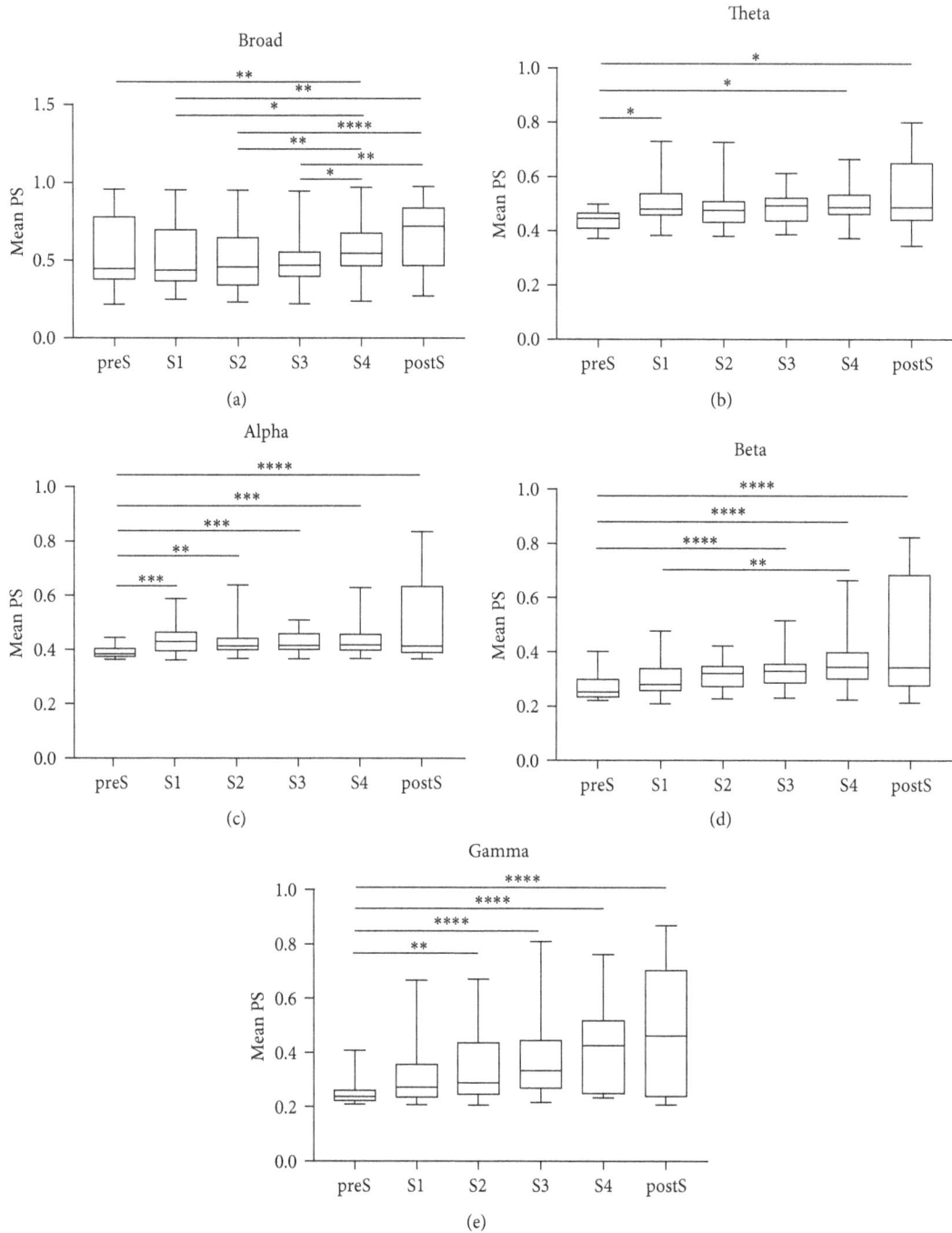

FIGURE 3: Statistical analysis results of mean phase synchronization of broadband signals and different frequency band signals (theta, alpha, beta, and gamma) are displayed in (a), (b), (c), (d), and (e), respectively. The middle line of the box corresponds to the median, and the 25% and 75% percentiles are the lower and upper borders of each box, respectively. The whiskers correspond to the total range of the data. (Friedman test with post hoc Dunn's multiple comparison test; $n = 22$, $^{*}p < 0.05$, $^{**}p < 0.01$, $^{***}p < 0.001$, and $^{****}p < 0.0001$).

The increasing synchronization of neural activities may be considered as an emergent self-regulatory mechanism of seizure termination [7]. Meanwhile, Sobayo and Mogul found that deep brain stimulation was more effective to terminate seizures when the frequency reflected the endogenous synchronization of naturally terminated seizures in a chronic rat epilepsy model [32], which supported that synchronization might cause seizure termination. However,

Majumdar et al. discussed the cause and effect relationship between the seizure termination and the increase of synchronization, and they concluded that the synchronization was an effect [33]. So far, it is not conclusive that the synchronization is the cause or effect of the seizure termination. In addition, the degree of synchronization was measured based on phase synchronization in this study, which characterized different aspects of synchronization

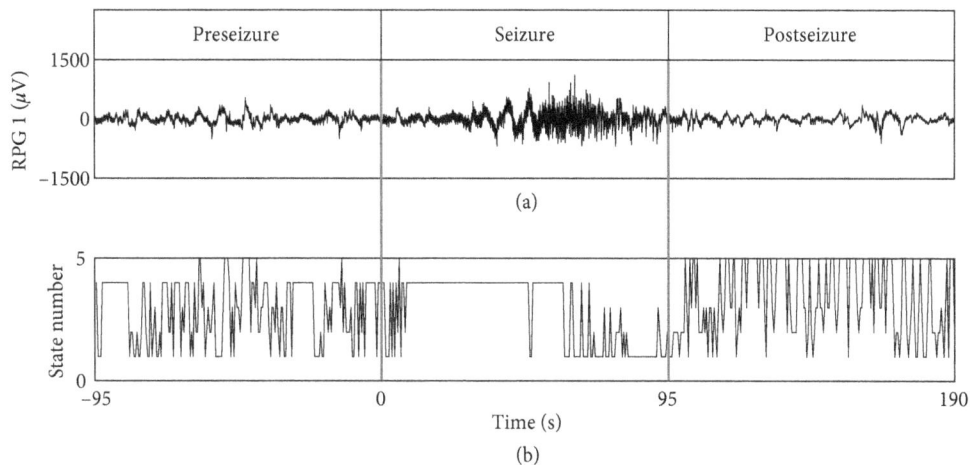

FIGURE 4: Transitions of network states of Study 037 during preseizure, seizure, and postseizure periods. The left red vertical line denotes the onset of this seizure, and the right red vertical line represents the termination of this seizure. (a) shows the #1 channel of the grid signals (RPG1) of the seizure of Study 037. The network states resulted from clustering of degree vectors are displayed in (b), in which each state number denotes a network state.

compared with other methods such as correlation and coherence. Further studies will be needed to explore the cause and effect relationship between the seizure termination and synchronization, and it should be more careful to apply synchronization to intervention of epilepsy especially.

3.2. No Significant Difference of Network State Change Rate during Periseizure. To investigate the transitions of network states, a set of network states were obtained by applying agglomerative hierarchical clustering to the set of degree vectors, which represented different brain connectivity patterns during preseizure, seizure, and postseizure periods. For example, the transitions of network states based on broadband signals during periseizure of Study 037 are shown in Figure 4(b), in which each state number denotes a network state. The network states switched among state 1, state 2, state 3, state 4, and state 5 frequently during the preseizure and postseizure periods. However, the frequency of network state changes decreased significantly during the seizure period, and the state 4 dominated the most of seizure periods.

The statistical analysis results across 22 seizures from 11 patients are shown in Figure 5. Although there is a downward trend of the network state change rate from the preseizure period to the seizure period and an upward trend of that from the seizure period to the postseizure period, no significant difference exists among the three periods.

Previous studies have demonstrated that brain network transitions existed in seizure periods based on measuring the coherence between each pair of ECoG signals [24], and the network reorganization was faster during preseizure periods than seizure periods by calculating correlation of the pairs of signals [25]. By computing time-variant partial-directed coherence, Liu et al. found there were two network states during the ictal-like discharges in hippocampal slices and those two states represented tonic and clonic phases, respectively [26].

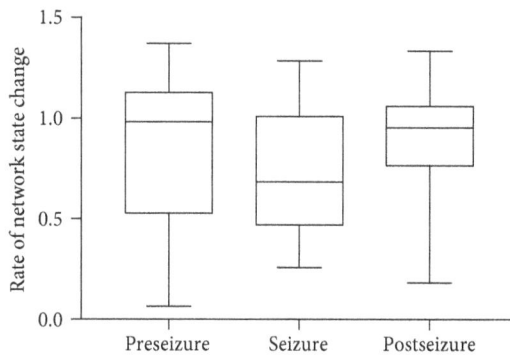

FIGURE 5: Statistical analysis results of network state change rate. The middle line of the box corresponds to the median, and the 25% and 75% percentiles are the lower and upper borders of each box, respectively. No significant difference exists among those pairs. (Friedman test with post hoc Dunn's multiple comparison test; $n = 22$).

Here, based on the phase synchronization, we also found the network transitions existed during the preseizure, seizure, and postseizure periods, and network state changes in the seizure period had a tendency to be less frequent compared with preseizure and postseizure periods. However, our statistical results did not show significant difference of the network state change rate among those periods, which might be due to that the networks were established by calculating the phase synchronization. Compared with those studies mentioned above, phase synchronization focused on measuring the difference of the instantaneous phase of rhythmic signals. So, our results were restricted to the network state changes based on phase synchronization, which did not dominate in evolution of seizure. Further research studies will be performed to track synchronization dynamics based on other methods such as partial-directed coherence and directed transfer function, which characterize the information flow direction and may be helpful to measure the interactions among signals.

4. Conclusions

In this study, phase synchronization was applied to measure the relationship between each pair of ECoG signals to establish the brain network, and the synchronization dynamics and network states evolution were tracked during preseizure, seizure, and postseizure periods. The results showed that synchronization increased prior to seizure termination and remained at the high level after seizure termination. Furthermore, there was no significant difference of the network states transition rate among the preseizure, seizure, and postseizure periods. Those results indicated that the phase synchronization might promote the seizure termination, and the role of network state transitions might not dominate the seizure evolution, which led to a deeper understanding of evolution of seizure. From a therapeutic perspective, these results might be helpful to explore new therapeutic methods focused on phase synchronization to terminate seizures.

Conflicts of Interest

The authors declare that there are no conflicts of interest regarding the publication of this paper.

Acknowledgments

This work was supported by the Key Basic Research Project of Science and Technology Commission of Shanghai (13DJ1400303).

References

[1] R. S. Fisher, C. Acevedo, A. Arzimanoglou et al., "ILAE official report: a practical clinical definition of epilepsy," *Epilepsia*, vol. 55, no. 4, pp. 475–482, 2014.

[2] Z. Haneef and S. Chiang, "Clinical correlates of graph theory findings in temporal lobe epilepsy," *Seizure*, vol. 23, no. 10, pp. 809–818, 2014.

[3] B. C. Bernhardt, L. Bonilha, and D. W. Gross, "Network analysis for a network disorder: the emerging role of graph theory in the study of epilepsy," *Epilepsy & Behavior*, vol. 50, pp. 162–170, 2015.

[4] M. A. Kramer and S. S. Cash, "Epilepsy as a disorder of cortical network organization," *The Neuroscientist*, vol. 18, no. 4, pp. 360–372, 2012.

[5] P. Jiruska, M. De Curtis, J. G. Jefferys et al., "Synchronization and desynchronization in epilepsy: controversies and hypotheses," *The Journal of Physiology*, vol. 591, no. 4, pp. 787–797, 2013.

[6] C. Schevon, J. Cappell, R. Emerson et al., "Cortical abnormalities in epilepsy revealed by local EEG synchrony," *Neuroimage*, vol. 35, no. 1, pp. 140–148, 2007.

[7] K. Schindler, C. E. Elger, and K. Lehnertz, "Increasing synchronization may promote seizure termination: Evidence from status epilepticus," *Clinical Neurophysiology*, vol. 118, no. 9, pp. 1955–1968, 2007.

[8] K. A. Schindler, S. Bialonski, M.-T. Horstmann, C. E. Elger, and K. Lehnertz, "Evolving functional network properties and

[9] E. Evangelista, C. Bénar, F. Bonini et al., "Does the thalamocortical synchrony play a role in seizure termination?," *Frontiers in Neurology*, vol. 6, p. 192, 2015.

[10] Z. Zhang, J.-J. Li, Q.-C. Lu, H.-Q. Gong, P.-J. Liang, and P.-M. Zhang, "Interaction between thalamus and hippocampus in termination of amygdala-kindled seizures in mice," *Computational and Mathematical Methods in Medicine*, vol. 2016, Article ID 9580724, 10 pages, 2016.

[11] P. Afra, C. C. Jouny, and G. K. Bergey, "Termination patterns of complex partial seizures: an intracranial EEG study," *Seizure*, vol. 32, pp. 9–15, 2015.

[12] P. L. Nunez, R. Srinivasan, A. F. Westdorp et al., "EEG coherency. I: statistics, reference electrode, volume conduction, laplacians, cortical imaging, and interpretation at multiple scales," *Electroencephalography and Clinical Neurophysiology*, vol. 103, no. 5, pp. 499–515, 1997.

[13] P. L. Nunez, R. B. Silberstein, Z. Shi et al., "EEG coherency II: experimental comparisons of multiple measures," *Clinical Neurophysiology*, vol. 110, no. 3, pp. 469–486, 1999.

[14] J. M. Hurtado, L. L. Rubchinsky, and K. A. Sigvardt, "Statistical method for detection of phase-locking episodes in neural oscillations," *Journal of Neurophysiology*, vol. 91, no. 4, pp. 1883–1898, 2004.

[15] Y.-H. Li, X.-L. Ye, Q.-Q. Liu et al., "Localization of epileptogenic zone based on graph analysis of stereo-EEG," *Epilepsy Research*, vol. 128, pp. 149–157, 2016.

[16] J.-W. Mao, X.-L. Ye, Y.-H. Li et al., "Dynamic network connectivity analysis to identify epileptogenic zones based on stereo-electroencephalography," *Frontiers in Computational Neuroscience*, vol. 10, p. 113, 2016.

[17] M. Ding, S. L. Bressler, W. Yang, and H. Liang, "Short-window spectral analysis of cortical event-related potentials by adaptive multivariate autoregressive modeling: data preprocessing, model validation, and variability assessment," *Biological Cybernetics*, vol. 83, no. 1, pp. 35–45, 2000.

[18] J.-Y. Kim, H.-C. Kang, J.-H. Cho et al., "Combined use of multiple computational intracranial EEG analysis techniques for the localization of epileptogenic zones in Lennox-Gastaut syndrome," *Clinical EEG and Neuroscience*, vol. 45, no. 3, pp. 169–178, 2014.

[19] Y. Lu, L. Yang, G. A. Worrell, and B. He, "Seizure source imaging by means of FINE spatio-temporal dipole localization and directed transfer function in partial epilepsy patients," *Clinical Neurophysiology*, vol. 123, no. 7, pp. 1275–1283, 2012.

[20] F. Mormann, T. Kreuz, R. G. Andrzejak et al., "Epileptic seizures are preceded by a decrease in synchronization," *Epilepsy Research*, vol. 53, no. 3, pp. 173–185, 2003.

[21] J.-J. Li, Y.-H. Li, H.-Q. Gong et al., "The spatiotemporal dynamics of phase synchronization during epileptogenesis in amygdala-kindling mice," *Plos One*, vol. 11, no. 4, Article ID e0153897, 2016.

[22] J. Kurths, A. Pikovsky, and M. Rosenblum, "Synchronization : a universal concept in nonlinear sciences," *Physics Today*, vol. 70, no. 1, p. 47, 2002.

[23] C. P. Warren, S. Hu, M. Stead et al., "Synchrony in normal and focal epileptic brain: the seizure onset zone is functionally disconnected," *Journal of Neurophysiology*, vol. 104, no. 6, pp. 3530–3539, 2010.

[24] S. P. Burns, S. Santaniello, R. B. Yaffe et al., "Network dynamics of the brain and influence of the epileptic seizure onset

zone," *Proceedings of the National Academy of Sciences*, vol. 111, no. 49, pp. E5321–E5330, 2014.

[25] A. N. Khambhati, K. A. Davis, B. S. Oommen et al., "Dynamic network drivers of seizure generation, propagation and termination in human neocortical epilepsy," *Plos Computational Biology*, vol. 11, no. 12, Article ID e1004608, 2015.

[26] B.-W. Liu, J.-W. Mao, Y.-J. Shi et al., "Dynamics in the neural network of an in vitro epilepsy model," *International Journal of Data Mining and Bioinformatics*, vol. 18, no. 2, pp. 125–143, 2017.

[27] A. Delorme and S. Makeig, "EEGLAB: an open source toolbox for analysis of single-trial EEG dynamics including independent component analysis," *Journal of neuroscience methods*, vol. 134, no. 1, pp. 9–21, 2004.

[28] J. Sun, X. Hong, and S. Tong, "Phase synchronization analysis of EEG signals: an evaluation based on surrogate tests," *IEEE Transactions on Biomedical Engineering*, vol. 59, no. 8, pp. 2254–2263, 2012.

[29] F. Mormann, K. Lehnertz, P. David, and C. E. Elger, "Mean phase coherence as a measure for phase synchronization and its application to the EEG of epilepsy patients," *Physica D: Nonlinear Phenomena*, vol. 144, no. 3–4, pp. 358–369, 2000.

[30] J. H. Ward Jr., "Hierarchical grouping to optimize an objective function," *Journal of the American Statistical Association*, vol. 58, no. 301, pp. 236–244, 1963.

[31] A. J. Trevelyan, D. Sussillo, B. O. Watson, and R. Yuste, "Modular propagation of epileptiform activity: evidence for an inhibitory veto in neocortex," *Journal of Neuroscience*, vol. 26, no. 48, pp. 12447–12455, 2006.

[32] T. Sobayo and D. J. Mogul, "Should stimulation parameters be individualized to stop seizures: evidence in support of this approach," *Epilepsia*, vol. 57, no. 1, pp. 131–140, 2016.

[33] K. Majumdar, P. D. Prasad, and S. Verma, "Synchronization implies seizure or seizure implies synchronization?," *Brain Topography*, vol. 27, no. 1, pp. 112–122, 2014.

Variable Selection and Joint Estimation of Mean and Covariance Models with an Application to eQTL Data

JungJun Lee [iD],[1] **SungHwan Kim** [iD],[2] **Jae-Hwan Jhong,**[1] **and Ja-Yong Koo** [iD][1]

[1]*Department of Statistics, Korea University, Seoul 02841, Republic of Korea*
[2]*Department of Applied Statistics, Konkuk University, Seoul 05029, Republic of Korea*

Correspondence should be addressed to SungHwan Kim; swiss747@gmail.com

Academic Editor: Nadia A. Chuzhanova

In genomic data analysis, it is commonplace that underlying regulatory relationship over multiple genes is hardly ascertained due to unknown genetic complexity and epigenetic regulations. In this paper, we consider a joint mean and constant covariance model (JMCCM) that elucidates conditional dependent structures of genes with controlling for potential genotype perturbations. To this end, the modified Cholesky decomposition is utilized to parametrize entries of a precision matrix. The JMCCM maximizes the likelihood function to estimate parameters involved in the model. We also develop a variable selection algorithm that selects explanatory variables and Cholesky factors by exploiting the combination of the GCV and BIC as benchmarks, together with Rao and Wald statistics. Importantly, we notice that sparse estimation of a precision matrix (or equivalently gene network) is effectively achieved via the proposed variable selection scheme and contributes to exploring significant hub genes shown to be concordant to *a priori* biological evidence. In simulation studies, we confirm that our model selection efficiently identifies the true underlying networks. With an application to miRNA and SNPs data from yeast (a.k.a. eQTL data), we demonstrate that constructed gene networks reproduce validated biological and clinical knowledge with regard to various pathways including the cell cycle pathway.

1. Introduction

Generally, joint estimation of mean and covariance has been developed to address problems related to biomedical data. In longitudinal data analysis, for instance, identifying correct correlation structures within each subject is a major focus and many studies come up with variants of joint mean and covariance estimation to enhance statistical efficiency (see Ye and Pan [1] and references therein). With regard to graphical models, particularly, conditional Gaussian graphical models (cGGM) aiming to elucidate conditional dependence structures subject to the mean have increasingly received much attention [2–5] and conceptually can also be viewed as examples of joint mean and covariance estimation in essence. On a methodological side, joint estimation has been found to be practically applicable in the sense that applications of joint estimation methods cover bioinformatics, such as hormone and transcriptome [1, 4, 6–8], and stock price analysis [9]. A majority of existing methods involve variable selection of covariates for the mean vector and sparsity of covariance

mainly based on the penalization methods. However, in this paper, we purposely focus on variable selection and joint estimation with a pure implementation of the likelihood-based method, unlike common penalization techniques, to better analyze eQTL data in light of genetic feature selection.

Over the decades, genomics research has focused on comprehensive understanding of regulatory networks in the context of system biology. Commonly we are interested in a gene network, which pictures the interplay among genetic factors (e.g., gene regulation and activation). Particularly, it is important to investigate how a given genotype (genetic variants) at a particular quantitative trait locus (QTL) affects measured phenotypes and traits at that locus. For instance, gene expression quantitative loci (eQTL) make use of gene expressions as quantitative traits. eQTL analysis has been widely applied to figure out the effect of genetic perturbations associated with diseases as well as to construct regulatory networks describing how genes regulate expressions of other genes [10, 11]. More precisely, the location of single nucleotide polymorphisms (SNPs) may affect multiple gene expression levels, and this accidentally causes misleading inference for dependency structure among genes [4]. Many popular methods [2–5, 12] have been introduced to identify gene networks, aiming at learning networks subject to perturbation effects by genetic variants on the basis of population gene expression and genotype data.

Yin and Li [4] proposed the sparse conditional graphical Gaussian model with ℓ_1 and the adaptive lasso penalty function. Li *et al.* [3] suggested the two-stage estimation framework: (1) estimating a nonsparse conditional covariance matrix of genes based on a conditional variance operator between the reproducing kernel Hilbert spaces of marker genes and then (2) using l_1 and adaptive lasso penalty to obtain sparse estimates of a precision matrix under the cGGM. Cai *et al.* [12] studied the covariate-adjusted precision matrix estimation (CAPME) method using the constrained ℓ_1 optimization.

While most recent studies encourage sparsity estimation of a precision matrix based on the penalized likelihood, we instead rely on classical variable methods based on the standard likelihood. Strictly speaking, the penalized likelihood, according to its definition, cannot be viewed as the likelihood. It naturally poses a question whether the likelihood-based method performs better than the penalized likelihood approaches. To address this question, we consider a joint mean and constant covariance model (JMCCM) inspired by Pourahmadi [13] and propose methods for variable selection which effectively identify sparse conditional gene networks and covariates relevant to gene regulations. We employ the modified Cholesky decomposition to guarantee positive definiteness of an estimated precision matrix [13]. With this reparametrization of the precision matrix, the log-likelihood function corresponding to our model can be decomposed into an additive form of each response in terms of Cholesky parameters. This facilitates a coordinate descent type implementation we adopt for the precision matrix estimation. The combination of both generalized cross-validation (GCV) and Bayesian information criterion (BIC) performs variable selection as a benchmark. Rao and Wald statistics are also utilized to add and delete genetic markers for each gene expression and the Cholesky factors for the precision matrix. To the best of our knowledge, only a few works use Rao and Wald statistics for variable selection in the joint estimation problem, particularly with an application to eQTL analysis.

In simulation studies, extensive simulation scenarios experimentally confirm improved estimation efficiency and precise variable selection of the proposed method. For real data applications, we perform eQTL analysis via the JMCCM with gene expressions and SNPs of yeast data, in pursuit of detecting the effects of variant perturbations and underlying gene regulations. We find that the JMCCM effectively uncovers biological pathways that may potentially account for known biological processes. Taken together, the JMCCM is shown to be effective in identifying conditional dependence structures among variables compared to the existing graphical models with penalization methods such as the sparse cGGM [5] and CAPME [12].

The paper is outlined as follows. In Section 2, we describe our JMCCM with modified Cholesky decomposition and

maximum likelihood estimates. The variable selection algorithm using Rao and Wald statistics for SNPs and Cholesky factors is explained in Section 3. Section 4 deals with simulation studies to demonstrate performance of variable selection and estimation of the proposed model. The yeast cell cycle pathway genes with SNPs data analysis are presented in Section 5. Concluding remarks and discussion in Section 6 are followed by the Appendix, which provides mathematical details of our method.

2. Model And Estimators

2.1. JMCCM with the Modified Cholesky Decomposition. Contrary to previous methods [3, 4], the JMCCM primarily aims at simultaneous estimation over the mean and precision matrix of the Gaussian graphical model. Suppose that (x, y) is a pair of the $p \times 1$ vector x of genetic markers and the $m \times 1$ random vector y of expression levels. Let x denote the vector of SNPs and let y denote the gene expression traits following m-variate multivariate normal distribution with the mean $\mu(x; \beta)$ and covariance matrix Σ as follows:

$$y \mid x \sim N_m \left(\mu \left(x; \beta \right), \Sigma \right), \qquad (1)$$

where the jth entry of $\mu(x; \beta)$ is $x^\top \beta_j$ for $j = 1, \ldots, m$, and $\beta_j = (\beta_j^1, \ldots, \beta_j^p)$ is the $p \times 1$ linear regression coefficient vector indicating effects of SNPs perturbations to gene expressions and $\beta = (\beta_1, \ldots, \beta_m)$. Importantly, note that Σ does not depend on x. The coefficient β is assumed to be sparse, since each gene is known to have only a few genetic regulators according to Cai *et al.* [12]. The precision matrix represents a gene network (graph), as in an undirected GGM, by corresponding the nonzero (i, j)th element of the precision matrix with an edge between two vertices i and j [14]. This edge represents conditional dependence of genes i and j given all other gene expression levels. Thus, our goal is to identify nonzero entries of the precision matrix in order to construct a conditional dependence genetic network after the effects of SNPs perturbations are removed. The precision matrix Σ^{-1} is also expected to be sparse [4].

One of our primary interests is to estimate the precision matrix Σ^{-1}, which is symmetrically positive definite, so we need to ensure that the estimate of the precision matrix also satisfies symmetrical positive definiteness. To this end, we apply the modified Cholesky decomposition [13] to the precision matrix, denoted by K, as follows:

$$K \left(\phi, \tau \right) = C \left(\phi \right)^\top D \left(\tau \right) C \left(\phi \right), \qquad (2)$$

where C is an upper triangular matrix with diagonal entries 1 and above-diagonal elements consisting of negative of $\phi = (\phi_{12}, \ldots, \phi_{1m}, \phi_{23}, \ldots, \phi_{2m}, \ldots, \phi_{m-1,m})$ and D is a diagonal matrix containing $\tau = (\tau_1, \ldots, \tau_m)$ with $\tau_j > 0$ for all $j = 1, \ldots, m$ as diagonal entries. Here, the superscript "⊤" denotes the transpose of a matrix. Positive definiteness of K is shown in Appendix A. Throughout this paper, a vector in the parenthesis is considered as a column vector. Let $\phi_j = (\phi_{j,j+1}, \ldots, \phi_{jm})$ for $j = 1, \ldots, m - 1$. Then we can write $\phi = (\phi_1, \ldots, \phi_{m-1})$. The parameter space for JMCCM is defined by

$\Theta = \{\theta = (\beta, \phi, \tau) : \beta \in \mathbb{R}^{mp}, \phi \in \mathbb{R}^{m(m-1)/2}$ and $\tau \in \mathbb{R}^m_+\}$, where $\mathbb{R}^m_+$ represents the set of m-dimensional vectors of positive real numbers.

2.2. Maximum Likelihood Estimation. Suppose that we have the N independent observations (x^i, y^i), $i = 1, \ldots, N$, sampled from (1), where $y^i = (y^i_1, \ldots, y^i_m)$ and $x^i = (x^i_1, \ldots, x^i_p)$ represent the ith observation of x and y, respectively. With $\Sigma^{-1} = K = K(\phi, \tau)$, $\mu(x) = \mu(x; \beta)$, and $\mu^i = \mu(x^i)$, the log-likelihood function corresponding to (1) is given by

$$\ell(\theta) = \frac{N}{2} \left\{ -m \log(2\pi) + \sum_{j=1}^m \log \tau_j - \mathrm{tr}\left(KV(\beta)\right) \right\}, \quad (3)$$

where $V(\beta) = (1/N) \sum_{i=1}^N (y^i - \mu^i)(y^i - \mu^i)^\top$ and "tr" denotes the trace of a matrix. A derivation of (3) can be found in Appendix B. The maximum likelihood estimator (MLE) of θ is defined by

$$\hat{\theta} = \underset{\theta \in \Theta}{\mathrm{argmax}}\, \ell(\theta). \quad (4)$$

Some notations are needed to express MLE of θ in conjunction with variable selection. For $j = 1, \ldots, m$, let G_j be an index set of active (or significant) coefficients of β_j and denote by g_j the number of elements in G_j. Let $G = \{G_1, \ldots, G_m\}$ and $g = g_1 + \cdots + g_m$. Obviously, $g \leq mp$ and if $g = mp$, then all variables are significant for all $y_1, \ldots, y_m$. Define $\beta(G) = (\beta_1(G_1), \ldots, \beta_m(G_m)) \in \mathbb{R}^g$ and $\beta_j(G_j) = \left[\beta_j^l\right]_{l \in G_j} \in \mathbb{R}^{g_j}$ for $j = 1, \ldots, m$. Write $y_k = (y_k^1, \ldots, y_k^N)$ for $k = 1, \ldots, m$, $X = (1/N)(x_1, \ldots, x_p)$, and $X(G_j) = [X_l]_{l \in G_j} \in \mathbb{R}^{N \times g_j}$, where X_l denotes lth column of X. Let $Y = (y_1^\top, \ldots, y_m^\top) \in \mathbb{R}^{mN}$, $\mathbb{X} = \oplus_{j=1}^m X(G_j) \in \mathbb{R}^{mN \times g}$, and $W = K \otimes I_N \in \mathbb{R}^{mN \times mN}$, where $\oplus$ and $\otimes$ represent direct sum and Kronecker product, respectively, and I_N is the $N \times N$ identity matrix. Then the MLE $\hat{\beta}(G)$ of $\beta(G)$ can be expressed as

$$\hat{\beta}(G) = \left(\mathbb{X}^\top W \mathbb{X}\right)^{-1} \mathbb{X}^\top W Y. \quad (5)$$

Observe that estimating $\beta(G)$ involves K.

We can estimate K by obtaining MLE of ϕ and τ. For $j = 1, \ldots, m-1$, let $\theta_j = (\beta, \phi_j, \tau_j)$ with $\theta_m = (\beta, \tau_m)$. Let V_{jj}, $V_{j,21}$, and $V_{j,22}$ represent the $(1, 1)$, $(2, 1)$, and $(2, 2)$ components of the lower jth principal submatrix $V_j(\beta)$ of $V(\beta)$. Then we can express

$$\ell(\theta) = \sum_{j=1}^m \ell_j(\theta_j), \quad (6)$$

where

$$\ell_j(\theta_j) = \frac{N}{2} \left\{ -\log(2\pi) + \log \tau_j \right.$$
$$\left. - \tau_j \left(V_{jj} - 2\phi_j^\top V_{j,21} + \phi_j^\top V_{j,22} \phi_j\right) \right\}. \quad (7)$$

By (6), we can obtain $(\hat{\phi}, \hat{\tau})$ from $(\hat{\phi}_j, \hat{\tau}_j)$ for each j with $\hat{\phi}_j = \mathrm{argmax}_{\phi_j} \ell_j(\theta_j)$ and $\hat{\tau}_j = \mathrm{argmax}_{\tau_j} \ell_j(\theta_j)$. Thus, instead of finding a solution to the optimization problem with (3), we optimize each $\ell_j(\theta_j)$ with respect to ϕ_j and τ_j. Thus, the MLE $\hat{\phi}_j$ and $\hat{\tau}_j$ are expressed in terms of $V(\beta)$ in a way that

$$\hat{\phi}_j = V_{j,22}^{-1} V_{j,21},$$

$$\frac{1}{\hat{\tau}_j} = V_{jj} - V_{j,12} V_{j,22}^{-1} V_{j,21} \quad (8)$$

$$\text{for } j = 1 \ldots, m-1$$

with $\hat{\beta}$ from (5) and $1/\hat{\tau}_m = V_{mm}$. We estimate Σ^{-1} by $\hat{K}$ and it is defined by

$$\hat{K} = K\left(\hat{\phi}, \hat{\tau}\right). \quad (9)$$

Derivations of (5), (6), and (8) are presented in Appendix C.

3. Consecutive Variable Selection Algorithm

As mentioned above, β and K are commonly believed to be sparse in genomic data analysis. To address sparsity, the lasso-type penalty imposed on both regression coefficients and precision matrix has been popularly applied to diverse graphical models [4, 5]. Stepping aside the lasso-type approach, we develop a variable selection technique that mainly relies on the combination of classical variable selection methods. Generally, the numbers of SNPs and genes tend to be considerably huge so that computational costs normally become prohibitive. In order to address this problem, the proposed variable selection algorithm proceeds with largely two stages: (1) preliminary variable selection for mean and precision matrix and (2) secondary variable selection in the middle of the joint model estimation. It is important to note that the first stage leads possible variables to be limited in scope (i.e., working parameters in the model) in order to circumvent high computational complexity.

3.1. Preliminary Variable Selection. Preliminary variable selection is largely twofold: variable selection for the mean part and covariance part. The idea behind that is to add variables (or equivalently parameters) to the joint model with the maximum Rao statistic and to delete ones with the minimum Wald statistic. You may refer to Koo [15] for the basis selection method or Kooperberg et al. [16] that explain variable selection schemes based on Rao and Wald statistics.

3.1.1. Mean Part. When it comes to the mean part, we carry out selecting predictor variables (i.e., SNPs) for each response variable (i.e., gene expression), dealing with a univariate multiple regression problem. In the addition stage, we start off with a model including only an intercept term. The MLE is used as estimator for β and maximum Rao statistic (Rao [17]) is the criterion for adding a predictor together with GCV (Friedman [18]) as a stopping rule. In the deletion stage, Wald statistic is calculated to exclude predictor variables such that

```
(1)  for j in 1 : m do
(2)      Set the minimal linear regression model: $Y_j = \beta_j^0$.
(3)      Compute $\widehat{\beta}_j^0$ and GCV.
(4)      while GCV decreases do
(5)          Among predictors not in the current model, add a predictor $X_b$ having the
             maximum Rao statistic.
(6)          Update $\widehat{\beta}_j(G_j)$ using (5) and compute GCV.
(7)      end while
(8)      while GCV decreases do
(9)          Among predictors in the current model, delete a predictor $X_{b'}$ having the
             minimum Wald statistic.
(10)         Update $\widehat{\beta}_j(G_j)$ using (5) and compute GCV.
(11)     end while
(12)     The optimal model is chosen by the minimum GCV.
(13) end for
```

ALGORITHM 1: Variable selection in the mean vector estimation.

the updated model minimizes Wald statistics. The final model for the mean regression is chosen by the minimum GCV. Details are summarized in Algorithm 1. Once Algorithm 1 is done, the number of predictor variables included in the joint model no longer increases, while variable reduction can happen in Algorithm 3 (Section 3.2).

3.1.2. Covariance Part. The rationale behind variable selection in the precision matrix estimation is that each Y_j, $j = 1, \ldots, m - 1$, is regressed on $Y_{j+1}, \ldots, Y_m$, and the regression coefficients are negative of off-diagonal entries of $C(\phi)$, the by-product of the modified Cholesky decomposition (2) [13, 19, 20]. Clearly, this is one of the major benefits of reparametrization via Cholesky decomposition [13] in pursuit of improved interpretation.

Subsequent to selection for predictor variables, we compute $V(\widehat{\beta}(G))$. Given initial $\widehat{\phi}_j^{(0)} = 0$, we start with computing $\widehat{\tau}_j$ for $j = 1, \ldots, m$ as in (8) using $V(\widehat{\beta}(G))$ obtained from Algorithm 1. Then compute Rao statistic to add one variable out of $Y_{j+1} \ldots, Y_m$ to the current model that builds on the response variable Y_j. We repeatedly update for Y_j, where $j = 1, \ldots, m - 1$. Next, we choose one variable, say ϕ_{lb}, for $l = 1, \ldots, m - 1$ and $b = l + 1, \ldots, m$, such that Rao statistic is maximized and thereby update $\widehat{\phi}_l$ and $\widehat{\tau}_l$, respectively. When calculating $\widehat{\tau}$ and $\widehat{\phi}$, the BIC is computed, and the addition process stops if the BIC no longer decreases. At the completion of addition, we build a model with all selected variables as a full model and subsequently begin deletion from a full model. Deletion process is similar to the addition process except that the minimum Wald statistic is used for deletion in place of the maximum Rao statistic. Successive deletion continues until the BIC stops decreasing. In the last stage, the final model is also selected by the BIC. Details are presented in Algorithm 2. Once Algorithm 2 is finished, the number of ϕ_{jk} included in the joint model no longer increases, while variable reduction could occur in the joint estimation (Algorithm 3, Section 3.2). Sparsity of $\widehat{K}$ is

achieved through this variable selection scheme along with Algorithm 3.

3.2. Secondary Variable Selection in the Middle of the Joint Model Estimation. With variables (i.e., parameters) selected by the preliminary stage above, we implement simultaneous parameter estimation for both mean and precision in the joint model and additional variable selection. Once $\widehat{K}$ is computed via Algorithm 2 with fixed $\widehat{\beta}(G)$, we start joint estimation by updating $\widehat{\beta}(G)$, which is formed with weight least square estimates as in (5) and weights coming from $\widehat{K}$. Then $\widehat{\phi}$ and $\widehat{\tau}$, ultimately $\widehat{K}$, are newly computed using updated $V(\widehat{\beta}(G))$, and again this updated $\widehat{K}$ serves as a weight for updating $\widehat{\beta}(G)$. Over the updates, the interplay between $V(\widehat{\beta}(G))$ and $\widehat{K}$ continues until the log-likelihood function converges. Afterwards, deletion to current parameters begins by Wald statistic, excluding one parameter with the minimum Wald statistic. Finally, the BIC is used as a stopping rule for deletion and selection to finalize model estimation. Algorithm 3 contains details about this procedure. While the preliminary variable selection works for each mean and covariance part under the assumption of $\widehat{\beta}(G)$ or $\widehat{K}$ are fixed, this joint estimation procedure is designed to improve estimation and selection accuracy by reflecting the changes of $\widehat{\beta}(G)$ and $\widehat{K}$.

4. Experimental Studies

In order to assess the performance of our proposed method, we carry out experimental simulations and compare the sparse conditional Gaussian graphical model (SCGGM), Zhang and Kim [5], covariate-adjusted precision matrix estimation (CAPME), Cai et al. [12] and joint model with lasso penalty (JML), and Jhong et al. [21], all of which are based on penalized likelihood approaches. The competing methods are run with their default setting regarding tuning parameters. To evaluate similarity, the estimated precision

---

(1) Compute $V(\widehat{\beta}(G))$ using $\widehat{\beta}(G)$ obtained from Algorithm 1.

(2) Compute $\widehat{\tau}_1, \ldots, \widehat{\tau}_m$ by (8).

(3) Combining initial $\phi_j^{(0)} = 0$ for all $j = 1, \ldots, m - 1$ with $\widehat{\tau}$, compute $\widehat{K}$ and BIC.

(4) **while** BIC decreases **do**

(5)   **for** j in $1 : (m - 1)$ **do**

(6)   **if** no elements of $\phi_j = (\phi_{j,j+1}, \ldots, \phi_{jm})$ are included in the joint model **then**

(7)   compute Rao statistics for ϕ_{jk} by $V_{kj}^2 / V_{kk}, k = j + 1, \ldots, m$.

(8)   **else**

(9)   Set a linear regression model with response Y_j and predictors Y_b's whose corresponding coefficients ϕ_{jb} are already included in the joint model. Here $b \in \{j + 1, \ldots, m\}$. Compute Rao statistic for adding one predictor among $Y_{j+1}, \ldots, Y_m$ whose corresponding ϕ_{jk}'s are not in this linear model.

(10)   **end if**

(11)   **end for**

(12)   Among all ϕ_{jk}'s not in the joint model, add one with the maximum Rao value. Denote this by ϕ_{lb} for $l = 1, \ldots, m - 1$ and $b = l + 1, \ldots, m$.

(13)   Update $\widehat{\phi}_l$, $\widehat{\tau}_l$ using (8) as well as $\widehat{K}$ and compute BIC.

(14) **end while**

(15) **while** BIC decreases **do**

(16)   Compute Wald statistics for all ϕ in the current model.

(17)   Delete one $\phi_{l'b'}$ with the minimum Wald.

(18)   Update $\widehat{\phi}_{l'}$, $\widehat{\tau}_{l'}$ using (8) as well as $\widehat{K}$ and compute BIC.

(19) **end while**

(20) The optimal model is chosen by the minimum BIC.

Algorithm 2: Variable selection in the precision matrix estimation.

---

(1) **repeat**

(2)   Update $\widehat{\beta}(G)$ by (5) and compute $V(\widehat{\beta}(G))$ with $\widehat{K}$ from Algorithm 2.

(3)   Update $\widehat{\tau}$, $\widehat{\phi}$ and $\widehat{K}$ using $V(\widehat{\beta}(G))$ obtained from the previous step.

(4) **until** the log-likelihood function converges.

(5) **while** BIC decreases **do**

(6)   Compute Wald statistic of deleting each β_j^p and ϕ_{jb} in the current model.

(7)   Delete one variable (i.e., parameter) with the minimum Wald statistic.

(8)   **repeat**

(9)   Update $\widehat{\beta}(G)$ by (5) and compute $V(\widehat{\beta}(G))$ with $\widehat{K}$ from the previous step.

(10)   Update $\widehat{\tau}$, $\widehat{\phi}$ and $\widehat{K}$ using $V(\widehat{\beta}(G))$ obtained from the previous step.

(11)   **until** the log-likelihood function converges.

(12) **end while**

(13) The optimal model is chosen by BIC.

Algorithm 3: Variable selection in the joint estimation.

---

matrix and true matrix are benchmarked by the Steins loss function:

$$\delta_{Stein}\left(K, \widehat{K}\right) = \mathrm{tr}\left(K\widehat{K}^{-1}\right) - \log\left|K\widehat{K}^{-1}\right| - m, \qquad (10)$$

where $\widehat{K}$ is an estimate of the true precision matrix K and $|\cdot|$ denotes the determinant of a matrix. The Frobenius norm of difference between K and $\widehat{K}$, denoted by $\|\Delta\|_F$, where $\Delta = K - \widehat{K}$, is also considered. In addition to the Steins loss function, to measure how efficiently our model recovers the true conditional dependent relationship among genes, specificity (SPE) and sensitivity (SEN) are used, as defined by

$$\begin{aligned} \mathrm{SPE} &= \frac{\mathrm{TN}}{\mathrm{TN} + \mathrm{FP}}, \\ \mathrm{SEN} &= \frac{\mathrm{TP}}{\mathrm{TP} + \mathrm{FN}}, \end{aligned} \qquad (11)$$

where TN, TP, FN, and FP are the numbers of true negatives, true positives, false negatives, and false positives with regard to off-diagonal elements of a precision matrix. Here, we treat a nonzero entry of a precision matrix as "positive." To combine sensitivity and specificity, Youden's index (=SPE + SEN − 1) is

TABLE 1: Six scenarios for small-scale experimental study.

Model	m	p	$\mathbb{P}(k_{ij} \neq 0)$	$\mathbb{P}(\beta_j^l \neq 0)$
1	10	10	$2/m$	$3.5/p$
2	20	10	$2/m$	$3.5/p$
3	40	10	$2/m$	$3.5/p$
4	20	20	$2/m$	$4/p$
5	30	30	$2/m$	$4/p$
6	40	40	$2/m$	$4/p$

TABLE 2: Three scenarios for large-scale experimental study.

Model	m	p	$\mathbb{P}(k_{ij} \neq 0)$	$\mathbb{P}(\beta_j^l \neq 0)$
7	100	100	$2/m$	$3/p$
8	200	200	$2.5/m$	$15/p$
9	400	200	$1.5/m$	$20/p$

used. The smaller values of δ_{Stein} and $\|\Delta\|_F$ are better, whereas the larger values of SPE, SEN, and Youden are better.

Inspired by Yin and Li [4], we generate simulation data sets in the form of eQTL data sets such that nonzero entries of a precision matrix, commonly called a link (or edge), are randomly assigned with probability c_1/m, where m is the number of genes and c_1 is some positive constant. For a link generated at the (i, j)th entry of the precision matrix, denoted by k_{ij}, the corresponding element is sampled from the uniform distribution over $[-1, 0.5] \cup [0.5, 1]$. For each row, off-diagonal elements are divided by the sum of their absolute values multiplied by 1.5. And we obtain the true precision matrix K by symmetrizing and setting diagonals as 1. To create the $p \times m$ regression coefficients matrix β, we first generate a $p \times m$ indicator matrix that has 1 as entry with probability c_2/p for some positive constant c_2. If the (l, j)th element of this indicator matrix is 1, β_j^l is randomly generated from $Unif([d_m, 1] \cup [-1, -d_m])$, where d_m is the smallest absolute value of K generated.

Producing β and K, we generate SNPs, $X = (X_1, \dots, X_p)$ with $X_l \sim$ Bernoulli$(1, 0.5)$ for $l = 1, \dots, p$. Finally, we simulated gene expressions by generating y from the multivariate normal distribution given x, $Y \mid X \sim N(X\beta, K^{-1})$. We generate a data set of N i.i.d. random vectors (X, Y), and simulations are repeated 50 times. In Table 1, we outline the six simulation scenarios of small-scale setup. Table 2 contains the three simulation scenarios of large-scale setup.

The small-scale simulation results in Table 3 suggest that the JMCCM produces better estimates than all other methods across all six models. Due to computational issues, we drop some results of JML from Table 3. By comparing the results of model 3 with 6 and 2 with 4, when $N = 1000$ and the number of genes is fixed, we can see that JMCCM and CAPME show less changes in δ_{Stein} and $\|\Delta\|_F$ than they appear in the SCGGM as the number of SNPs increases. This indicates that JMCCM and CAPME are less subject to the increment of the number of SNPs than SCGGM, when modest size of genes is involved. Estimation performance of CAPME seems to be affected by the number of genes more easily than JMCCM because Stein loss and Frobenius norm of CAPME for models

1, 2, and 3 with fixed p increase more rapidly than those of JMCCM do. For identifying structures of the precision matrix, JMCCM surpasses SCGGM in discovering nonzero elements (higher sensitivity) as complexity of the model rises. This is possibly due to the fact that SCGGM tends to produce sparse estimates more than the true precision matrix. Higher sensitivity implies that our proposed model is less likely to miss the influential conditional dependency among genes. While CAPME and JML score near 1 in sensitivity, they mark poor number in specificity because 5-fold cross-validation for CAPME and validation approach for JML with default setting for tuning parameters selection tend to choose small ones, leading to dense estimates. JMCCM produces higher Youden's index across all simulation scenarios compared to all other methods, and the performance gap between JMCCM and others is increasingly widened as the models increase in sample size and complexity. The results for the large-scale simulations (models 7–9) are summarized in Table 4 and Table S3. Due to long computing time, the results of CAPME for models 8 and 9 are not reported. Overall, the results are consistent with the small-scale simulations. The gap between JMCCM and SCGGM in estimation performance widened as the complexity of the model increases (Table 4).

We also simulate SNPs to mimic the linkage disequilibrium (LD) which is known to be a common phenomenon in DNA sequence and to assess the performance of our approach. We randomly generate two groups of SNPs which lie on LD, each of which contains LD block including 10 correlated SNPs such that correlation is greater than 0.9. Together with these SNPs, 10 SNPs are generated independently from Bernoulli trials with probability of 0.5 for a total of 20 SNPs and 20 genes: $m = 20$ and $p = 20$. Table 5 presents the simulation results using these data of sample size $N = 500$ and $N = 1000$ with 50 repetitions. Compared to the results of model 4 in Table 3, which is based on 20 independent SNPs with $N = 500$, LD is found to have little impact on all methods, except for slight decreases in Stein loss and Frobenius norm of SCGGM.

5. eQTL Analysis of Yeast Data

In this section, we apply the proposed algorithm to genomic eQTL (i.e., expression quantitative trait loci) data in order to examine whether the proposed method effectively recovers true dependency of gene expressions, which builds on known molecular mechanisms. To this end, we collect a set of yeast data [22], including polymorphic genotypes and mRNA expressions. The yeast data have been widely applied to elucidate the biological interactions between nucleotide polymorphisms and their responding genes (e.g., perturbation effects) [23–26]. Thus, our primary goal is to identify conditional dependency among genes with an adjustment of SNPs perturbations to each gene expression level.

The data sets are collected for two yeast parent strains, BY4716 (BY) and RM11-1a (RM), and their 112 segregants. We obtain SNPs for 1,260 loci to the exclusion of the redundant SNPs observed in neighboring genetic regions and leave 3,684 expression genes after screening out genes of missing more than 5%. In order to validate whether or

TABLE 3: Comparisons of the performance of JMCCM with SCGGM, CAPME, and JML for models 1–6. Standard errors are presented in parenthesis.

Model	Method	δ_{Stein}	$\|\Delta\|_F$	SPE	SEN	Youden
			$N = 500$			
1	JMCCM	0.139 (0.004)	0.519 (0.008)	0.864 (0.010)	0.723 (0.014)	0.587 (0.012)
	SCGGM	0.171 (0.007)	0.556 (0.010)	0.865 (0.030)	0.624 (0.027)	0.506 (0.014)
	CAPME	0.113 (0.003)	0.512 (0.008)	0.002 (0.001)	1.000 (0.000)	0.002 (0.001)
	JML	0.099 (0.003)	0.450 (0.005)	0.160 (0.026)	0.980 (0.005)	0.140 (0.024)
			$N = 500$			
2	JMCCM	0.241 (0.005)	0.677 (0.009)	0.915 (0.004)	0.801 (0.007)	0.716 (0.006)
	SCGGM	0.349 (0.008)	0.821 (0.012)	0.661 (0.029)	0.882 (0.016)	0.542 (0.017)
	CAPME	0.430 (0.007)	1.028 (0.011)	0.005 (0.001)	1.000 (0.000)	0.005 (0.001)
	JML	0.232 (0.004)	0.670 (0.008)	0.210 (0.009)	0.980 (0.003)	0.200 (0.009)
			$N = 500$			
3	JMCCM	0.705 (0.011)	1.145 (0.009)	0.947 (0.002)	0.653 (0.006)	0.600 (0.005)
	SCGGM	1.158 (0.034)	1.506 (0.032)	0.716 (0.036)	0.706 (0.029)	0.422 (0.010)
	CAPME	1.703 (0.012)	2.217 (0.015)	0.005 (0.000)	1.000 (0.000)	0.005 (0.000)
	JML	-	-	-	-	-
			$N = 500$			
4	JMCCM	0.239 (0.006)	0.678 (0.011)	0.910 (0.004)	0.802 (0.007)	0.712 (0.007)
	SCGGM	0.402 (0.010)	0.869 (0.011)	0.825 (0.031)	0.772 (0.017)	0.597 (0.019)
	CAPME	0.447 (0.007)	1.081 (0.010)	0.004 (0.001)	1.000 (0.000)	0.004 (0.001)
	JML	0.284 (0.005)	0.793 (0.008)	0.110 (0.006)	1.000 (0.001)	0.100 (0.006)
			$N = 500$			
5	JMCCM	0.463 (0.007)	0.953 (0.007)	0.941 (0.003)	0.731 (0.007)	0.672 (0.006)
	SCGGM	0.743 (0.011)	1.188 (0.010)	0.978 (0.002)	0.567 (0.007)	0.545 (0.007)
	CAPME	0.983 (0.008)	1.683 (0.012)	0.005 (0.001)	1.000 (0.000)	0.005 (0.001)
	JML	0.524 (0.524)	1.074 (0.009)	0.140 (0.006)	0.980 (0.002)	0.120 (0.006)
			$N = 500$			
6	JMCCM	0.711 (0.010)	1.153 (0.010)	0.951 (0.002)	0.639 (0.006)	0.590 (0.005)
	SCGGM	1.126 (0.011)	1.438 (0.007)	0.988 (0.001)	0.440 (0.004)	0.428 (0.004)
	CAPME	1.781 (0.013)	2.406 (0.013)	0.006 (0.000)	0.999 (0.000)	0.006 (0.000)
	JML	-	-	-	-	-
			$N = 1000$			
1	JMCCM	0.068 (0.002)	0.364 (0.006)	0.814 (0.007)	0.886 (0.009)	0.700 (0.009)
	SCGGM	0.139 (0.010)	0.483 (0.018)	0.888 (0.024)	0.668 (0.031)	0.556 (0.016)
	CAPME	0.055 (0.002)	0.346 (0.006)	0.003 (0.001)	1.000 (0.000)	0.003 (0.001)
	JML	0.046 (0.001)	0.301 (0.005)	0.150 (0.015)	1.000 (0.001)	0.150 (0.015)
			$N = 1000$			
2	JMCCM	0.117 (0.003)	0.466 (0.006)	0.894 (0.003)	0.898 (0.005)	0.793 (0.004)
	SCGGM	0.168 (0.007)	0.550 (0.010)	0.652 (0.018)	0.960 (0.006)	0.612 (0.016)
	CAPME	0.215 (0.003)	0.696 (0.007)	0.003 (0.001)	1.000 (0.000)	0.003 (0.001)
	JML	0.119 (0.002)	0.459 (0.006)	0.320 (0.120)	0.990 (0.003)	0.310 (0.012)
			$N = 1000$			
3	JMCCM	0.321 (0.006)	0.766 (0.007)	0.916 (0.002)	0.808 (0.004)	0.724 (0.003)
	SCGGM	0.645 (0.015)	1.107 (0.011)	0.674 (0.021)	0.847 (0.024)	0.521 (0.008)
	CAPME	0.824 (0.006)	1.405 (0.007)	0.005 (0.000)	1.000 (0.000)	0.005 (0.000)
	JML	-	-	-	-	-
			$N = 1000$			
4	JMCCM	0.115 (0.003)	0.467 (0.006)	0.893 (0.003)	0.904 (0.006)	0.797 (0.005)
	SCGGM	0.286 (0.009)	0.745 (0.012)	0.786 (0.028)	0.822 (0.019)	0.609 (0.015)
	CAPME	0.215 (0.003)	0.703 (0.006)	0.003 (0.001)	1.000 (0.000)	0.003 (0.001)
	JML	0.123 (0.002)	0.486 (0.005)	0.160 (0.006)	1.000 (0.002)	0.150 (0.005)

TABLE 3: Continued.

Model	Method	δ_{Stein}	$\|\Delta\|_F$	SPE	SEN	Youden
			$N = 1000$			
5	JMCCM	0.217 (0.004)	0.643 (0.006)	0.924 (0.002)	0.867 (0.005)	0.792 (0.004)
	SCGGM	0.671 (0.011)	1.141 (0.001)	0.995 (0.002)	0.542 (0.009)	0.536 (0.008)
	CAPME	0.473 (0.004)	1.065 (0.007)	0.004 (0.000)	1.000 (0.000)	0.004 (0.000)
	JML	-	-	-	-	-
			$N = 1000$			
6	JMCCM	0.331 (0.005)	0.781 (0.006)	0.926 (0.002)	0.789 (0.005)	0.715 (0.004)
	SCGGM	1.024 (0.010)	1.380 (0.006)	0.998 (0.000)	0.414 (0.003)	0.412 (0.003)
	CAPME	0.844 (0.006)	1.466 (0.008)	0.005 (0.000)	0.999 (0.000)	0.004 (0.000)
	JML	-	-	-	-	-

TABLE 4: Comparisons of the performance of JMCCM with SCGGM and CAPME for models 7–9. Standard errors are presented in parenthesis.

Model	Method	δ_{Stein}	$\|\Delta\|_F$	SPE	SEN	Youden
			$N = 500$			
7	JMCCM	2.234 (0.021)	2.071 (0.011)	0.969 (0.001)	0.638 (0.004)	0.608 (0.003)
	SCGGM	2.670 (0.017)	2.160 (0.007)	0.994 (0.000)	0.512 (0.002)	0.506 (0.002)
	CAPME	12.914 (0.038)	9.257 (0.028)	0.002 (0.000)	1.000 (0.000)	0.002 (0.000)
			$N = 500$			
8	JMCCM	6.560 (0.073)	3.669 (0.028)	0.982 (0.001)	0.475 (0.004)	0.457 (0.003)
	SCGGM	10.687 (0.035)	4.318 (0.006)	0.925 (0.000)	0.430 (0.002)	0.355 (0.002)
	CAPME	-	-	-	-	-
			$N = 500$			
9	JMCCM	16.703 (0.254)	5.998 (0.062)	0.986 (0.001)	0.466 (0.003)	0.452 (0.002)
	SCGGM	34.025 (0.722)	7.277 (0.048)	0.874 (0.005)	0.453 (0.003)	0.328 (0.003)
	CAPME	-	-	-	-	-

TABLE 5: Comparisons of the performance of JMCCM with SCGGM and CAPME for the experiment with highly correlated SNPs. 20 genes (m) and 20 SNPs (p) are involved. Standard errors are presented in parenthesis.

Method	δ_{Stein}	$\|\Delta\|_F$	SPE	SEN	Youden
			$N = 500$		
JMCCM	0.239 (0.006)	0.678 (0.011)	0.910 (0.004)	0.802 (0.007)	0.712 (0.007)
SCGGM	0.402 (0.010)	0.869 (0.011)	0.825 (0.031)	0.772 (0.017)	0.597 (0.019)
CAPME	0.447 (0.007)	1.081 (0.010)	0.004 (0.001)	1.000 (0.000)	0.0004 (0.001)
			$N = 1000$		
JMCCM	0.115 (0.003)	0.467 (0.006)	0.893 (0.003)	0.904 (0.006)	0.797 (0.005)
SCGGM	0.286 (0.009)	0.745 (0.012)	0.786 (0.028)	0.822 (0.019)	0.609 (0.015)
CAPME	0.215 (0.003)	0.703 (0.006)	0.003 (0.001)	1.000 (0.000)	0.003 (0.001)

not the estimated gene network is consistent with unknown biological knowledge, we take the true signaling pathway for comparison. Out of 3,684 yeast genes, we purposely focus on a set of 64 genes that are ascertained in the cell cycle yeast pathway available in the KEGG database [24]. Together with 1,260 SNPs as predictors, we construct a gene network model of 64 genes. JMCCM selects 222 nonzero elements of the precision matrix and leaves nonzero regression coefficients, for a total of 111 links among genes. A total of 489 regression coefficients of SNPs over gene expression levels are included in the final model. Figure 2 displays the conditional gene

network estimated by the proposed joint model. A pair of two genes is linked if an off-diagonal element of the estimated precision matrix is nonzero, and so 51 genes are shown to be linked and assemble in a module.

Given this estimated gene network, we notice that the gene network is found to be concordant with the true cell cycle pathway. For instance, according to the true cell cycle pathway in Figure 1, MCM3 is linked to ORC3, ORC5, MCM7, and MCM4. MCM5 is connected to TAH11 and ORC1. PHO4 is closely linked to CLN2 and SIC1, whose molecular function is related to MAP kinase orthologs (i.e., MAPK pathway

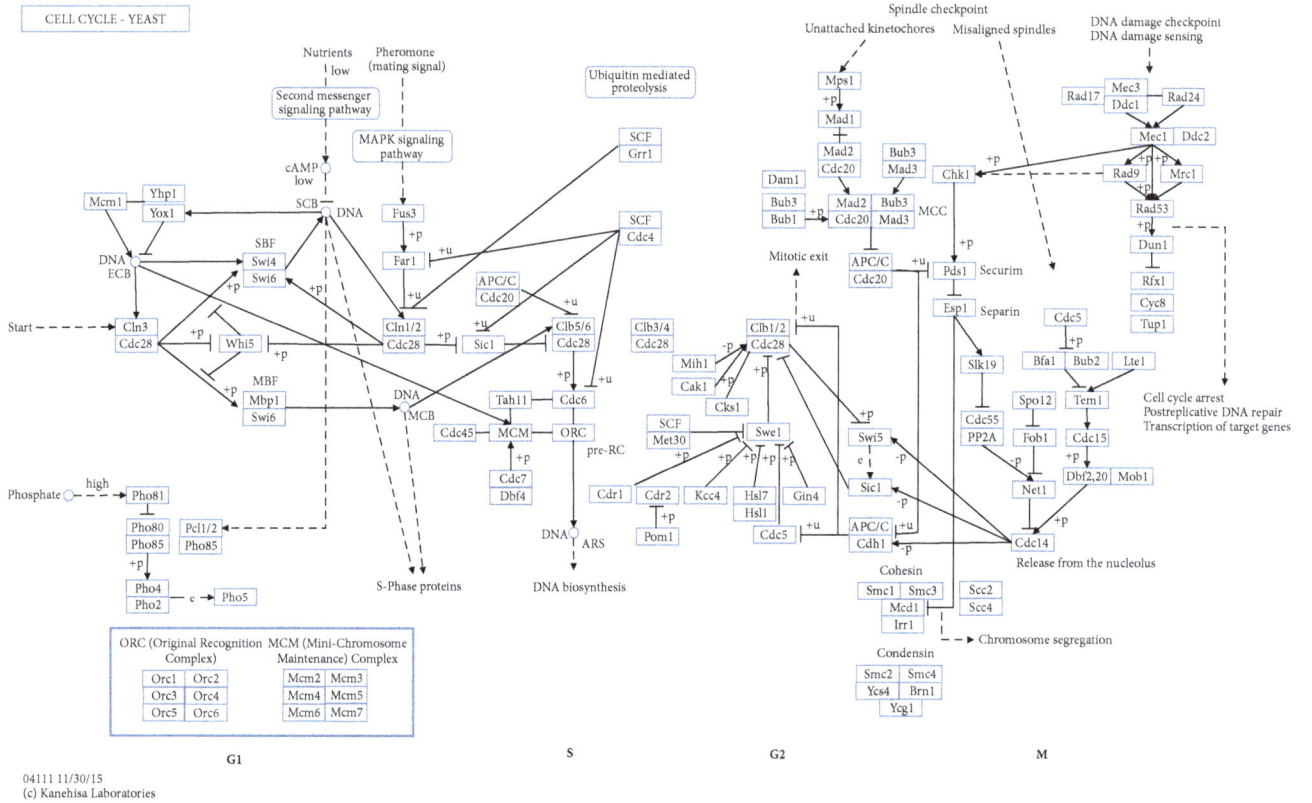

FIGURE 1: The yeast cell cycle pathway from the KEGG database. Source: http://www.kegg.jp/kegg-bin/highlight_pathway?scale=1.0&map=map04111&keyword=cell%20cycle.

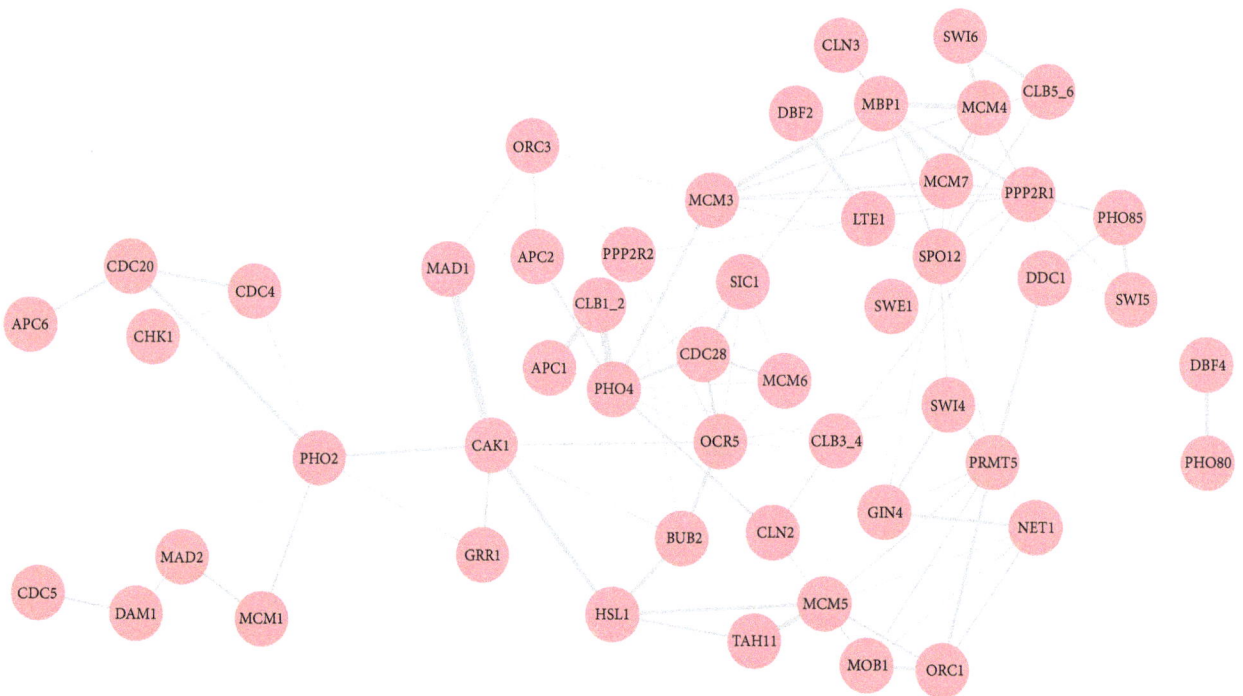

FIGURE 2: The gene network of the yeast data related to the cell cycle pathway via the JMCCM.

TABLE 6: Gene ontology (GO) enrichment analysis over the genes in detected module from the JMCCM.

Module	Module size	GO category	GO enrichment p value
		Carboxylic acid metabolic process	0.00101
		Carboxypeptidase activity	0.00904
		Catabolic process	0.00101
		Cellular catabolic process	0.00101
Module 1	94	Exopeptidase activity	0.00904
		Metalloexopeptidase activity	0.00904
		Metallopeptidase activity	0.00904
		Organic acid metabolic process	0.00101
		Peptidase activity	0.00904

genes). It is interesting to note that CLN3 and SWI4 are mutually connected together, linking to their downstream gene MBP1. Hence, this undirected graph contributes to recovering lots of links among the 64 genes of the pathway.

With regard to genetic variant effects, JMCCM is shown to effectively identify some of the well-known direct genetic perturbations. Gene expressions are regulated by some genetic variants, which, unless otherwise taken into account, may falsely capture the interplay of genes in a network. Our founding includes Clb-specific Cdk inhibitor (SIC1) as influencing the molecular interface between cyclin-Cdk complexes (e.g., binding to and blocking Cdk1/Clb activity, ultimately to maneuver the timing of DNA replication (see Table S1 in Supplementary Materials; [27]). In addition, our gene networks demonstrate that SIC1 is strongly perturbed by CLB3, while SCGGM did not detect any perturbation effects. More interestingly, many previous experiments validated the association between SIC1 and CLB3 to uncover the underlying mechanism of the cell cycle [28–30]. Clearly, this implies that JMCCM does a better job in accounting for SNPs perturbation as compared to SCGGM.

Moreover, the gene module detected from JMCCM is shown in Table 6. Pertaining to these gene modules, we hypothesize if gene modules, each containing hub genes and their neighboring genes, are enriched with common biological processes or not. To test this hypothesis, we conduct the gene ontology (GO) enrichment analysis [31] over the detected gene network modules (see Table S2 in Supplementary Materials) from both JMCCM and SCGGM using Fisher's exact tests. Table 6 demonstrates that the proposed method outstandingly performs detecting modules biologically associated with many molecular processes, while none is detected by SCGGM. More importantly, the pathway of the organic acid metabolic process enriched in gene module 1 is also reported and validated on the basis of the network modules constructed with large-scale integration of yeast data in Zhu et al. [32].

Putting all things together, we conclude that the proposed method facilitates recovering the true SNPs perturbations in the midst of gene regulations and elucidating the underlying interplay of gene interactions. These fortes of the proposed algorithm are favored for reinforcing a priori biological knowledge and address a novel hypothesis related to clinical and translational potential.

6. Conclusion and Discussion

In this paper, we propose JMCCM to efficiently identify conditional dependent structures of gene expressions with adjustments to perturbation effects of SNPs. Contrary to the existing conditional graphical models, the precision matrix commonly used to reveal the true relationship among genes is parameterized via the modified Cholesky decomposition. The maximum likelihood estimates of the precision matrix were computed, while variable selection of SNPs and Cholesky factors are carried out separately and jointly by the GCV and BIC criterion. From experimental studies, it is clearly shown that JMCCM performs better than the existing penalization methods. Besides, JMCCM in the application to yeast cell cycle data successfully recovers many parts of the cell cycle pathway with adjustments of SNPs to each gene expressions level. Notably, the model entails the estimation of precision matrix, of which components are assumed to be constant. So, in the future, we may relax this somewhat strong assumption in the way that the model can parametrize over τ and ϕ in pursuit of more accurate estimation [13]. We leave this for next study.

Appendix

A. Positive Definiteness of K

The matrix representation of the modified Cholesky decomposition (2) is given by

$$
C(\phi) = \begin{bmatrix} 1 & -\phi_{12} & \cdots & -\phi_{1m} \\ & 1 & \cdots & -\phi_{2m} \\ & & \ddots & \vdots \\ & & & 1 \end{bmatrix},
$$

$$
D(\tau) = \begin{bmatrix} \tau_1 & & & \\ & \tau_2 & & \\ & & \ddots & \\ & & & \tau_m \end{bmatrix}.
$$

(A.1)

For simplicity, write $C = C(\phi)$ and $D = D(\tau)$. For any nonzero vector $u \in \mathbb{R}^m$,

$$u^\top K u = u^\top C^\top D C u = (Cu)^\top D (Cu)$$

$$= \sum_{j=1}^{m} \left((Cu)_j \right)^2 \tau_j > 0. \qquad \text{(A.2)}$$

Since $\tau_j > 0$ for all $j = 1, \ldots, m$, $\sum_{j=1}^{m} ((Cu)_j)^2 \tau_j = 0$ if and only if $Cu = 0$, which cannot happen here because u is a nonzero vector. Thus K is a positive definite matrix.

B. A Derivation of the Log-Likelihood Function

The probability density function of (1) is given by

$$f(y \mid x; \theta)$$

$$= \frac{|K|^{1/2}}{(2\pi)^{m/2}} \exp \left\{ -\frac{1}{2} (y - \mu(x))^\top K (y - \mu(x)) \right\}, \qquad \text{(B.1)}$$

where $\theta = (\beta, \phi, \tau)$. The log-likelihood function corresponding to JMCCM can be derived as follows:

$$\ell(\theta) = \log \sum_{i=1}^{N} f\left(y^i \mid x^i; \theta\right)$$

$$= \frac{-mN}{2} \log(2\pi) + \frac{N}{2} \log |K|$$

$$- \frac{1}{2} \sum_{i=1}^{N} \left(y^i - \mu^i\right)^\top K \left(y^i - \mu^i\right) \qquad \text{(B.2)}$$

$$= \frac{N}{2} \left\{ -m \log(2\pi) + \sum_{j=1}^{m} \log \tau_j - \operatorname{tr}(KV(\beta)) \right\}$$

where the last equality comes from $|C| = |C^\top| = 1$, $|D| = \tau_1 \tau_2 \cdots \tau_m$, and

$$\log |K| = \log \left| C^\top \right| |D| |C| = \log |D| = \sum_{j=1}^{m} \log \tau_j. \qquad \text{(B.3)}$$

C. Derivations of MLE $\widehat{\beta}$, $\widehat{\phi}$, and $\widehat{\tau}$

Using notations presented in Section 2.2, optimization problem for $\widehat{\beta}(G)$ is expressed as

$$\max \left\{ \frac{1}{2} \left[\log |K| - (Y - X\beta(G))^\top W (Y - X\beta(G)) \right] \right\}. \qquad \text{(C.1)}$$

Denote the score function of $\beta(G)$ by $S(\beta(G))$. Observe that

$$S(\beta(G)) = \frac{\partial}{\partial \beta(G)} \left\{ -\frac{1}{2} \left(Y^\top W Y \right. \right.$$

$$- 2\beta(G)^\top X^\top W Y + \beta(G)^\top X^\top W X \beta(G) \qquad \text{(C.2)}$$

$$\left. \left. - \sum_{j=1}^{m} \log \tau_j \right) \right\} = X^\top W Y - X^\top W X \beta(G)$$

By solving the normal equation $S(\beta(G)) = 0$, we have (5).

To derive (6), let $C(\phi_j) = (0, \ldots, 0, 1, \phi_{j,j+1}, \ldots, \phi_{jm})$, jth row of C. Then we can see that $C^\top D C = \sum_{j=1}^{m} \tau_j C(\phi_j) C(\phi_j)^\top$. The log-likelihood function (3) can be expressed as the sum of $\ell_j(\theta_j)$ as follows:

$$\ell(\theta) = \frac{N}{2} \left\{ -\log(2\pi) + \sum_{j=1}^{m} \log \tau_j - \operatorname{tr}(KV(\beta)) \right\}$$

$$= \frac{N}{2} \left\{ -m \log(2\pi) + \sum_{j=1}^{m} \log \tau_j \right.$$

$$\left. - \operatorname{tr} \left(\sum_{j=1}^{m} \tau_j C(\phi_j) C(\phi_j)^\top V(\beta) \right) \right\}$$

$$= \frac{N}{2} \left\{ -m \log(2\pi) + \sum_{j=1}^{m} \log \tau_j \right. \qquad \text{(C.3)}$$

$$\left. - \sum_{j=1}^{m} \tau_j C(\phi_j)^\top V(\beta) C(\phi_j) \right\}$$

$$= \frac{N}{2} \left\{ -m \log(2\pi) + \sum_{j=1}^{m} \log \tau_j \right.$$

$$\left. - \sum_{j=1}^{m} \tau_j \left(V_{jj} - 2\phi_j^\top V_{j,21} + \phi_j^\top V_{j,22} \phi_j \right) \right\}$$

$$= \sum_{j=1}^{m} \ell_j(\theta_j).$$

Finally, for any given $j = 1, \ldots, m - 1$, the gradient of log-likelihood function with respect to ϕ_j and τ_j is given by

$$\nabla \ell_j(\theta_j)$$

$$= \left[\begin{array}{c} N\tau_j \left(V_{j,21} - V_{j,22} \phi_j \right) \\ \frac{N}{2} \left\{ \frac{1}{\tau_j} - \left(V_{jj} - 2\phi_j^\top V_{j,21} + \phi_j^\top V_{j,22} \phi_j \right) \right\} \end{array} \right]. \qquad \text{(C.4)}$$

Then (8) is obtained by solving $\nabla \ell_j(\theta_j) = 0$ with respect to ϕ_j and τ_j.

Disclosure

A part of results from the earlier version of this research were presented in the poster session at 2016 Spring Seminar held by the Korean Statistical Society.

Conflicts of Interest

The authors declare that there are no conflicts of interest regarding the publication of this manuscript.

Acknowledgments

This research is supported by the Basic Science Research Program through the National Research Foundation of Korea (NRF) funded by the Ministry of Education, Science and Technology (NRF-2015R1D1A1A01057747 and NRF-2017R1C1B5017528).

References

[1] H. Ye and J. Pan, "Modelling of covariance structures in generalised estimating equations for longitudinal data," *Biometrika,* vol. 93, no. 4, pp. 927–941, 2006.

[2] H. Chun, M. Chen, B. Li, and H. Zhao, "Joint conditional Gaussian graphical models with multiple sources of genomic data," *Frontiers in Genetics*, vol. 4, article 294, 2013.

[3] B. Li, H. Chun, and H. Zhao, "Sparse estimation of conditional graphical models with application to gene networks," *Journal of the American Statistical Association*, vol. 107, no. 497, pp. 152–167, 2012.

[4] J. Yin and H. Li, "A sparse conditional Gaussian graphical model for analysis of genetical genomics data," *The Annals of Applied Statistics*, vol. 5, no. 4, pp. 2630–2650, 2011.

[5] L. Zhang and S. Kim, "Learning gene networks under SNP perturbations using eQTL datasets," *PLoS Computational Biology,* vol. 10, no. 2, Article ID e1003420, 2014.

[6] X. He, Z.-Y. Zhu, and W.-K. Fung, "Estimation in a semiparametric model for longitudinal data with unspecified dependence structure," *Biometrika*, vol. 89, no. 3, pp. 579–590, 2002.

[7] D. Xu, Z. Zhang, and L. Wu, "Joint Variable Selection of Mean-Covariance Model for Longitudinal Data," *Open Journal of Statistics*, vol. 03, no. 01, pp. 27–35, 2013.

[8] X. Zheng, W. K. Fung, and Z. Zhu, "Variable selection in robust joint mean and covariance model for longitudinal data analysis," *Statistica Sinica*, vol. 24, no. 2, pp. 515–531, 2014.

[9] K. A. Sohn and S. Kim, "Joint Estimation of Structured Sparsity and Output Structure in Multiple-Output Regression via Inverse-Convariance Regularization," in *Proceedings of the in Proceedings of the 15th International Conference on Artificial Intelligence and Statistics (AISTATS,* vol. XX, pp. 1081–1089, 2012.

[10] M. Morloy, C. M. Molony, T. M. Weber et al., "Genetic analysis of genome-wide variation in human gene expression," *Nature*, vol. 430, no. 7001, pp. 743–747, 2004.

[11] B. E. Stranger, M. S. Forrest, A. G. Clark et al., "Genome-wide associations of gene expression variation in humans." *PLoS Genetics*, vol. 1, no. 6, p. e78, 2005.

[12] T. T. Cai, H. Li, W. Liu, and J. Xie, "Covariate-adjusted precision matrix estimation with an application in genetical genomics," *Biometrika*, vol. 100, no. 1, pp. 139–156, 2013.

[13] M. Pourahmadi, "Joint mean-covariance models with applications to longitudinal data: unconstrained parameterisation," *Biometrika*, vol. 86, no. 3, pp. 677–690, 1999.

[14] S. r. Hojsgaard, D. Edwards, and S. Lauritzen, *Graphical models with R*, Springe, New York, NY, USA, 2012.

[15] J.-Y. Koo, "Spline estimation of discontinuous regression functions," *Journal of Computational and Graphical Statistics*, vol. 6, no. 3, pp. 266–284, 1997.

[16] C. Kooperberg, S. Bose, and C. J. Stone, "Polychotomous Regression," *Journal of the American Statistical Association*, vol. 92, no. 437, pp. 117–127, 1997.

[17] C. R. Rao, *Linear Methods of Statistical Induction and their Applications*, Wiley, New York, NY, USA, 2nd edition, 1973.

[18] J. H. Friedman, "Multivariate adaptive regression splines," *The Annals of Statistics*, vol. 19, no. 1, pp. 1–67, 1991.

[19] M. Pourahmadi, *High-Dimensional Covariance Estimation*, Wiley Series in Probability and Statistics, John Wiley & Sons, Hoboken, NJ, USA, 2013.

[20] N. Verzelen, "Adaptive estimation of covariance matrices via Cholesky decomposition," *Electronic Journal of Statistics*, vol. 4, pp. 1113–1150, 2010.

[21] J. H. Jhong, J. Lee, S. Kim, and J. Y. Koo, "Joint Modeling for Mean Vector and Covariance Estimation with l1-Penalty," *Quantitative Bio-Science*, vol. 36, no. 1, pp. 33–38, 2017.

[22] R. B. Brem and L. Kruglyak, "The landscape of genetic complexity across 5,700 gene expression traits in yeast," *Proceedings of the National Acadamy of Sciences of the United States of America*, vol. 102, no. 5, pp. 1572–1577, 2005.

[23] S.-S. C. Huang and E. Fraenkel, "Integrating proteomic, transcriptional, and interactome data reveals hidden components of signaling and regulatory networks," *Science Signaling*, vol. 2, no. 81, p. ra40, 2009.

[24] M. Kanehisa, S. Goto, M. Furumichi, M. Tanabe, and M. Hirakawa, "KEGG for representation and analysis of molecular networks involving diseases and drugs," *Nucleic Acids Research*, vol. 38, no. 1, pp. D355–D360, 2009.

[25] F. Markowetz, D. Kostka, O. G. Troyanskaya, and R. Spang, "Nested effects models for high-dimensional phenotyping screens," *Bioinformatics*, vol. 23, no. 13, pp. i305–i312, 2007.

[26] E. Yeger-Lotem, L. Riva, L. J. Su et al., "Bridging high-throughput genetic and transcriptional data reveals cellular responses to alpha-synuclein toxicity," *Nature Genetics*, vol. 41, no. 3, pp. 316–323, 2009.

[27] M. Barberis, "Sic1 as a timer of Clb cyclin waves in the yeast cell cycle - Design principle of not just an inhibitor," *FEBS Journal*, vol. 279, no. 18, pp. 3386–3410, 2012.

[28] V. Archambault, E. J. Chang, B. J. Drapkin, F. R. Cross, B. T. Chait, and M. P. Rout, "Targeted proteomic study of the cyclin-Cdk module," *Molecular Cell*, vol. 14, no. 6, pp. 699–711, 2004.

[29] A. Breitkreutz, H. Choi, J. R. Sharom et al., "A global protein kinase and phosphatase interaction network in yeast," *Science*, vol. 328, no. 5981, pp. 1043–1046, 2010.

[30] N. J. Krogan, G. Cagney, H. Yu et al., "Global landscape of protein complexes in the yeast saccharomyces cerevisiae," *Nature*, vol. 44, p. 0, 2006.

[31] S. Carbon, A. Ireland, C. J. Mungall et al., "AmiGO: Online access to ontology and annotation data," *Bioinformatics*, vol. 25, no. 2, pp. 288-289, 2009.

Computational Techniques for Eye Movements Analysis towards Supporting Early Diagnosis of Alzheimer's Disease

Jessica Beltrán [iD],[1,2] Mireya S. García-Vázquez,[1] Jenny Benois-Pineau,[3]
Luis Miguel Gutierrez-Robledo,[4] and Jean-François Dartigues[5]

[1]Instituto Politécnico Nacional-CITEDI, Tijuana, BC, Mexico
[2]CONACYT, Ciudad de México, Mexico
[3]LaBRI, University of Bordeaux, Bordeaux, France
[4]Instituto Nacional de Geriatría, Ciudad de México, Mexico
[5]INSERM, University of Bordeaux, Bordeaux, France

Correspondence should be addressed to Jessica Beltrán; jessicabeltran@gmail.com

Academic Editor: Hyuntae Park

An opportune early diagnosis of Alzheimer's disease (AD) would help to overcome symptoms and improve the quality of life for AD patients. Research studies have identified early manifestations of AD that occur years before the diagnosis. For instance, eye movements of people with AD in different tasks differ from eye movements of control subjects. In this review, we present a summary and evolution of research approaches that use eye tracking technology and computational analysis to measure and compare eye movements under different tasks and experiments. Furthermore, this review is targeted to the feasibility of pioneer work on developing computational tools and techniques to analyze eye movements under naturalistic scenarios. We describe the progress in technology that can enhance the analysis of eye movements everywhere while subjects perform their daily activities and give future research directions to develop tools to support early AD diagnosis through analysis of eye movements.

1. Introduction

Neurodegenerative diseases are a group of disorders characterized by the progressive degeneration of the neurons of the central or peripheral nervous systems. The degeneration affects neuron synapsis or produces neuron death [1]. The most frequent neurodegenerative diseases are Alzheimer's disease (AD) and Parkinson disease (PD) [2, 3]. According to the Alzheimer's Association (https://www.alz.org/), currently there are 5.7 million people living with AD only in the US and it is expected that this number would increase to 13.8 million by 2050 [4]. Although there is no cure for AD [5], several treatments have been tested [6], for example, currently approved drugs such as donepezil, galantamine, and rivastigmine [7] and nonpharmacologic therapies [4].

Alzheimer' disease is frequently diagnosed at late stages when symptoms have become evident, which occurs after a process of months or years of neuron degeneration [6].

However, when diagnosed at early stages, treatment helps to overcome the symptoms and improves the quality of life [2, 6] and offers to caregivers the opportunity to adapt and prepare the characteristics changes of dementia [8]. Also, the early diagnosis would allow testing the administration of more aggressive therapy to prevent AD development [9]. Despite many efforts, the noninvasive diagnosis of AD at early stages remains unsolved [5, 10].

Recent literature reviews have outlined robust findings demonstrating that eye movements abnormalities are sign of cognitive decline [11, 12] and can eventually be used to assess AD disease progression. Furthermore, current technology provides noninvasive equipment and methods to assess visual deficits ubiquitously and objectively in naturalistic scenarios [13]. An example is the use of eye trackers, which are devices that measure gaze fixation and saccadic motions of eyes. Eye trackers have been used in experiments of oculomotor performance related to AD diagnosis [14]. However, currently eye trackers have been used only in controlled laboratory settings. To analyze eye movements in naturalistic scenarios, such as in activities of daily living (ADL), besides the gaze fixation points, understanding the scene is required. The understanding of the scene can be achieved through analysis of recorded video with computer vision techniques. The computational analysis of the video, supported by the areas of psychology and neurology, allows distinguishing the items from the scenes that grab the attention of the viewer [15, 16]. This information can be used to compare the areas of interest from people with AD (PwAD) and control groups (people without AD) when observing natural scenes with a potential use in early detection.

In this paper, we firstly describe technological tools and methods that have been used to gather eye movements data. Then, we review existing research that has encountered relation between eye movements and AD. This section also describes a evolution of research on eye movements and AD since earliest research towards naturalistic scenarios more suitable for early detection. Section 4 describes computational techniques that are useful for complementing the analysis of eye movements and AD in naturalistic scenarios. Finally, Section 5 includes the conclusion and future directions.

2. Data Collection

To collect data, an important step is choosing a proper eye tracker device according to a planned research study. Eye trackers are devices that measure the point of gaze or eye movements from an individual [17]. The availability of eye movements recordings allows researchers to gather and analyze ground truth data about visual exploration [18]. This feature makes eye trackers a useful tool to study changes in cognition through eye movements analysis [19, 20]. The cognitive process are not directly measured with eye trackers. We can manipulate independent variables according to experimental design setups and measure the behavioral response from participants with eye movements measures [21].

Eye tracking provides a noninvasive tool without contraindications suitable for potential screening and tracking of AD [22]. Eye trackers provide data sensitivity that makes them suitable for analyzing oculomotor abnormalities in AD. However, there are different technological approaches for the construction of eye trackers [21]. For this reason, it is important to choose properly the adequate eye tracker features that fit the study.

Eye trackers can be static or provide mobility. For example, there are screen-based eye trackers, as the one used in [23]. These types of eye trackers are desktop mounted and collect fixation points only from the gaze towards the content displayed on a screen. Another type of eye trackers is head mounted, as the "ExpressEye" used in [19]. In this case the device allows capturing gaze fixations not limited to a specific screen; however, the user can not freely move because the apparatus is cumbersome. Nowadays, there are available commercial mobile eye trackers, such as Tobbi© (https://www.tobiipro.com) or SMI© (https://www.smivision.com) that provide continuous, remote, and pervasive capture capabilities. These capabilities are desirable to analyze eye movements from PwAD in naturalistic scenarios.

Despite capabilities provided by eye trackers, there are concerns about the use of eye trackers when participants are unrestrained [24]. The concerns are about the reliability of gaze recording when capturing data when participants take a nonoptimal pose. This later might represent a challenge in naturalistic experimental setups.

To gather data from participants in AD studies, researches divide participants into groups. Usually, the groups reported in the literature are young controls, elder controls, and PwAD. However, there are studies that also include a group people with Mild Cognitive Decline (MCI) to differentiate between persons in a more advanced stage of AD. The cognitive status from participants is usually evaluated through neuropsychological tests, such as the Mini Mental State Examination (MMSE) [12]. However, some studies have used other techniques such as thyroid function test and magnetic resonance images [11] among others.

The participants perform instructed oculomotor tasks while observing visual stimuli, such as images or video. The fixation points from the participants are collected using the chosen eye tracking device. Then, statistical tests and other modeling techniques are applied for data analysis. Finally, results are presented correlating outcome measures with a cognitive status and by showing differences among control groups and PwAD if present. In the next section different approaches that have encountered relation between eye movements and AD under different experimental setups are described.

3. Eye Movements and Alzheimer's Disease

Several researches on predementia have reported manifestations of visual symptoms produced by senile plaques and tangles located in the visual regions of the brain [38, 39]. The pathological changes in the visual system caused by neurodegenerative diseases are reviewed in [40–43]. Examples of these pathological changes are visual acuity changes, atypical pupillary responses, and alteration in the oculomotor performance [44].

Eye movements involve a complex oculomotor control system formed by extensive cerebral regions [45]. Through post mortem studies, there is evidence that pathologies associated with AD affect the oculomotor brain regions [46, 47]. Altered eye movements patterns reflect the resulting underlying visuospatial and executive function impairments. Thus, movement patterns are related to higher cognitive control processes [48]. That is why, for example, eye movements allow exploring the cognitive process underlying visual search, providing information about how people forage and plan when performing visual search tasks [49].

Typically, the studies dedicated to explore relationships between eye movements and AD compare certain outcome measures between persons with AD (PwAD) and control groups when they accomplish a specific oculomotor tasks.

Examples of these tasks are fixating on a given point [19] or watching a picture [12]. An example of a dependent variable on these studies is the reaction time to perform the given tasks.

To examine the research involving eye movements and Alzheimer's disease, we searched in the PubMed© (https://www.ncbi.nlm.nih.gov/pubmed) database with the keywords "Alzheimer's disease" and "Eye movements". The database included 165 articles from 1979 to 2017. From the 165 articles, 14 are review articles and 80 articles are not related to AD; focus on atypical subsets of AD or eye movements are not part of the study. From the 165 results, we found that 71 articles are relevant to the research of oculomotor performance of AD patients. The 19.7% (14 articles) from the relevant articles were published in the last 3 years. This shows that research analyzing eye movements is gaining importance in AD studies. Furthermore, recent research shows that the analysis of oculomotor deficits is useful in early detection of AD and also has the potential to be used to assess disease progression [43, 50].

Table 1 shows a summary of the research indexed in PubMed since the last 5 years related to eye movements analysis and AD. The summary includes the references and years, the methods used by the researches, the main findings from the studies and information about the participants, and apparatus if present. In the following sections, we describe and categorize conducted research showing an evolution from early attempts towards more naturalistic scenarios.

3.1. Saccadic Eye Movements and Alzheimer's Disease. Traditional studies using saccadic eye movements (SEM) tasks have reported differences between PwAD and control groups. A saccade is a rapid motion of the eye (typically lasting between 30 to 80 ms to complete) [21]. Example of these studies includes prosaccades and antisaccades analysis [19, 51]. To study prosaccades, a participant has to saccade from a initial point to an appearing peripheral target. Then, the reaction time or latency is measured from the subject to fixate on the presented peripheral target. The research described in [37, 52, 53] reports increased latency of saccades from PwAD when compared to control groups that can be associated with cognitive process. On the other hand, to study antisaccades, the participant must fixate an opposite direction from a presented peripheral target [54]. As the participants have to inhibit the automatic saccade towards the stimulus, the antisaccade task requires additional executive processing from participants [55]. The nature of antisaccades can be associated with executive attention and research results indicate that patients with AD have shown more antisaccade errors with fewer corrections than control groups [56]. The papers [14, 44, 48, 50] review work conducted on eye movements and their relationship with AD.

There are different challenges regarding eye movements studies and AD. The first challenge arises because oculomotor abnormalities are not exclusive from AD and it is important to develop techniques that properly distinguish AD from other diseases. For example, SEM abnormalities have been encountered in Multiple System Atrophy, such as slower prosaccade and increased antisaccade errors [57].

Furthermore, SEM abnormalities might be related to aging. For example, in [58] it is reported that latencies uncorrected or increased time to correct error in antisaccades increase with aging. Older adults appear to have stronger difficulty ignoring distractions during day-to-day activities than younger adults. It seems that any variable that reduces the strength of the top-down neural signal to produce a voluntary saccade, or that increases saccade speed, will enhance the likelihood that a reflexive saccade to a stimulus with an abrupt onset will occur [59]. So, what is the effect of "normal" aging on eye saccade speed? It has been shown [60] that the Digit Symbol Substitution Test can be altered as far as 20 years before AD in older individuals with a high level of study is manifest. The performance in this test is related to the speed of eye saccades. This decline in performance speed and executive functions might be nonspecific prodromal Alzheimer's but could as well characterize a state of cerebral vulnerability on which the illness would progress more easily. Despite the relationship between age related cognitive decline and saccadic eye movements (SEM) deficits has been outlined, specific cognitive alterations underlying age-related changes in saccadic performance remain unclear. The nature of aging effects on SEMs has been only rarely approached. The progressive age-related decline of processing speed and executive attention is associated with and can be highlighted through saccadic age movement deficits as well in prosaccade and antisaccade tasks.

As can be see from Table 1, research from five years ago mainly focused in studying prosaccades and antisaccades. Indeed, the study of SEM was dominant since the earliest approaches dedicated to analyze eye movements and its relation to AD [52, 61–64]. As described, in SEM experiments the participants must fixate to a target. Although SEM studies have reported significant difference between persons with AD and control groups, there is still a research gap to fill in order to use SEM analysis as a marker for AD. Differentiate SEM abnormalities from AD, "normal" aging, and other conditions are among the main challenges from SEM analysis.

Prosaccade and antisaccade tasks have been popular in research studies due to their simplicity [58]. These tasks require a controlled scenario to conduct the evaluations. As research has evolved, more complex tasks have been studied towards associating eye movements deficits to support AD diagnosis. In Section 3.2 studies involving the execution of more complex tasks than attending to single target points are described. However, this research still lies in a category of controlled scenarios.

3.2. Eye Movements Analysis in Controlled Scenarios. Since the past years, research studies have moved forward to conduct other types of experiments aiming to identify eye movements abnormalities related to AD. For example, in [12] the participants performed a more complex task that only attend a target point that consisted in detecting and categorizing a specific object within a natural scene. The participants observed two visual stimuli in a monitor, one including an image with an animal and the other including a distractor image. The participants were asked to saccade to

TABLE 1: Research on eye movements and Alzheimer disease on pubmed since 2013.

Cite	Methods	Findings	Participants/Apparatus
2016 [25]	Subjects responded to targets presented on a hemispherical screen with diverse eccentricity.	PwAD recognized less targets in the center. No difference was found with CG on the peripheral targets.	AD: 18 CG: 20 Apparatus: Hemispherical screen Octupus 900 with camera used for eye tracking.
2017 [26]	The King-Devick test (with saccadic and other movements) was applied to subjects.	The King-Devick test may a tool to detect cognitive impairment associated with AD.	AD: 32 CG: 135 MCI: 39 Apparatus: N/A
2016 [27]	Subjects looked a series of slides containing four images of different emotional themes.	PwAD with apathy had diminished attentional bias toward social-themed stimuli.	AD: 36 (Apathy: 17 Not apathy: 19) Apparatus: Binocular eye tracking system developed by EL-MAR Inc.
2016 [11]	Eye movements from subjects were examined during reading regular and high predictable sentences.	PwAD gaze was longer than CG gaze. CG decreased gaze duration with high predictable sentences suggesting reading enhancement using stored information.	AD: 35 CG: 35 Apparatus: EyeLink 1000. Chinrest to control eye movements.
2015 [28]	Subjects performed a variety of tasks: walking, through stairs, through a room with and without obstacles.	The Posterior Cortical Atrophy (PCA) patient had longer mean fixation durations than PwAD and CG. Mean fixation duration between PwAD and CG was similar.	AD: 1 CG:1 PCA: 1 Apparatus: SMI mobile eye tracker
2015 [29]	Eye movements from subjects were examined while read sentences.	PwAD had more fixations on regular and high predictable sentences. PwAD spend more time reading the sentence. CG had less frequent second pass fixation over sentences.	AD: 35 CG-elderly: 35 Apparatus: EyeLink 1000. Chinrest to control eye movements.
2015 [19]	Longitudinal study with Gap and overlap paradigms.	PwAD had slower reaction times than CG. Prosaccades did not deteriorate after the 12-month longitudinal study in AD.	AD: 11 CG elderly: 25 Apparatus: ExpressEye
2015 [30]	Subjects made saccadic movement to photographs to target instructed scenes (natural vs urban, indoor vs outdoor)	Were found differences between controls and PwAD on accuracy but not saccadic latency.	AD: 24 CG age-matched: 28 CG young: 26 Apparatus: Eye tracker (Red-M, Senso-Motoric Instruments)
2015 [23]	Eye movements from subjects were examined while read proverbs.	PwAD have less word predictability than CG.	AD: 20 CG: 40 Apparatus: EyeLink 1000. Chinrest to control eye movements.

TABLE 1: Continued.

Cite	Methods	Findings	Participants/Apparatus
2014 [31]	Eye movements from subjects were examined while read low and high predictable sentences.	CG have shorter gaze duration on high predictable sentences. PwAD have similar gaze duration on both low and high predictable sentences. PwAD gaze duration is longer than CG.	AD: 20 CG age-matched: 40 Apparatus: EyeLink 1000. Chinrest to control eye movements.
2014 [32]	Eye movements from subjects were examined while read sentences	PwAD have altered visual exploration and absence on contextual predictability.	AD: 18 HC age-matched: 40 Apparatus: EyeLink 2K. Chinrest to control eye movements.
2013 [33]	Eye movements from subjects were examined while read sentences	PwAD evidences marked alterations in eye movement behavior during reading.	AD: 20 CG age-matched: 25 Apparatus: EyeLink 1000. Chinrest to control eye movements.
2014 [12]	Subjects were asked to spot an animal target contained in Colored photographs along with other distracting items.	PwAD were significate less accurate than elderly controls. Elder were less accurate than young controls.	AD: 17 mild AD. CG elderly: 23 CG young: 24. Apparatus: Eye tracker (Senso-Motoric Instruments)
2014 [34]	Subjects were required to look to a small fixation cross for 20 seconds on the center of a screen.	CG and PwAD showed significantly differences of microsaccade direction.	AD: 18 MCI: 15 CG age-matched: 21 Apparatus: Eye See Cam
2013 [35]	Visual targets were presented to subjects in a dim room. Prosaccade and antisaccade trials.	The antisaccade taks performance serves as a measure of executive function on PwAD.	AD: 28 MCI: 36 CG elderly: 118 Apparatus: Dual Purkinje Image Tracker. Heads stabilized on a chinrest.
2013 [36]	Pro-saccade and anti-saccade tasks. Gap and overlap paradigms.	PwAD have an excessive proportion of uncorrected errors in the antisaccade test.	AD: 18 Parkinson disease: 25 CG-young: 17 CG elderly: 18. Apparatus: Head mounted device ExpressEye eyetracker.
2013 [37]	Horizontal and vertical saccades. Gap and overlap paradigms on a black computer screen.	A link between MMSE and saccade latency.	AD: 25 Amnestic MCI: 18 CG elderly: 30 Apparatus: Head mounted Eyeseecam

CG: Control Group; MCI: Mild Cognitive Impairment; MMSE: Mini Mental State Examination.

the image that contained the animal while their success to fixate to the animal and to the correct image was measured. The results from this study show that persons with AD, even in a mild stage of the disease, when compared with control groups have difficulties to select the relevant targets.

Another example is given by the work in [11] that focuses on the analysis of reading behavior of PwAD. Reading is an ADL that involves the use of working memory and memory retrieval function. Thus, the experiments in [11] involve analysis of more complex task than usual SEM studies. The experiment consisted in a comparison of the eye gaze position of PwAD and control participants when reading sentences. The findings from [11] show that PwAD have a longer gaze duration than controls. Additionally, they found that a predictability degree on the sentences is accounted by control subjects but not by PwAD. This suggests that PwAD have impairments with their working memory and memory retrieval functions. Although the work in [11] is towards analysis of eye movements in ADL, the current experiments are under controlled scenarios in the sense that use screen based eye trackers and even use a chin rest to constrain head movements. Another research studies the attention to repeated and novel stimuli [65] that is related to cognition and attention. The experiments consist in presenting slides to mild-to-moderate PwAD that contain novel and repeated images. The researchers report that fixations on the images serve to evaluate attendance to repeated and novel content providing the potential to be used to measure disease progression.

Another study analyzes the effects of AD on visual exploration [25]. The study focuses on visual search performance for target detection in the far periphery. The participants, AD patients, and control subjects explore a hemispherical screen and respond to presented targets. The results from this study show differences in AD patients and control subjects when identifying targets on different eccentricities from the screen. Researchers also report differences on target detection times and number of fixations. The work in [66] uses eye movements analysis during video watching to infer people's cognitive function. Researches defined 13 features from fixations and found correlations between the features and memory capability. Example of these features include mean fixation duration, fixation count, and mean saccade amplitude. Different from other specific laboratory tasks, in these experiments the participants freely watch videos from different scenarios while features from eye movements are extracted.

A pilot study in France, LYLO [67], focused on measuring the rigidity and lack of curiosity of PwAD. In this study, the patients were screened in laboratory settings with static images displayed. And statistical parameters computed from recordings of saccades and fixations were compared. A step forward measuring visual impairments in a naturalistic situation consists in using everyday visual content such as colour video content for patients screening. The lack of curiosity hence can be induced from gaze recordings of intentionally degraded natural video content. The baseline model of automatic prediction of attention for normal control subjects was developed in [67, 68]. Contrarily to [69] where

the first step to make the observation "natural" was done by using video in free viewing conditions, in [68, 69] video was intentionally degraded.

While studying visual deficits on laboratory tasks has been productive for AD assessment, its application requires cooperative scenarios. That is, subjects must cooperate consciously performing the oculomotor tasks to get their assessment. Thus, this type of assessment is adequate when there is already an evident manifestation of dementia that requires evaluation. In addition, the manifestation cannot be severe enough so the subject is not able to cooperate. To achieve early diagnosis, it is necessary to have techniques that allow the evaluation of eye movements abnormalities on scenarios that allow naturalistic assessment without the explicit cooperation from subjects, for example, to analyze how AD affects eye movements in ADL, such as cooking or gardening. In the following section we describe the work related to analysis of eye movements in naturalistic scenarios.

3.3. Eye Movements Analysis in Naturalistic Tasks. When performing daily activities such as cooking or gardening, subjects interact with several objects, for example knifes, pans, or remote controls. During these interactions, a succession of different actions is involved, for example, cutting a vegetable or watering a plant. While executing these actions, humans use their vision to locate the objects and to manipulate them [70]. Indeed, the eye movements during everyday tasks provide relevant information about complex cognitive process related to object identification, place memory, tasks execution, and monitoring [71].

Studies attempt to understand the relation between activity execution and eye movements by investigating the eye patterns and eye-hand coordination on actions [72, 73]. For example, results support that people shift their gaze to target sites anticipating actions [74]. Also, results indicate that subjects rarely fixate on objects irrelevant to a performed action [73]. In fact, almost all eye movements during activities are targeted to fixation of task relevant objects, suggesting that visual attention can be modelled as "top-down" having little influence of the "intrinsic saliency" of the scene [72]. Top-down modelling refers to aspects of attention and gaze that are under executive control and may be influenced by tasks' directives and working memory [75]. Thus, top-down models require prior knowledge from the context [15]. On the other hand, bottom-up modelling refers to attention that is driven by properties of the visual stimulus being independent from tasks or semantic [75].

The described findings so far have arisen from experiments with healthy subjects. While the results are important to understand the eye movements in ADL, experiments with AD patients are scarce. This later is critical to support the diagnosis in early stages and to monitor changes of the disease. Healthy subjects have demonstrated different results when conducting specific oculomotor task when compared with PwAD and we expect the same in naturalistic scenarios.

In the work by Forde et al. [76] the eye movements in an ADL task are analyzed from a patient with action disorganization syndrome (ADS), from a PwAD, and from control subjects. The results show difference in the visual behavior from the participants while they were preparing a cup of tea. For example, the ADS patient made no glances to objects anticipating their use and had an increased number of fixations to irrelevant objects during the task. This shows different results from those stated in [73, 74]. The AD patient showed fewer fixations overall than control subjects and the ADS patients. In addition, the PwAD showed a lower proportion of relevant fixations compared to control subjects. In the work by Suzuki et al. [28] eye movement is investigated during locomotion. One AD patient, one Posterior Cortical Atrophy (PCA) patient, and one healthy subject used an eye tracking device while performing locomotion activities (walking along corridors, up and down stairs, and across a room with or without obstacles). The results show that the PCA patients were the slowest in performing the locomotion activities. Also, the PCA patient had longer fixation than the PwAD and the healthy subject. The PwAD required prompting during task competition showing memory impairment. Both studies show important findings toward understanding eye movements from PwAD; however more experiments with more participants are required.

A research goal is to understand eye movements abnormalities when performing ADL that serve to identify early signs of AD and to alert about a possible development of the disease. However, several challenges must be addressed first. For example, despite finding differences between PwAD and control groups, several abnormalities on visual deficits are not unique to AD but they are also present in other pathologies. In addition, it is important to find a visual marker that can be used to measure the progression of the disease; that is, the longitudinal studies must be conducted. Additionally, the clinical and personal history of each patient must be considered. PwAD might have differences in their visual behavior due to their physiological and personal context. Such is the case, for example, if they have sensorial impairments or a determining event in their lives. For example, a manual worker might have a different behavior than a white-collar worker.

The analysis of visual behavior during ADL has the potential to become a tool for AD assessment and for monitoring progression. Its success strongly relies on the development of technology able to measure eye movements. To be a pervasive tool it has to measure eye movements easily and in a noninvasive way allowing subjects to perform their activities in a natural manner.

Currently, there are clinical trials registers describing ongoing research with the objective to analyze eye movements in naturalistic tasks. For example, by doing a search with the terms "Alzheimer's disease" and "eye movements" in the database ClinicalTrials.gov provided by the US National Library of Medicine, there are 10 results currently recruiting participants. We identified 2 as relevant ongoing studies of eye movements in naturalistic scenarios for AD. In [77], researchers aim to analyze eye movements when reading sentences. In [78], researchers aim to analyze deficits in visual exploration in ADL.

Researchers in [78] expect to encounter that persons with AD have less ability of using scene semantic when locating objects. In this sense, the understanding of scene is paramount. In the next section we describe how the use of computational techniques can leverage the analysis of eye movements and AD by scene understanding.

4. Towards Early Detection Leveraging on Computational Attention Modelling

As we mentioned before, the identification of abnormalities in eye movements to support the early diagnosis or progression of an eventual dementia disease in elderly population during performance of ADL is a real scientific challenge. In this sense, some interesting approaches propose to predict human visual attention emulating the Human Visual Systems performance [79]. Indeed, computational visual attention models (CVSM) attempt to explain and describe the process of perceptual behavior and are compared with ground truth measured by eye trackers in psychovisual experiments [80–82]. Several exciting CVSM such as visual saliency techniques on egocentric video are useful for the use in naturalistic scenarios to estimate the areas from the video that are more likely to become the focus of human visual attention [15]. The egocentric video provides a first-person view from the individual who "wears" an egocentric camera giving visual information about objects, locations, and interactions.

Visual saliency techniques have been already combined with eye tracking in the field of Autism Spectrum Disorder (ASD) to screen differences between people with ASD and controls [83]. Researchers compare eye movements from both groups when freely viewing natural scenes images. In the analysis fixations towards visually salient regions, such as color, intensity, orientation, objects, and faces, are considered. To the best of our knowledge, research regarding the combination of data from eye trackers and visual saliency modeling to analyze eye movements abnormalities from PwAD is scarce. As we show earlier in Section 3.2 the work in [67] approaches with the analysis of fixations to degraded images, but more research is missing.

Suitable devices identified to be appropriated for monitoring ADLs with egocentric vision capabilities are mobile eye trackers [20], such as Tobbi© or SMI©. Additionally, egocentric cameras such as GoPro, Samsung Glass, and Microsoft Sense Cam [84] would allow scene understanding. Certainly, they record egocentric video giving a first-person view or in other words, what the camera wearer sees [85]. This captured information can be useful to analyze or predict some or all of visual attentive behavior through visual saliency computation. In this section, the main characteristics from the research on visual saliency are described, the techniques used and how this research field can be applied in the context of eye movements analysis.

(1) Computational Visual Saliency Models. The research field that analyzes video computationally to estimate the image regions that attract visual attention is called visual saliency detection [86, 87]. This research field matches the areas of neuroscience, psychology, and computer vision [16].

Early work on visual saliency modelling uses handcrafted low-level features such as contrast [88], color [89], edges [90], and orientation. It is funded on feature integration theory by Treisman and Gelade [91]. In addition, there is work that performs higher-level features extraction such as objects [92] and faces [93] in order to incorporate, into the low-level features, semantic elements of the observed scenes. Moreover, since the boom of deep learning, there are different proposals of configuration and arrangements of these supervised classification tools such as the convolutional neural networks [94–96] that report increased results for saliency estimation tasks. However, as deep learning requires a huge amount of data, more annotated information on diverse scenarios is still required. The works in [15, 97, 98] review techniques used for visual saliency detection.

According to the method used for modeling attention, there are two main categories of methods followed in the research of visual saliency: bottom-up modelling and top-down modelling. Bottom-up methods use information such as color, contrast, orientation, and texture [99]; they predict stimuli driven attention. And top-down models require prior knowledge on the visual search task and the context [15]. Currently, most of the work in visual saliency enters in the category of bottom-up methods.

The visual saliency modelling outputs a saliency map S, which is a two-dimensional topographically arranged map that encodes stimulus conspicuity of the visual scene [100]. The pixel values in the map indicate the saliency degree of the corresponding regions in the visual scene [15]. The maps are compared against ground truth maps built upon gaze fixations recorded by eye trackers when subjects are performing visual tasks. The ground truth might include synthetic stimuli or come from natural scenes including still images and video [101].

Pioneer research on visual saliency studied saliency from a third-person perspective, for instance, using still images [102] or video [103] coming from nonegocentric cameras. In the scenario of understanding scene for AD studies, the interest is nevertheless in saliency from the point of view of the subject performing activities. Hence, building saliency maps in egocentric video content and from the point of view of the subjects wearing recording device is required. However, the analysis of egocentric video brings new challenges. For instance, motion cues are significant in third-person video but camera motion is inherent to egocentric recordings [104]. Therefore, a residual motion in image plane of egocentric video has to be computed after motion of camera wearer has been compensated [105]. Egocentric video allows better introducing contextual knowledge from the subject because egocentric video follows the field of view of the subject's action. In this sense, this paradigm can support top-down attention modeling [106] in naturalistic scenarios such as in ADLs execution.

Egocentric video, beside the bottom-up image cues, provides context about the manipulation of objects [107, 108], about hands positions [106, 109], ego-motion [110], actions [111, 112], and activities [113, 114]. The egocentric video supports top-down attention modelling by the ensemble of these diverse contextual information. For example, a model assumes that gaze goes towards a given object currently held by the subject's hands. In addition, the ego-motion that occurs in visual exploration towards locating a specific object that is required in a given activity also serves for gaze estimation [115].

Top-down and bottom-up computational visual attention modelling show correlation between human fixations and predicted saliency maps. However, most of the results arise from experiments including healthy participants while scarce studies involve PwAD. In this review, we focus on the scenario for early AD detection. Thus, we address the relevant work relating computational attention modelling applied to AD in the next section.

(2) Computational Visual Saliency Models and Diagnosis. Progress in prediction of visual saliency including in egocentric content makes it possible to build robust prediction models for regions of high expectancy for the fixations of the test subject. Therefore, if a subject executing an ADL does not fixate the predicted areas properly, then it can be supposed that this subject has to undergo further tests to diagnose AD or not. For healthy subjects, visual saliency techniques assume that the subject will execute the activity fixating toward relevant objects or with coherent visual exploration. However, as mentioned in the work by Forde et al. [76], the participant with AD had lower proportion of relevant fixations compared to healthy subjects in ADL settings.

Another relevant feature about gaze measuring in patients with AD is the sensitivity. For example, the diagnosis performed with SEM tasks requires saccadic sensitivity. However, current visual saliency techniques addressing saccadic estimation are in early stages [116].

Although top-down mechanisms dominate the attention modelling from healthy subjects, it has been suggested that the visual behavior from persons with cognitive problems might rely on bottom-up mechanisms and saliency driven with less fixations on objects relevant to the task [71]. The work in [117] suggests that visual attention problems from AD patients are more notorious when the target item is not salient and shares common features with the background. The study in [118] analyzes the visual search task performance from AD patients by conducting experiments using salient and not salient search conditions. The researchers measure the reaction times when PwAD and control participants search for target elements. The PwAD show longer reaction times than control participants. However, the gap between both groups is bigger when searching for nonsalient target items. This suggests that salient elements attract PwAD.

The research in [105] on egocentric video acknowledges the potential to use visual saliency techniques to develop a tool for medical practitioners in realistic ADL scenarios. The researchers perform gaze comparison from an actor and a viewer. The actor is a person performing an activity (potentially a PwAD) while the viewer is a person watching egocentric video recordings from the actor (the medical practitioner). The paper suggests a relation between the gaze from the actor and the viewer. This relation consists in a time shift between the points of attention from the actor and the viewer. In other words, the viewer looks at the same place in the visual scene compared to the (healthy) actor but a few milliseconds later. The potential of this tool relies on the ability of a system to determine if the gaze from the actor is normal or abnormal according to the perspective from a medical practitioner. Additionally, the settings from the tool, like the use of egocentric camera, allow the use of computational attention-modelling techniques.

Computational attention-modelling techniques can be complemented with other contextual information in order to know more about the subject oculomotor behavior. For example, the amount of time that a participant takes to complete an activity can be explored. As literature shows, people with cognitive deficits take longer to complete tasks.

5. Conclusions and Future Directions

Neurodegenerative diseases, specifically Alzheimer's disease, are a problem that affects population worldwide. Currently, AD has no cure, but it has been demonstrated that treatment is helpful to delay the progression and improve quality of life. The diagnosis occurs frequently at late stages of the disease, when symptoms are evident. Nevertheless, research has found that AD is present up to 20 years before the disease is manifested. To have better treatment outcomes, it is desirable to have an early diagnosis. Understanding contextual differences that might influence the course of the disease would also be helpful. Among the current diagnostic techniques, visual behavior has the potential to become useful in early stages and to be a pervasive tool. Several investigations have explored the relations of eye movements with AD through specific oculomotor tasks demonstrating visual features that can be used for early diagnosis and progression measurement. However, more experiments are necessary under naturalistic scenarios to develop a useful tool that can be used in early stages. Nevertheless, changes happening in older individuals without cognitive impairment must also be taken into consideration and eventually they have to be approached by means of further research in normal individuals. Eye movements abnormalities have been measured mostly using eye tracking technology. Nevertheless, computer vision techniques, such as visual saliency and object detections in ADL performance settings, could be a good means to measure visual attention of PwAD to diagnose in terms of its difference to normal control attention in naturalistic scenarios when performing ADLs. Several challenges must be addressed, such as estimating gaze on top-down driven mechanisms and relating bottom-up mechanisms with the activities. Also, it is important to conduct experiments with persons with different cognitive problems in order to learn the features that differentiate among healthy subjects, people with different diseases, and persons with AD.

Conflicts of Interest

The authors declare that there are no conflicts of interest regarding the publication of this paper.

Acknowledgments

This review was supported by the projects CATEDRAS CONACYT numbers 672 and IPN-SIP2018.

References

[1] G. Díaz, E. Romero, J. A. Hernández-Tamames, V. Molina, and N. Malpica, "Automatic classification of structural MRI for diagnosis of neurodegenerative diseases," *Acta Biologica Colombiana*, vol. 15, no. 3, pp. 165–180, 2010.

[2] J. Koikkalainen, H. Rhodius-Meester, A. Tolonen et al., "Differential diagnosis of neurodegenerative diseases using structural MRI data," *NeuroImage: Clinical*, vol. 11, pp. 435–449, 2016.

[3] A. J. Stoessl, "Neuroimaging in the early diagnosis of neurodegenerative disease," *Translational Neurodegeneration*, vol. 1, article no. 5, 2012.

[4] A. Association, "2018 Alzheimers disease facts and figures," *Alzheimer's & Dementia*, vol. 14, no. 3, pp. 367–429, 2018.

[5] J. Dauwels and S. Kannan, "Diagnosis of alzheimer's disease using electric signals of the brain—a grand challenge," *Asia-Pacific Biotech News*, vol. 16, no. 10n11, pp. 22–38, 2012.

[6] A. Nordberg, J. O. Rinne, A. Kadir, and B. Långström, "The use of PET in Alzheimer disease," *Nature Reviews Neurology*, vol. 6, no. 2, pp. 78–87, 2010.

[7] W. V. Graham, A. Bonito-Oliva, and T. P. Sakmar, "Update on alzheimer's disease therapy and prevention strategies," *Annual Review of Medicine*, vol. 68, no. 1, pp. 413–430, 2017.

[8] M. E. De Vugt and F. R. J. Verhey, "The impact of early dementia diagnosis and intervention on informal caregivers," *Progress in Neurobiology*, vol. 110, pp. 54–62, 2013.

[9] K. Pietrzak, K. Czarnecka, E. Mikiciuk-Olasik, and P. Szymanski, "New Perspectives of Alzheimer Disease Diagnosis – the Most Popular and Future Methods," *Medicinal Chemistry*, 2017.

[10] J. Weuve, C. Proust-Lima, M. C. Power et al., "Guidelines for reporting methodological challenges and evaluating potential bias in dementia research," *Alzheimer's & Dementia*, vol. 11, no. 9, article no. 2048, pp. 1098–1109, 2015.

[11] G. Fernández, F. Manes, L. E. Politi et al., "Patients with Mild Alzheimer's Disease Fail When Using Their Working Memory: Evidence from the Eye Tracking Technique," *Journal of Alzheimer's Disease*, vol. 50, no. 3, pp. 827–838, 2016.

[12] M. Boucart, G. Bubbico, S. Szaffarczyk, and F. Pasquier, "Animal spotting in Alzheimer's disease: An eye tracking study of object categorization," *Journal of Alzheimer's Disease*, vol. 39, no. 1, pp. 181–189, 2014.

[13] A. König, G. Sacco, G. Bensadoun et al., "The role of information and communication technologies in clinical trials with patients with Alzheimer's disease and related disorders," *Frontiers in Aging Neuroscience*, vol. 7, p. 110, 2015.

[14] R. J. Molitor, P. C. Ko, and B. A. Ally, "Eye movements in alzheimers disease," *Journal of Alzheimers Disease*, vol. 44, no. 1, pp. 1–12, 2015.

[15] M. Runxin, Y. Yu, and X. Yue, "Survey on Image Saliency Detection Methods," in *Proceedings of the 7th International Conference on Cyber-Enabled Distributed Computing and Knowledge Discovery, CyberC 2015*, pp. 329–338, September 2015.

[16] L. Huo, L. Jiao, S. Wang, and S. Yang, "Object-level saliency detection with color attributes," *Pattern Recognition*, vol. 49, pp. 162–173, 2016.

[17] P. K. Muthumanickam, C. Forsell, K. Vrotsou, J. Johansson, and M. Cooper, "Supporting exploration of eye tracking data: Identifying changing behaviour over long durations," in *Proceedings of the 6th Workshop Beyond Time and Errors on Novel Evaluation Methods for Visualization, BELIV 2016*, pp. 70–77.

[18] V. Pallarés, M. Hernández, and L. Dempere-Marco, "Eye-Tracking Data in Visual Search Tasks: A, Hallmark of Cognitive Function," *Biosystems and Biorobotics*, vol. 15, pp. 873–877, 2017.

[19] T. J. Crawford, A. Devereaux, S. Higham, and C. Kelly, "The disengagement of visual attention in Alzheimer's disease: A longitudinal eye-tracking study," *Frontiers in Aging Neuroscience*, vol. 7, article no. 118, 2015.

[20] L. Itti, "New Eye-Tracking Techniques May Revolutionize Mental Health Screening," *Neuron*, vol. 88, no. 3, pp. 442–444, 2015.

[21] K. Holmqvist, M. Nyström, R. Andersson et al., *Eye tracking: A comprehensive guide to methods and measures*, OUP Oxford, 2011.

[22] I. M. Pavisic, N. C. Firth, S. Parsons et al., "Eyetracking metrics in young onset alzheimer's disease: a window into cognitive visual functions," *Frontiers in Neurology*, vol. 8, article 377, 2017.

[23] G. Fernández, L. R. Castro, M. Schumacher, and O. E. Agamennoni, "Diagnosis of mild Alzheimer disease through the analysis of eye movements during reading," *Journal of integrative neuroscience*, vol. 14, no. 1, pp. 121–133, 2015.

[24] D. C. Niehorster, T. H. W. Cornelissen, K. Holmqvist, I. T. C. Hooge, and R. S. Hessels, "What to expect from your remote eye-tracker when participants are unrestrained," *Behavior Research Methods*, pp. 1–15, 2017.

[25] V. Vallejo, D. Cazzoli, L. Rampa et al., "Effects of Alzheimer's disease on visual target detection: A "peripheral bias"," *Frontiers in Aging Neuroscience*, vol. 8, article no. 200, 2016.

[26] K. M. Galetta, K. R. Chapman, M. D. Essis et al., "Screening Utility of the King-Devick Test in Mild Cognitive Impairment and Alzheimer Disease Dementia," *Alzheimer Disease & Associated Disorders*, vol. 31, no. 2, pp. 152–158, 2017.

[27] S. A. Chau, J. Chung, N. Herrmann, M. Eizenman, and K. L. Lanctôt, "Apathy and Attentional Biases in Alzheimer's Disease," *Journal of Alzheimer's Disease*, vol. 51, no. 3, pp. 837–846, 2016.

[28] T. Suzuki, K. Yong, B. Yang et al., "Locomotion and eye behaviour under controlled environment in individuals with Alzheimer's disease," in *Proceedings of the 37th Annual International Conference of the IEEE Engineering in Medicine and Biology Society, EMBC 2015*, pp. 6594–6597, August 2015.

[29] G. Fernández, M. Schumacher, L. Castro, D. Orozco, and O. Agamennoni, "Patients with mild Alzheimer's disease produced shorter outgoing saccades when reading sentences," *Psychiatry Research*, vol. 229, no. 1-2, pp. 470–478, 2015.

[30] Q. Lenoble, G. Bubbico, S. Szaffarczyk, F. Pasquier, and M. Boucart, "Scene categorization in Alzheimer's disease: A saccadic choice task," *Dementia and Geriatric Cognitive Disorders Extra*, vol. 5, no. 1, pp. 1–12, 2015.

[31] G. Fernández, F. Manes, N. P. Rotstein et al., "Lack of contextual-word predictability during reading in patients with mild Alzheimer disease," *Neuropsychologia*, vol. 62, no. 1, pp. 143–151, 2014.

[32] G. Fernández, J. Laubrock, P. Mandolesi, O. Colombo, and O. Agamennoni, "Registering eye movements during reading in Alzheimers disease: Difficulties in predicting upcoming words," *Journal of Clinical and Experimental Neuropsychology*, vol. 36, no. 3, pp. 302–316, 2014.

[33] G. Fernández, P. Mandolesi, N. P. Rotstein, O. Colombo, O. Agamennoni, and L. E. Politi, "Eye movement alterations during reading in patients with early Alzheimer disease.," *Investigative ophthalmology & visual science*, vol. 54, no. 13, pp. 8345–8352, 2013.

[34] Z. Kapoula, Q. Yang, J. Otero-Millan et al., "Distinctive features of microsaccades in Alzheimer's disease and in mild cognitive impairment," *AGE*, vol. 36, no. 2, pp. 535–543, 2014.

[35] H. W. Heuer, J. B. Mirsky, E. L. Kong et al., "Antisaccade task reflects cortical involvement in mild cognitive impairment," *Neurology*, vol. 81, no. 14, pp. 1235–1243, 2013.

[36] T. J. Crawford, S. Higham, J. Mayes, M. Dale, S. Shaunak, and G. Lekwuwa, "The role of working memory and attentional disengagement on inhibitory control: Effects of aging and Alzheimer's disease," *AGE*, vol. 35, no. 5, pp. 1637–1650, 2013.

[37] Q. Yang, T. Wang, N. Su, S. Xiao, and Z. Kapoula, "Specific saccade deficits in patients with Alzheimer's disease at mild to moderate stage and in patients with amnestic mild cognitive impairment," *AGE*, vol. 35, no. 4, pp. 1287–1298, 2013.

[38] A. C. McKee, R. Au, H. J. Cabral et al., "Visual association pathology in preclinical Alzheimer disease," *Journal of Neuropathology & Experimental Neurology*, vol. 65, no. 6, pp. 621–630, 2006.

[39] A. A. Brewer and B. Barton, "Visual cortex in aging and Alzheimer's disease: Changes in visual field maps and population receptive fields," *Frontiers in Psychology*, vol. 5, Article ID Article 74, 2014.

[40] Y. Kusne, A. B. Wolf, K. Townley, M. Conway, and G. A. Peyman, "Visual system manifestations of Alzheimer's disease," *Acta Ophthalmologica*, 2016.

[41] J. K. H. Lim, Q.-X. Li, Z. He et al., "The eye as a biomarker for Alzheimer's disease," *Frontiers in Neuroscience*, vol. 10, article no. 536, 2016.

[42] R. A. Armstrong, "Alzheimer's disease and the eye," *Journal of Optometry*, vol. 2, no. 3, pp. 103–111, 2009.

[43] F. Z. Javaid, J. Brenton, L. Guo, and M. F. Cordeiro, "Visual and ocular manifestations of Alzheimer's disease and their use as biomarkers for diagnosis and progression," *Frontiers in Neurology*, vol. 7, article no. 55, 2016.

[44] M. R. MacAskill and T. J. Anderson, "Eye movements in neurodegenerative diseases," *Current Opinion in Neurology*, vol. 29, no. 1, pp. 61–68, 2016.

[45] R. Tzekov and M. Mullan, "Vision function abnormalities in Alzheimer disease," *Survey of Ophthalmology*, vol. 59, no. 4, pp. 414–433, 2014.

[46] U. Rüb, K. Del Tredici, C. Schultz, J. A. Büttner-EnneVer, and H. Braak, "The premotor region essential for rapid vertical eye movements shows early involvement in Alzheimer's disease-related cytoskeletal pathology," *Vision Research*, vol. 41, no. 16, pp. 2149–2156, 2001.

[47] A. L. Boxer, S. Garbutt, W. W. Seeley et al., "Saccade abnormalities in autopsy-confirmed frontotemporal lobar degeneration and alzheimer disease," *JAMA Neurology*, vol. 69, no. 4, pp. 509–517, 2012.

[48] M. L. G. Freitas Pereira, M. von Zuben A Camargo, I. Aprahamian, and O. V. Forlenza, "Eye movement analysis and cognitive processing: Detecting indicators of conversion to Alzheimer's disease," *Neuropsychiatric Disease and Treatment*, vol. 10, pp. 1273–1285, 2014.

[49] T. A. Amor, S. D. S. Reis, D. Campos, H. J. Herrmann, and J. S. Andrade, "Persistence in eye movement during visual search," *Scientific Reports*, vol. 6, Article ID 20815, 2016.

[50] O. A. Coubard, "What do we know about eye movements in Alzheimer's disease? The past 37 years and future directions," *Biomarkers in Medicine*, vol. 10, no. 7, pp. 677–680, 2016.

[51] T. J. Crawford and S. Higham, "Distinguishing between impairments of working memory and inhibitory control in cases of early dementia," *Neuropsychologia*, vol. 81, pp. 61–67, 2016.

[52] Q. Yang, T. Wang, N. Su, Y. Liu, S. Xiao, and Z. Kapoula, "Long Latency and High Variability in Accuracy-Speed of Prosaccades in Alzheimer's Disease at Mild to Moderate Stage," *Dementia and Geriatric Cognitive Disorders Extra*, vol. 1, no. 1, pp. 318–329, 2011.

[53] S. Garbutt, A. Matlin, J. Hellmuth et al., "Oculomotor function in frontotemporal lobar degeneration, related disorders and Alzheimer's disease," *Brain*, vol. 131, no. 5, pp. 1268–1281, 2008.

[54] L. D. Kaufman, J. Pratt, B. Levine, and S. E. Black, "Antisaccades: A probe into the dorsolateral prefrontal cortex in Alzheimer's disease. A critical review," *Journal of Alzheimer's Disease*, vol. 19, no. 3, pp. 781–793, 2010.

[55] A. Peltsch, A. Hemraj, A. Garcia, and D. P. Munoz, "Saccade deficits in amnestic mild cognitive impairment resemble mild Alzheimer's disease," *European Journal of Neuroscience*, vol. 39, no. 11, pp. 2000–2013, 2014.

[56] L. D. Kaufman, J. Pratt, B. Levine, and S. E. Black, "Executive deficits detected in mild Alzheimer's disease using the antisaccade task," *Brain and Behavior*, vol. 2, no. 1, pp. 15–21, 2012.

[57] S. H. Brooks, E. M. Klier, S. D. Red et al., "Slowed prosaccades and increased antisaccade errors as a potential behavioral biomarker of multiple system atrophy," *Frontiers in Neurology*, vol. 8, article no. 261, 2017.

[58] N. Noiret, N. Carvalho, É. Laurent et al., "Saccadic Eye Movements and Attentional Control in Alzheimer's Disease," *Archives of Clinical Neuropsychology*, vol. 33, no. 1, pp. 1–13, 2018.

[59] A. C. Bowling, P. Lindsay, B. G. Smith, and K. Storok, "Saccadic eye movements as indicators of cognitive function in older adults," *Aging, Neuropsychology, and Cognition*, vol. 22, no. 2, pp. 201–219, 2015.

[60] H. Amieva, H. Mokri, M. Le Goff et al., "Compensatory mechanisms in higher-educated subjects with Alzheimer's disease: A study of 20 years of cognitive decline," *Brain*, vol. 137, no. 4, pp. 1167–1175, 2014.

[61] F. W. Bylsma, D. X. Rasmusson, G. W. Rebok, P. M. Keyl, L. Tune, and J. Brandt, "Changes in visual fixation and saccadic eye movements in Alzheimer's disease," *International Journal of Psychophysiology*, vol. 19, no. 1, pp. 33–40, 1995.

[62] L. A. Hershey, L. Whicker, L. A. Abel, L. F. Dell'osso, S. Traccis, and D. Grossniklaus, "Saccadic Latency Measurements in Dementia," *JAMA Neurology*, vol. 40, no. 9, pp. 592-593, 1983.

[63] W. A. Fletcher and J. A. Sharpe, "Saccadic eye movement dysfunction in Alzheimer's disease," *Annals of Neurology*, vol. 20, no. 4, pp. 464–471, 1986.

[64] F. J. Pirozzolo and E. C. Hansch, "Oculomotor reaction time in dementia reflects degree of cerebral dysfunction," *Science*, vol. 214, no. 4518, pp. 349–351, 1981.

[65] S. A. Chau, N. Herrmann, C. Sherman et al., "Visual Selective Attention Toward Novel Stimuli Predicts Cognitive Decline in Alzheimer's Disease Patients," *Journal of Alzheimer's Disease*, vol. 55, no. 4, pp. 1–11, 2017.

[66] Y. Zhang, T. Wilcockson, K. I. Kim, T. Crawford, H. Gellersen, and P. Sawyer, "Monitoring dementia with automatic eye movements analysis," *Smart Innovation, Systems and Technologies*, vol. 57, pp. 299–309, 2016.

[67] S. Chaabouni, J. Benois-pineau, F. Tison, C. Ben Amar, and A. Zemmari, "Prediction of visual attention with deep CNN on artificially degraded videos for studies of attention of patients with Dementia," *Multimedia Tools and Applications*, vol. 76, no. 21, pp. 1–20, 2017.

[68] S. Chaabouni, F. Tison, J. Benois-Pineau, and C. Ben Amar, "Prediction of visual attention with Deep CNN for studies of neurodegenerative diseases," in *Proceedings of the 14th International Workshop on Content-Based Multimedia Indexing, CBMI 2016*, pp. 1–6, June 2016.

[69] P.-H. Tseng, I. G. M. Cameron, G. Pari, J. N. Reynolds, D. P. Munoz, and L. Itti, "High-throughput classification of clinical populations from natural viewing eye movements," *Journal of Neurology*, vol. 260, no. 1, pp. 275–284, 2013.

[70] M. Land, N. Mennie, and J. Rusted, "The roles of vision and eye movements in the control of activities of daily living," *Perception*, vol. 28, no. 11, pp. 1311–1328, 1999.

[71] S. C. Seligman and T. Giovannetti, "The Potential Utility of Eye Movements in the Detection and Characterization of Everyday Functional Difficulties in Mild Cognitive Impairment," *Neuropsychology Review*, vol. 25, no. 2, pp. 199–215, 2015.

[72] M. F. Land and M. Hayhoe, "In what ways do eye movements contribute to everyday activities?" *Vision Research*, vol. 41, no. 25-26, pp. 3559–3565, 2001.

[73] M. F. Land, "Eye movements and the control of actions in everyday life," *Progress in Retinal and Eye Research*, vol. 25, no. 3, pp. 296–324, 2006.

[74] F. Donnarumma, M. Costantini, E. Ambrosini, K. Friston, and G. Pezzulo, "Action perception as hypothesis testing," *Cortex*, vol. 89, pp. 45–60, 2017.

[75] J. F. G. Boisvert and N. D. B. Bruce, "Predicting task from eye movements: On the importance of spatial distribution, dynamics, and image features," *Neurocomputing*, vol. 207, pp. 653–668, 2016.

[76] E. M. E. Forde, J. Rusted, N. Mennie, M. Land, and G. W. Humphreys, "The eyes have it: An exploration of eye movements in action disorganisation syndrome," *Neuropsychologia*, vol. 48, no. 7, pp. 1895–1900, 2010.

[77] ClinicalTrials.gov [Internet], National Library of Medicine (US), Centre Hospitalier Universitaire de Nice, Identifier NCT02557464, "Identification of early markers of alzheimer's disease by using eye tracking in reading. (adal)," 2015, this study is currently recruiting participants. Available: https://clinicaltrials.gov/ct2/show/NCT02557464?term=eye&cond=Alzheimer+Disease&cntry=FR&rank=1.

[78] ClinicalTrials.gov [Internet], National Library of Medicine (US), Centre Hospitalier Universitaire de Nice, Identifier NCT02941289 , "Visuospatial attention, eye movements and instrumental activities of daily living (iadls) in alzheimer's disease (arva-ma)," 2016, this study is currently recruiting participants. Available: https://clinicaltrials.gov/ct2/show/NCT02941289?term=Eye+movements&recrs=ab&cond=Alzheimer+Disease&rank=1.

[79] M. Mancas, V. P. Ferrera, N. Riche, and J. G. Taylor, *From Human Attention to Computational Attention: A Multidisciplinary Approach*, vol. 10, Springer, 2016.

[80] S. Frintrop, "Computational visual attention," in *Computer Analysis of Human Behavior*, pp. 69–101, Springer, 2011.

[81] L. Itti and C. Koch, "Computational modelling of visual attention," *Nature Reviews Neuroscience*, vol. 2, no. 3, pp. 194–203, 2001.

[82] J. K. Tsotsos and A. Rothenstein, "Computational models of visual attention," *Scholarpedia*, vol. 6, no. 1, article 6201, 2011.

[83] S. Wang, M. Jiang, X. M. Duchesne et al., "Atypical Visual Saliency in Autism Spectrum Disorder Quantified through Model-Based Eye Tracking," *Neuron*, vol. 88, no. 3, pp. 604–616, 2015.

[84] S. Singh, C. Arora, and C. V. Jawahar, "First person action recognition using deep learned descriptors," in *Proceedings of the 2016 IEEE Conference on Computer Vision and Pattern Recognition, CVPR 2016*, pp. 2620–2628, July 2016.

[85] A. Betancourt, P. Morerio, C. S. Regazzoni, and M. Rauterberg, "The evolution of first person vision methods: A survey," *IEEE Transactions on Circuits and Systems for Video Technology*, vol. 25, no. 5, pp. 744–760, 2015.

[86] J. Pan, C. Canton-Ferrer, K. McGuinness et al., "Salgan: Visual saliency prediction with generative adversarial networks," *CoRR*, https://arxiv.org/abs/1701.01081v2.

[87] M. Cornia, L. Baraldi, G. Serra, and R. Cucchiara, "Predicting human eye fixations via an lstm-based saliency attentive model," *CoRR*, https://arxiv.org/abs/1611.09571v3.

[88] P. Reinagel and A. M. Zador, "Natural scene statistics at the centre of gaze," *Network: Computation in Neural Systems*, vol. 10, no. 1-10, article 4, 1999.

[89] T. Jost, N. Ouerhani, R. V. Wartburg, R. Müri, and H. Hügli, "Assessing the contribution of color in visual attention," *Computer Vision and Image Understanding*, vol. 100, no. 1-2, pp. 107–123, 2005.

[90] R. J. Baddeley and B. W. Tatler, "High frequency edges (but not contrast) predict where we fixate: A Bayesian system identification analysis," *Vision Research*, vol. 46, no. 18, pp. 2824–2833, 2006.

[91] A. M. Treisman and G. Gelade, "A feature-integration theory of attention," *Cognitive Psychology*, vol. 12, no. 1, pp. 97–136, 1980.

[92] A. Borji, M. Cheng, H. Jiang, and J. Li, "Salient object detection: a survey," *CoRR*, https://arxiv.org/abs/1411.5878.

[93] M. Cerf, E. P. Frady, and C. Koch, "Faces and text attract gaze independent of the task: Experimental data and computer model," *Journal of vision*, vol. 9, no. 12, pp. 10-10, 2009.

[94] S. S. S. Kruthiventi, V. Gudisa, J. H. Dholakiya, and R. V. Babu, "Saliency unified: A deep architecture for simultaneous eye fixation prediction and salient object segmentation," in *Proceedings of the 2016 IEEE Conference on Computer Vision and Pattern Recognition, CVPR 2016*, pp. 5781–5790, July 2016.

[95] G. Li and Y. Yu, "Deep contrast learning for salient object detection," in *Proceedings of the 2016 IEEE Conference on Computer Vision and Pattern Recognition, CVPR 2016*, pp. 478–487, July 2016.

[96] N. Liu and J. Han, "DHSNet: Deep hierarchical saliency network for salient object detection," in *Proceedings of the 2016 IEEE Conference on Computer Vision and Pattern Recognition, CVPR 2016*, pp. 678–686, July 2016.

[97] Q. Zhao and C. Koch, "Learning saliency-based visual attention: A review," *Signal Processing*, vol. 93, no. 6, pp. 1401–1407, 2013.

[98] A. Borji and L. Itti, "State-of-the-art in visual attention modeling," *IEEE Transactions on Pattern Analysis and Machine Intelligence*, vol. 35, no. 1, pp. 185–207, 2013.

[99] J. Kuen, Z. Wang, and G. Wang, "Recurrent attentional networks for saliency detection," in *Proceedings of the 2016 IEEE Conference on Computer Vision and Pattern Recognition, CVPR 2016*, pp. 3668–3677, July 2016.

[100] R. Veale, Z. M. Hafed, and M. Yoshida, "How is visual salience computed in the brain? Insights from behaviour, neurobiology and modeling," *Philosophical Transactions of the Royal Society B: Biological Sciences*, vol. 372, no. 1714, Article ID 20160113, 2017.

[101] A. Borji, D. N. Sihite, and L. Itti, "Quantitative analysis of human-model agreement in visual saliency modeling: a comparative study," *IEEE Transactions on Image Processing*, vol. 22, no. 1, pp. 55–69, 2013.

[102] L. Duan, J. Gu, Z. Yang, J. Miao, W. Ma, and C. Wu, "Bio-inspired Visual Attention Model and Saliency Guided Object Segmentation," in *Genetic and Evolutionary Computing*, vol. 238 of *Advances in Intelligent Systems and Computing*, pp. 291–298, Springer, 2014.

[103] W.-T. Li, H.-S. Chang, K.-C. Lien, H.-T. Chang, and Y.-C. F. Wang, "Exploring visual and motion saliency for automatic video object extraction," *IEEE Transactions on Image Processing*, vol. 22, no. 7, pp. 2600–2610, 2013.

[104] Y.-C. Su and K. Grauman, "Detecting engagement in egocentric video," in *Proceedings of the European Conference on Computer Vision*, pp. 454–471, Springer, 2016.

[105] H. Boujut, V. Buso, J. Benois-Pineau et al., "Visual saliency maps for studies of behavior of patients with neurodegenerative diseases: Observer's versus actor's points of view," in *Innovation in Medicine & Healthcare*, KES, 2013.

[106] V. Buso, I. González-Díaz, and J. Benois-Pineau, "Goal-oriented top-down probabilistic visual attention model for recognition of manipulated objects in egocentric videos," *Signal Processing: Image Communication*, vol. 39, pp. 418–431, 2015.

[107] A. Fathi, X. Ren, and J. M. Rehg, "Learning to recognize objects in egocentric activities," in *Proceedings of the 2011 IEEE Conference on Computer Vision and Pattern Recognition, CVPR 2011*, pp. 3281–3288, June 2011.

[108] X. Ren and M. Philipose, "Egocentric recognition of handled objects: Benchmark and analysis," in *Proceedings of the IEEE Computer Society Conference on Computer Vision and Pattern Recognition Workshops, CVPR Workshops 2009*, pp. 1–8, IEEE, 2009.

[109] Y. Li, A. Fathi, and J. M. Rehg, "Learning to predict gaze in egocentric video," in *Proceedings of the 2013 14th IEEE International Conference on Computer Vision, ICCV 2013*, pp. 3216–3223, December 2013.

[110] K. Matsuo, K. Yamada, S. Ueno, and S. Naito, "An attention-based activity recognition for egocentric video," in *Proceedings of the 2014 IEEE Conference on Computer Vision and Pattern Recognition Workshops, CVPRW 2014*, pp. 551–556, USA, June 2014.

[111] P. Le Bek, *Learning to recognise actions in egocentric video, [MSc, thesis]*, University Glasgow, School of Computing Science, 2014.

[112] S. Singh, C. Arora, and C. V. Jawahar, "Trajectory aligned features for first person action recognition," *Pattern Recognition*, vol. 62, pp. 45–55, 2017.

[113] M. Ma, H. Fan, and K. M. Kitani, "Going deeper into first-person activity recognition," in *Proceedings of the 2016 IEEE Conference on Computer Vision and Pattern Recognition, CVPR 2016*, pp. 1894–1903, July 2016.

[114] T.-H. Nguyen, J.-C. Nebel, and F. Florez-Revuelta, "Recognition of activities of daily living with egocentric vision: A review," *Sensors*, vol. 16, no. 1, article no. 72, 2016.

[115] K. Yamada, Y. Sugano, T. Okabe et al., "Attention prediction in egocentric video using motion and visual saliency," *Advances in Image and Video Technology*, pp. 277–288, 2012.

[116] X. Sun, H. Yao, R. Ji, and X.-M. Liu, "Toward statistical modeling of saccadic eye-movement and visual saliency," *IEEE Transactions on Image Processing*, vol. 23, no. 11, pp. 4649–4662, 2014.

[117] J. K. Foster, M. Behrmann, and D. T. Stuss, "Visual attention deficits in Alzheimer's disease: Simple versus conjoined feature search," *Neuropsychology*, vol. 13, no. 2, pp. 223–245, 1999.

[118] A. Tales, J. Muir, R. Jones, A. Bayer, and R. J. Snowden, "The effects of saliency and task difficulty on visual search performance in ageing and Alzheimer's disease," *Neuropsychologia*, vol. 42, no. 3, pp. 335–345, 2004.

4

Parallel Computing Sparse Wavelet Feature Extraction for P300 Speller BCI

Zhihua Huang [iD],[1] **Minghong Li,**[2] **and Yuanye Ma**[3]

[1]*College of Mathematics and Computer Science, Fuzhou University, Fuzhou, China*
[2]*Department of Physiology, Yunnan University of Traditional Chinese Medicine, Kunming, China*
[3]*Kunming Institute of Zoology, CAS, Kunming, China*

Correspondence should be addressed to Zhihua Huang; hzh@fzu.edu.cn

Academic Editor: Luminita Moraru

This work is intended to increase the classification accuracy of single EEG epoch, reduce the number of repeated stimuli, and improve the information transfer rate (ITR) of P300 Speller. Target EEG epochs and nontarget EEG ones are both mapped to a space by Wavelet. In this space, Fisher Criterion is used to measure the difference between target and nontarget ones. Only a few Daubechies wavelet bases corresponding to big differences are selected to construct a matrix, by which EEG epochs are transformed to feature vectors. To ensure the online experiments, the computation tasks are distributed to several computers that are managed and integrated by Storm so that they could be parallelly carried out. The proposed feature extraction was compared with the typical methods by testing its performance of classifying single EEG epoch and detecting characters. Our method achieved higher accuracies of classification and detection. The ITRs also reflected the superiority of our method. The parallel computing scheme of our method was deployed on a small scale Storm cluster containing three desktop computers. The average feedback time for one round of EEG epochs was 1.57 ms. The proposed method can improve the performance of P300 Speller BCI. Its parallel computing scheme is able to support fast feedback required by online experiments. The number of repeated stimuli can be significantly reduced by our method. The parallel computing scheme not only supports our wavelet feature extraction but also provides a framework for other algorithms developed for P300 Speller.

1. Introduction

The advances in the field of brain-computer interfaces (BCIs) are encouraging researchers to explore its various possibilities of benefiting the studies of neuroscience, artificial intelligence, biomedical engineering, and so on. A BCI is a system that measures the activity of central nervous system (CNS) and converts it to artificial output which can change the interactions between the brain and its environment [1]. Although the activity of CNS can be measured by all kinds of brain signals, most BCIs rely on electrical measures because they can be acquired easily [1, 2]. Electroencephalogram (EEG) is the electrical measure of the activity of CNS from electrodes placed on the scalp. BCIs based on EEG are noninvasive. Because of this, the prospective applications of this kind of BCI on persons, including special patients and everyman, impress the researchers in the area.

The EEG-based BCIs could be fulfilled in diverse ways, which mainly include P300 Speller, sensorimotor rhythm (SMR), steady-state visual evoked potential (SSVEP), and slow cortical potential (SCP) [1–4]. They rely on different neuroscience principles and have different features. P300 Speller BCIs were first proposed in [3] and constructed on the basis of P300 event-related potentials (ERP) that are evoked by the target stimulus in an oddball paradigm and mean that the subjects are paying attention to the target [1–4]. An advantage of P300 Speller BCIs is that only a few trainings enable subjects to use them to spell words to a computer and achieve a stable performance [1, 2]. Many researchers are attracted by the potential of P300 Speller BCIs to seek the possible improvements and their applications [1, 5–10]. In the research [5], an asynchronous BCI, which is able to automatically detect the intention of subjects starting to spell words, was designed by combining P300 and SSVEP. It was reported that a system using dynamic P300 Speller matrix can facilitate the access of severely motor-impaired persons to the World Wide Web and multimedia content [6]. According to [7], some researchers explored the approach to improving the P300 Speller performance by using a green family faces paradigm. Krumpe and colleagues considered the situation where a stimulus-locked classification cannot be used. They evaluated the feasibility of detecting a P300 in a reactive EEG-based BCI through an asynchronous classification in their study [8]. Jin et al. observed the decrease of subjects' attention during the presentation of stimuli in P300 Speller BCI and proposed to use honey-comb-shaped figures with 1–3 red points as stimuli to catch subjects' attention [9]. According to [10], Mao et al. reviewed the progress of the application of EEG-based BCI to interaction with robots and enumerated many promising examples of applying P300-based BCI.

To implement P300-based BCI, the key is the detection of P300 ERP. As for ERP estimation, averaging many EEG epochs is the most common practice. Although this method can serve the implementation of P300-based BCI, it faces very big challenges because the stimulus is needed to be repeated many times. It is hard to improve the response time and information transfer rate (ITR) of P300-based BCI if averaging EEG epochs underlies the detection of P300 ERP. As a result, many approaches based on machine learning have been developed for P300 detection in this kind of BCIs. They usually consist of a few important steps such as extracting the features from EEG and training an appropriate classifier. Since EEG or ERP are the signals acquired from the scalp, wavelet analysis, one of excellent signal processing tools [11], is very suitable to be used to handle the problem of extracting the features from EEG.

According to [11], unlike the Fourier transform, whose basis functions, sine or cosine, are all in a frequency and extend infinitely in time, wavelet analysis is based on completely different basis functions that are localized in time and frequency. The ability of wavelet analysis to highlight specific time and frequency components of signals makes itself very useful for processing EEG or ERP [12, 13]. Some examples of applying wavelet analysis in the field include EEG spike detection, ERP component separation, denoising EEG or ERP, etc [12, 13]. Demiralp et al. discovered that the delta response dominates the P300 component in their research and then used the wavelet coefficients of EEG epochs in the frequency range of 0.5–4 Hz during the time period of 310–430 ms after stimulus onset to detect P300 and found that the cognitive state could influence the presence of P300 [14, 15]. Perseh and Sharafat developed a scheme that extracts the features from EEG epochs for P300 Speller BCI by applying wavelet transform [16]. In [17], Robinson and colleagues showed that the wavelet-common spatial pattern algorithm could effectively extract informative features from EEG data for classifying the two different speeds of the right-hand movement. Aniyan et al. designed an algorithm to separate ERP components in single-trial EEG data by

making use of the asymmetry of wavelet [18]. Huang and Zheng [19] presented a method to process P300 ERP on the basis of the combination of autoregression model and wavelet representation.

Wavelet methodology has had a significant impact in the area of time series [11] and has been extensively used to deal with all kinds of problems on EEG and ERP [12–19]. In this paper, we use wavelet analysis to address the issue of EEG feature extraction in P300 Speller BCI. According to [3, 20], in P300 Speller BCI, a target EEG epoch is among the consecutive EEG epochs that are overlapped on one another so that nontarget EEG epochs could also contain P300 waveform just in a bit different time range, compared to target EEG epochs. Hence, it is still difficult to highlight the difference between target EEG epochs and nontarget EEG epochs simply using wavelet in P300 Speller BCI. Here, we proposed an algorithm to extract informative features from EEG epochs for P300 Speller BCI by combining wavelet analysis with Fisher Criterion [21]. The idea underlying this algorithm is that the ERP evoked in P300 Speller is a kind of sparse signal in the wavelet domain. So, we call it sparse wavelet feature extraction. Considering the speed requirement of the online experiments, we also designed and implemented the parallel computing scheme of the algorithm based on our previous work [22] and the real-time distributed computation platform of storm [23, 24]. We tested our algorithm in the experiment, and the results demonstrated its effectiveness. This work was partly presented in the conferences [25, 26].

2. Materials and Methods

The P300 Speller paradigm [3, 20] intuitively tells us that the difference between target EEG epochs and nontarget EEG epochs is not obvious. Averaging enough EEG epochs could highlight the difference. However, it would be accomplished only at the cost of time and efficiency. Our intention is to seek a way in which the features substantially reflecting the difference could be extracted from single-trial EEG epochs. The key of our method is to find the sparse wavelet bases for P300 Speller BCI. The algorithm is implemented on Matlab.

2.1. Wavelet Transform. Wavelet transform can explore the details of a signal in different scales at any time position. Formally, the wavelet transform of a time signal $f(t)$ is defined as following [11]:

$$C(a, b) = \int_{-\infty}^{+\infty} f(t) \psi_{a,b}^*(t) \, \mathrm{dt}, \qquad (1)$$

where $\psi_{a,b}(t) = 1/\sqrt{a}\psi((t - b)/a)$, $a > 0$, $b \in R$, and $*$ means complex conjugation.

Equation (1) shows that wavelet transform maps a function of time to another function of a and b, which, respectively, represent scale and time location. So, local frequency information of signals can be reflected clearly by wavelet transform. This is very import to P300 Speller BCI that need to find the time and frequency range of EEG epochs during which the differences between target and nontarget exist. The direct numerical implementation of Equation (1) usually is called continuous wavelet transform (CWT) [11]. However, CWT involves too many closely spaced scales and time points that are highly correlated. The information provided by CWT is unnecessarily redundant and CWT is not very efficient. A computationally simpler implementation is discrete wavelet transform (DWT) that is constructed on a set of orthogonal wavelet bases [11], such as Daubechies Wavelet [12]. DWT algorithm is based on a simple recursive filter scheme. The result of DWT algorithm is not redundant but sufficient for reconstruction of the time function.

In P300 Speller BCI, the $f(t)$ would be digitally sampled, and in the time window following the stimulus onset, be extracted into an EEG epoch that can be denoted as a vector e. DWT transforms e to another vector in same dimension. It can be formally written as follows:

$$b = We, \tag{2}$$

where W is an orthogonal matrix representing DWT, b as a vector in same dimension as e, is the result of DWT. In P300 Speller BCI, the difference between target and nontarget EEG epochs is that P300 component appears at different positions of the EEG epochs, so only a few elements reflecting the difference benefit the recognition of target EEG epochs. Selecting them from all elements is helpful.

2.2. Fisher Criterion.

Clearly, it is not efficient to use all elements of b in recognizing target EEG epochs. The next problem we face is to find a way in which only the best elements are selected to be passed to classifiers.

Aniyan et al. [18] reported a wavelet-based method carrying out the detection and isolation of special ERP component. The method is a fully automated algorithm that selects the best scale analysis from CWT for separating ERP components from single-trial EEG epochs. Although the problem handled by [18] is different, it at least demonstrates the feasibility of developing an algorithm for the issue that we need to solve.

According to [21], Fisher Criterion is a discriminant criterion function that is defined by the ratio of the between-class scatter to the within-class scatter. By maximizing the criterion function, one can get a projection axis. After the samples are projected on the axis, the between-class scatter is maximized and the within-class scatter is minimized.

In P300 Speller BCI, the aim is discriminating target EEG epochs and nontarget EEG epochs. We denote an EEG epoch on a channel by a vector e. Further, a e^+ represents a target EEG epoch and a e^- means a nontarget epoch. DWT, respectively, transforms e^+ and e^- to b^+ and b^-. Some elements of b are useful for discriminating b^+ and b^- but others not. We need to use Fisher Criterion to optimize DWT for P300 Speller BCI. In the optimized DWT, only the elements that clearly benefit the discrimination of the two classes remain in the results of transformation.

2.3. EEG Feature Extraction Algorithm.

In Equation (2), the matrix represents DWT. In fact, our optimization means

removing some rows from W in Equation (2). In accordance with Fisher Criterion, we need to maximize a function described by Equation (3) to seek a solution.

$$J(\omega) = \frac{\left(\omega^T \overline{b^+} - \omega^T \overline{b^-}\right)^2}{\omega^T \Sigma^+ \omega + \omega^T \Sigma^- \omega}, \tag{3}$$

where $\overline{b^+}$ and $\overline{b^-}$, respectively, represent the means of b^+ and b^- and Σ^+ and Σ^- are the covariance matrix of b^+ and b^-.

According to [21], the direction of the expected unit vector can be obtained by the following equation:

$$\omega = \left(\Sigma^+ + \Sigma^-\right)^{-1}\left(\overline{b^+} - \overline{b^-}\right). \tag{4}$$

In the vector ω, the absolute values of the elements mean their importance to discriminating b^+ and b^-. Each element of ω corresponds to a row of W. This shows that we can sort the elements of ω by their absolute values, remove some rows of W corresponding to the elements of small absolute values, and then get a new transform matrix M. In fact, M is a set of optimal wavelet bases for the channel of the subject. On the basis of the above analysis, we propose our EEG feature extraction algorithm for P300 Speller BCI. The algorithm includes two stages. In short, the first stage is to get M and the second stage is to use M.

The goal of the first stage is to determine an M for each channel. After training a subject, we can collect some target EEG epochs and nontarget EEG epochs. By them, a data set comprising many e^+ and e^- can be built for every valuable channel. According to Equation (2), the data set can be transformed to another data set containing many b^+ and b^-. From this new data set, ω can be obtained by Equation (4). In light of the absolute value of ω elements, the rows of W that are important to discriminating the target EEG epochs and nontarget EEG epochs are selected to construct M. The first stage of EEG feature extraction algorithm is depicted as Algorithm 1. In this, N means that we need to transform EEG epochs on the channel to N-dimension feature vectors, Matrix W represents the DWT for the data set comprising many e^+ and e^-, and Matrix M would be used to compute the feature vectors of EEG epochs on same channel.

In the second stage, every valuable channel of EEG epochs can be transformed to a low dimension vector by the following equation:

$$r = Me. \tag{5}$$

All r of an EEG epoch can be concatenated into a feature vector, which is in much lower dimension than the EEG epoch but has the most information in the EEG epoch that is helpful to the discrimination of target and nontarget. The feature vector is the result of EEG feature extraction algorithm.

2.4. Parallel Computing Scheme.

In a P300 Speller BCI, the classifiers are always trained offline when the subjects are in rest. Therefore, the first stage is also carried out offline if EEG feature extraction algorithm is applied in a P300 Speller BCI. Its speed is not a critical factor. As for the second stage, it is performed online when a P300 Speller BCI using the

---

Input: N, a data set comprising many e^+ and e^-
Output: Matrix M
  Construct Matrix W
  Compute $b^+ = We^+$ for all e^+
  Compute $b^- = We^-$ for all e^-
  Compute $\omega = (\Sigma^+ + \Sigma^-)^{-1} (\overline{b^+} - \overline{b^-})$
  Construct Matrix M with the rows of W associated with the N largest absolute values of ω elements

---

ALGORITHM 1: Stage 1 of EEG feature extraction.

algorithm is running. Every EEG epoch is needed to be computed when it is gotten, and the computation is expected to be completed as soon as possible. So, the speed is very important for the second stage of EEG feature extraction algorithm.

In fact, we have met the speed trouble. Originally, we implemented the algorithm in BCI2000 and tried online P300 Speller experiments of the algorithm. BCI2000 often stopped the experiments since the computation could not keep up with the steps of the experiments.

Although the speed problem can be solved by replacing the desktop computer with a high-performance hardware system, it is not a good solution in view of the cost and convenience. A preliminary parallel computing framework was proposed to increase the computation speed of P300 Speller in our previous work [22]. Here, we also seek to distribute the computing tasks of the algorithm to several desktop computers that are cooperating with one another. A very good mechanism for this problem is Storm, an open source real-time distributed stream data processing system [23, 24]. Its performances of low latency and fault-tolerance have been verified by many famous applications. We designed a parallel computing scheme of EEG feature extraction algorithm on the basis of Storm.

The parallel computing scheme of the algorithm based on Storm is shown in Figure 1. The scheme includes four kinds of computing units: DataSpout, ExtractBolt, ClassifyBolt, and SynthesizeBolt. They are built in accordance with the standard of Spout or Bolt in Storm [23, 24]. There is only one DataSpout in the scheme. DataSpout is connected to the EEG acquirement system and receives the signal segments from it. DataSpout assembles an EEG epoch and sends it to an ExtractBolt when the segments that have come are enough for an EEG epoch. The task of ExtractBolt is to conduct the computation described in Equation (5) for each channel of an EEG epoch. There are many ExtractBolts in the scheme. The number of them depends on how many computers and what kind of computer is included in this scheme. All ExtractBolts simultaneously operate but, respectively, compute different EEG epochs. An ExtractBolt outputs a feature vector to a ClassifyBolt when it completes the computation of an EEG epoch. Every ClassifyBolt is a computing unit of classifying a feature vector. Although the classification is not the focus in this paper, the scheme should contain the classification from the perspective of the computation integrity. In this scheme, all ClassifyBolts implement the same classifier. Similar to the ExtractBolts,

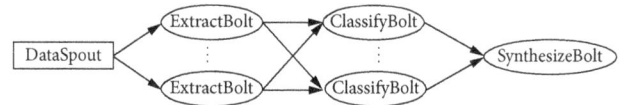

FIGURE 1: Parallel computing scheme.

many ClassifyBolts run at the same time but handle different feature vectors. Every ClassifyBolt transmits the score of classifying the feature vector to SynthesizeBolt. There is only one SynthesizeBolt in the scheme. SynthesizeBolt simply picks the row and column corresponding to the biggest the scores and feedbacks them to other parts of the BCI system.

Usually, one round of stimuli is not sufficient for a satisfactory detection of characters. The scores of a few rounds are necessarily accumulated to enhance the reliability. SynthesizeBolt does not give out the feedbacks until the gap between the biggest score and the second biggest one exceeds a threshold. Since the scores of a few rounds are summed, the computing units in ExtractBolt and ClassifyBolt are required to be linear. Equation (5) shows that the computing units in ExtractBolt are linear. As for ClassifyBolt, nonlinear classifiers are not acceptable. On the contrary, this scheme does not have a preference for any linear classifier. The scheme is flexible at this point.

3. Results and Discussion

3.1. Preliminary Work

3.1.1. Experiment Design. Our main aim is verifying whether EEG feature extraction algorithm can improve the performance of P300 Speller BCI by reducing the number of repeated stimuli. We designed the experiment procedure according to the P300 speller paradigm [1, 3, 4, 20]. The subjects were instructed to quietly sit in front of a screen and gaze at the screen. A 6×6 matrix of characters was presented on this screen. The six rows and six columns of the character matrix were randomly highlighted. The duration of highlighting was 120 ms, and the interval between the two consecutive highlighting was 80 ms. Each of the six rows and six columns was highlighted once in a round. This kind of flash was conducted fifteen rounds, called a sequence, for a wanted character. The subjects were asked to silently count when the wanted characters were being highlighted.

The experiments involved three phases. The first phase aimed to provide the subjects with practice opportunities so that they could adapt themselves to operating P300 speller. The intention of the second phase was to construct a training set for each subject. The goal of the third phase was to build a test set for each subject.

3.1.2. Subject and Instrument.

Nine subjects (three males and six females) took part in the experiments. Eight of them were university students (the average age was 24 years old), and one was a university staff (43 years old). All subjects were right-handed, and their eyesight varied in the degree of myopia. All subjects had sufficient rest between the experiments. For convenience, the nine subjects were denoted by S1 to S9.

The instrument for EEG signal acquisition was the 64-channel Neuroscan system, including the EEG cap, the amplifier, and the signal acquisition software. The sampling rate was set to 1000 Hz. BCI2000 [20] was used to present the character matrix and the stimuli, and it was integrated with the Neuroscan signal acquisition software to process the signals and save them to the data files.

3.1.3. Data Set.

In the second phase, the following steps were taken to construct the training sets. All characters in the character matrix were randomly divided into four groups. Every subject was arranged to input the characters group by group by the means of P300 speller. The course during which a subject input one group of characters is defined as a run. Between the two consecutive runs, the subjects all had a chance to sufficiently rest.

EEG signals were acquired when the subjects were working. First, the signals were filtered by such preliminary processes such as common average reference (CAR). Next, the signals except those from the electrodes of FZ, CZ, PZ, PO7, PO8, and OZ were removed. The reason for doing so is that the signals from these electrodes evidently have the main effect on P300 speller [1]. Every signal epoch of 800 ms following a stimulus onset was cut out. A stimulus onset corresponds to six 800 ms signal epochs from the six electrodes. The epochs corresponding to the wanted characters were labeled as positive examples and others as negative examples. All positive examples and negative ones belonging to one subject were added into the training set of the subject.

Before the third phase, every signal epoch was downsampled to a 15-dimension vector, then the six vectors corresponding to one stimulus onset were concatenated to be a feature vector, and a linear discriminant function was trained on the set of feature vectors for each subject. In the third phase, the subjects were instructed to formally use P300 Speller. BCI2000 was configured to use the trained linear discriminant functions to recognize the targets. As mentioned before, the subjects input about 10 characters in a run and had a rest after a run. Meanwhile, the EEG signals were stored into the data files for the subsequent analyses.

The most experiments in the third phase achieved the run accuracy of 100% for the character recognition. Although the accuracies of the remaining runs were close to 100%, only the runs with the accuracy of 100% were selected into the test sets. This ensured that the test sets were composed of the best data, and the adverse influence of dirty data could be excluded as much as possible.

3.2. Procedure and Performance of Classifying.

The proposed method involves both Wavelet Transform and Fisher Criterion, so we call it WF in a brief form. The question on whether or not WF could improve the performance of classifying EEG epochs in P300 Speller BCI is needed to be tested. Since WF does not focus on classifier but feature extraction, WF, downsampling (DS), and xDAWN (xD) [27] were, respectively, combined with the stepwise linear discriminant analysis (SWLDA), the default classifier in BCI2000, to classify the EEG epochs in the test data sets. According to [28], DS and xD are the typical feature extractions used to classify ERP in BCI. We evaluated WF by comparing the three kinds of classification results.

For WF, all kinds of mother wavelets are available. According to [12], the wave shapes of mother wavelets play an important role in this kind of tasks. On basis of this opinion, we got the difference wave shape by subtracting the averaged EEG epoch corresponding to target stimuli from the averaged EEG epoch corresponding to nontarget stimuli and compared it with a variety of mother wavelets. Finally, we chose the Daubechies 4 (DB4) in the study to construct a matrix for each channel of one subject. As for the dimension of feature vector, WF and DS both transformed a channel of one epoch to a 15-dimension vector. The reason for 15-dimension is that, by default, BCI2000 gets a 15-dimension vector from a channel of one epoch. As six channels were used, the final feature vectors were of 90-dimension. For consistency, xD also transformed each epoch into a 90-dimension feature vector. The three different algorithms produced the feature vectors of same dimension. It is to eliminate the possibility that the difference of their performances stems from the dimension distinction of feature vector.

The experiment design has shown that a sequence, through which a subject input a character, includes $15 * 12$ EEG epochs. We investigated the classification performance by using WF, DS, and xD to classify all epochs of each sequence. For a sequence, three receiver operating characteristics (ROC) [29] curves were drawn, respectively, for WF, DS, and xD, and the areas under the ROC curve (AUC) [29] were also worked out. Figure 2 demonstrates a ROC graph for each subject. TPR means true positive rate, and FPR means false positive rate. Every graph contains three ROC curves: WF, DS, and xD. They are the results of classification performance of WF, DS, and xD in a sequence of the subjects.

For a ROC curve, the AUC indicates the performance of classification. Bigger means better. In Figure 2, it is obvious that the WF curves have bigger AUC than those of DS and xD for S1, S3, S4, S5, S7, and S9. Their AUCs are very similar for S2, S6, and S8. Clearly, WF performs better in the example.

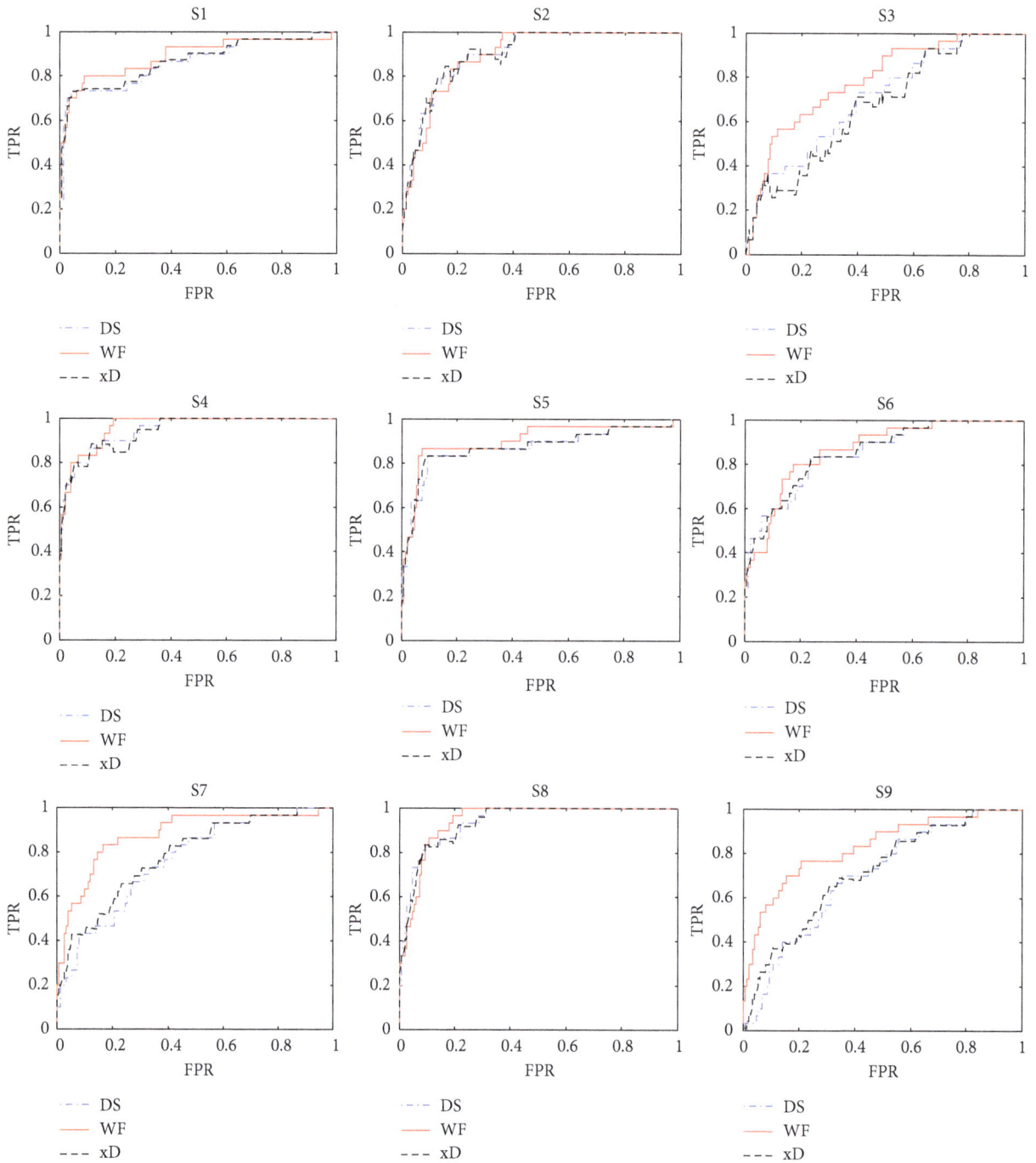

FIGURE 2: ROC curves of subject 1–9.

However, an example is not enough. We figured out all sequences AUCs of each subject. Their means and standard deviations are shown in Figure 3. The heights of the bars are the means of AUCs of Subject 1–9. The error bars represent the standard deviations of the AUCs. For S1, S2, S3, S6, S7, S8, and S9, WF AUC means are bigger than those of DS and xD. For S4 and S5, WF AUC means are similar to those of DS and xD. As for the standard deviations, no significant difference appears. Figure 3 shows that, in general, WF did better than DS and xD in classifying the EEG epochs of single trial from P300 Speller BCI. Furthermore, the WF, DS,

and xD AUC of each sequence were, respectively, paired, and paired t-tests were conducted over the data sets of the paired AUCs. P value of the pair of WF and DS is 1.38E-62, that of WF and xD 1.43E-60, and that of DS and xD 0.15. It is very obvious that WF is superior to DS and xD in the task of classification. On the contrary, DS and xD had similar performance in the task.

3.3. Detection of Characters and Statistic Analysis. For P300 Speller BCI, the wanted character is recognized by selecting

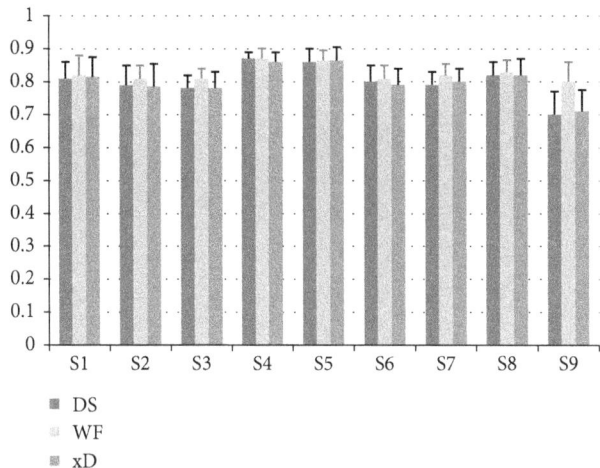

FIGURE 3: AUC means and standard deviations.

the most possible row and column of the character matrix through the synthesis of the classification results. The accuracy of classification is not that of detecting characters. As shown in Figure 4, the accuracy of detecting characters varies basically from 20% to 75% when only the first round of EEG epochs are used. Round = n means that the detection of characters is the result of synthesizing the classification of the first n-round EEG epochs. The accuracy of detecting characters changes with the round. The curves reflect the trend that a higher accuracy could be achieved when more rounds are used. Therefore, one round of stimuli is usually not sufficient for P300 Speller BCI. By default, BCI2000 presents 15 rounds of stimuli for a wanted character. We did the experiments in the condition of BCI2000 default configuration and constructed the test data set in which every sequence contains 15 rounds of EEG epochs. Thus, we can observe how the performances of detecting characters change when the rounds vary from 1 to 15.

In Figure 4, the DS, WF, and xD curves, respectively, imply the trends that their performances change with the rounds. They can get higher accuracies when more rounds are processed. For S2, S3, S6, S7, S8, and S9, the WF curves are above the DS and xD ones, indicating that WF did better than DS and xD for these subjects. Especially, there is a big gap between the WF curves and the other two for S9, meaning that WF achieved much higher accuracies of detecting characters than DS and xD for S9. For S1, S4, and S5, the three curves are very similar, implying that they performed similarly. For the three subjects, the accuracies exceed 60% when only one round of EEG epochs is used. It is good enough. So, it is difficult for WF to obviously perform better than DS and xD for these subjects. In general, WF can clearly achieve higher accuracies of detecting characters than the other two.

Although more rounds mean higher accuracies of detecting characters, fewer rounds are expected from the perspective of efficiency. There is a trade-off between the accuracy and efficiency. To seek a good balance,

we turned to the information transfer rate (ITR), a measure about the amount of communication in unit time [4]. Equation (6) and (7) show how ITR should be calculated:

$$\text{ITR} = \frac{B}{t}, \tag{6}$$

$$B = \log_2 N + P \log_2 P + (1 - P)\log_2 \frac{1 - P}{N - 1}, \tag{7}$$

where N is the number of the characters in the character matrix, P is the accuracy of recognizing characters, and t is calculated, respectively, for round = $1, 2, \ldots, 15$ according to Equation (8). In Equation (8), the time unit is millisecond, and gap means the interval between the consecutive sequences. Here, we figured out t by setting gap as 2000 and converted the unit of t to minute before using t in the following equation:

$$t = 12 \times 200 \times (\text{round} - 1) + 11 \times 200 + 800 + \text{gap}. \tag{8}$$

The results of ITR are shown in Figure 5. The meaning of round = n is same as that in Figure 4. The curves reflect the trends that the ITRs change with the increase of round. Similarly, WF has higher ITRs than DS and xD for S2, S3, S6, S7, S8, and S9, and their ITRs are very high and close for S1, S4, and S5. This also means that WF is mostly superior to DS and xD. Additionally, the ITR curves can help seek the trade-off between accuracy and efficiency. We can see a peak in the ITR curves for the subjects except S4. For the WF curves, the peak is at round = 2 for S1, round = 3 for S2, round = 4 for S3, round = 2 for S5, round = 5 for S6, round = 5 for S7, round = 4 for S8, and round = 3 for S9. The peaks are the biggest ITRs for the subjects. More rounds do not lead to higher ITRs. The round numbers corresponding to the peaks are the best choices for the subjects. As for the exception of S4, the reason that no peak exists is that the accuracies of detecting characters are very high at round = 1. So, round = 1, 2, or 3 is suitable for S4 according to its accuracy curve. To sum up, WF not only significantly increases the accuracy of detecting characters but also reduces the round numbers to 2–5.

3.4. Speed of Parallel Computing. The parallel computing scheme is shown as Figure 1. WF was implemented in the ExtractBolts and SWLDA in the ClassifyBolts. The four kinds of computing units in the scheme were deployed on a Storm platform based on three ordinary desktop computers. The configurations of the three computers were, respectively: Intel Pentium dual core E6600 3.06 GHz, Intel Pentium CPU G850 2.90 GHz, and Intel core i5-4590 3.30 GHz. The Storm was supported by 1 G RAM on each of the three computers. The parallel computing scheme substituted for the signal processing module of BCI2000 and was connected to the other parts of BCI2000 during our online experiments. No delay cues emerged in our online experiments.

When our method is applied in P300 Speller, the system extracts the feature vector from each EEG epoch,

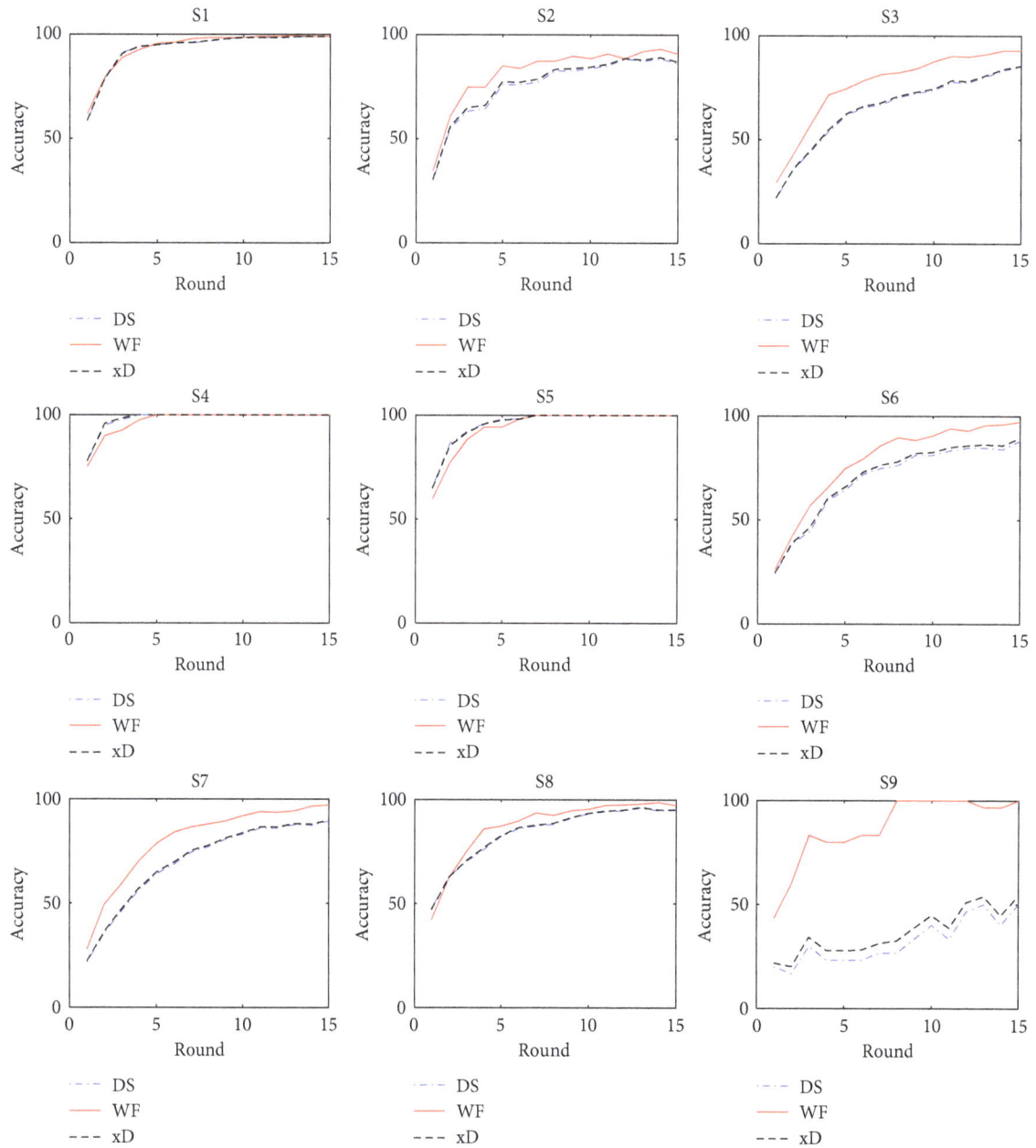

FIGURE 4: Accuracy of detecting characters.

classifies it, and begins to synthesize the classification results of all EEG epochs at the end of one round of stimuli. According to the synthesization, the system can give out the detected character or continue to present the stimuli. Whether or not the synthesization is completed in time is an important factor of the performance of our method.

Under the conditions mentioned above, we tested the time from the end of one round of stimuli to the moment when the response to the round is given out. The probability distribution of the time value is shown as Figure 6. The maximum response time is 16 ms, and the mean is 1.57 ms. In P300 Speller, every stimulus lasts 200 ms. All the responses were given out before the next stimulus occurred.

4. Conclusions

BCI not only brings people a lot of visions about the future but also has many practical applications in the fields of rehabilitation therapy. Among all kinds of BCIs, the reliability of P300 Speller has been attracting the attention of researchers. Many efforts were made to improve P300 Speller. This work aims at developing a new feature extraction and its parallel computing scheme for P300 Speller.

The proposed feature extraction is based on Wavelet Transform, which has been proved by many researches to be a good tool for analyzing P300 component. In P300 Speller, both target EEG epochs and nontarget EEG ones contain P300 component. The difference between the two is not obvious. We mapped the EEG epochs to the wavelet space

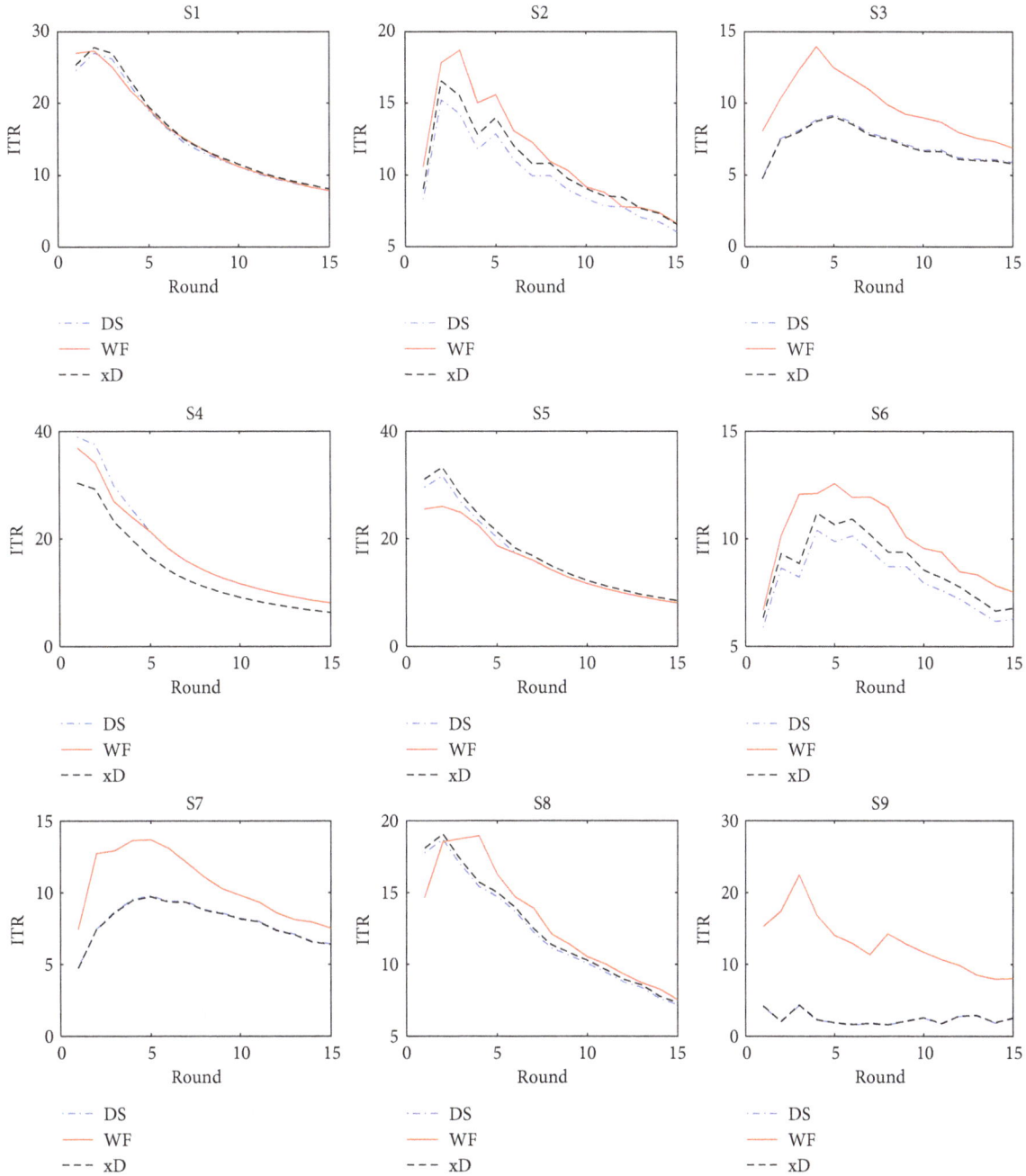

FIGURE 5: ITR curves.

and measured the differences between target and nontarget in the space according to Fisher Criterion. The wavelet bases corresponding to small differences were filtered, and a sparse wavelet space was constructed for each subject. The feature extraction algorithm based on the sparse wavelet spaces was developed for P300 Speller.

The test results show the superiority of the proposed feature extraction. Firstly, WF, DS, and xD were applied in the classification of single-trial epochs from P300 Speller. Their performances of classifying single trial epochs were measured by AUC. The comparison of AUC between the methods indicated that WF outperformed the other two in classifying single trial epochs from P300

Speller. Secondly, WF, DS, and xD were further compared by detecting the wanted characters. For most subjects, the accuracy curves of WF are above the ones of the other two, implying that WF achieved better performance in the detection of characters of P300 Speller than DS and xD did. Finally, ITRs were calculated on basis of the detection accuracies. The comparison of ITRs demonstrated the result that is consistent with the comparison of the detection accuracies.

Additionally, the parallel computing scheme of the feature extraction was designed and implemented to ensure the fast feedback for online P300 Speller experiments. It is worth mentioning that the parallel computing scheme is able

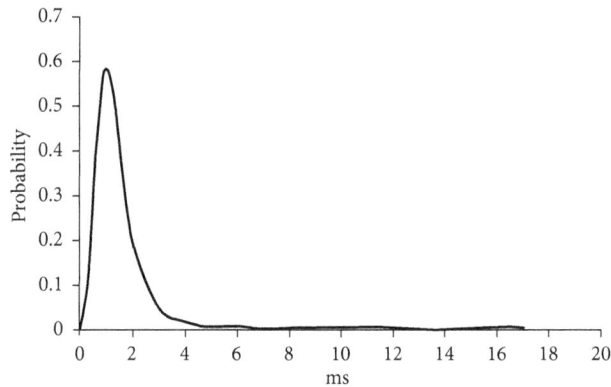

FIGURE 6: Probability distribution of the feedback time.

to support any other algorithms for P300 Speller. An algorithm can be implemented on our parallel computing scheme to extract the features or classify the EEG epochs for online P300 Speller experiments, even though it is computationally complex.

On the contrary, something should be further handled. The problem on which kind of wavelet bases is the best choice for our method is needed to be systematically studied. The matrix used to extract features in WF is obtained by a supervised training. Some issues on the supervised training remain unknown. For example, how much data is enough for the supervised training? When the supervised training is needed to be conducted again to adapt to the change of EEG. We plan to study such interesting problems in the future.

Conflicts of Interest

The authors declare that they have no conflicts of interest.

Acknowledgments

The experiment had been approved by the Ethics Committee of Kunming Institute of Zoology, and all participants had read and filled in the informed consent and all procedures complied with the Helsinki declaration. This work was supported in part by Key Project of Science and Technology Plan of Fujian Province, China (2014H0025) and Science and Technology Foundation of Fuzhou University (2013-XQ-30). Shunying Guo, Suyun Lin, Yukun Wen, and Wei Huang participated in this work when they studied at Fuzhou University. The authors thank them for their contributions.

References

[1] J. R. Wolpaw and E. W. Wolpaw, *Brain-Computer Interfaces: Principles and Practice*, Oxford University Press, New York, NY, USA, 2012.

[2] B. Graiman, B. Allison, and G. Pfurtscheller, *Brain-Computer Interfaces: A Gentle Introduction in Brain-Computer Interfaces: Revolutionizing Human-Computer Interaction*, Springer, Berlin, Germany, 2010.

[3] L. A. Farwell and E. Donchin, "Talking off the top of your head: toward a mental prosthesis utilizing event-related brain potentials," *Electroencephalography and Clinical Neurophysiology*, vol. 70, no. 6, pp. 510–523, 1988.

[4] J. R. Wolpaw, N. Birbaumer, D. J. McFarland, G. Pfurtscheller, and T. M. Vaughan, "Brain computer interfaces for communication and control," *Clinical Neurophysiology*, vol. 113, no. 6, pp. 767–791, 2002.

[5] R. C. Panicker, S. Puthusserypady, and Y. Sun, "An asynchronous P300 BCI With SSVEP-based control state detection," *IEEE Transactions on Biomedical Engineering*, vol. 58, no. 6, pp. 1781–1788, 2011.

[6] S. Halder, A. Pinegger, I. Kathner et al., "Brain-controlled applications using dynamic P300 speller matrices," *Artificial Intelligence in Medicine*, vol. 63, no. 1, pp. 7–17, 2015.

[7] Q. Li, S. Liu, J. Li, and O. Bai, "Use of a green familiar faces paradigm improves p300-speller brain-computer interface performance," *PLoS One*, vol. 10, no. 6, Article ID e0130325, 2015.

[8] T. Krumpe, C. Walter, W. Rosenstiel, and M. Spuler, "Asynchronous P300 classification in a reactive brain-computer interface during an outlier detection task," *Journal of Neural Engineering*, vol. 13, no. 4, article 046015, 2016.

[9] J. Jin, H. Zhang, I. Daly, X. Wang, and A. Cichocki, "An improved P300 pattern in BCI to catch users attention," *Journal of Neural Engineering*, vol. 14, no. 3, article 036001, 2017.

[10] X. Mao, M. Li, W. Li et al., "Progress in EEG-based brain robot interaction systems," *Computational Intelligence and Neuroscience*, vol. 2017, Article ID 1742862, 25 pages, 2017.

[11] D. B. Percival and A. T. Walden, *Wavelet Methods for Time Series Analysis*, Cambridge University Press, New York, NY, USA, 2006.

[12] V. J. Samar, K. P. Swartz, and M. R. Raghuveer, "Multiresolution analysis of event-related potentials by wavelet decomposition," *Brain and Cognition*, vol. 27, no. 3, pp. 398–438, 1995.

[13] V. J. Samar, A. Bopardikar, R. Rao, and K. Swartz, "Wavelet analysis of neuroelectric waveforms: a conceptual tutorial," *Brain and Language*, vol. 66, no. 1, pp. 7–60, 1999.

[14] T. Demiralp, A. Ademoglu, M. Schrmann, C. Basar-Eroglu, and E. Basar, "Detection of P300 waves in single trials by the wavelet transform (WT)," *Brain and Language*, vol. 66, no. 1, pp. 108–128, 1999.

[15] T. Demiralp, A. Ademoglu, Y. Istefanopulos, C. Basar-Eroglu, and E. Basar, "Wavelet analysis of oddball P300," *International Journal of Psychophysiology*, vol. 39, no. 2-3, pp. 221–227, 2001.

[16] B. Perseh and A. R. Sharafat, "An efficient P300-based BCI using wavelet features and IBPSO-based channel selection," *Journal of Medical Signals and Sensors*, vol. 2, no. 3, pp. 128–143, 2012.

[17] N. Robinson, A. P. Vinod, K. K. Ang, K. P. Tee, and C. T. Guan, "EEG-based classification of fast and slow hand movements using wavelet-CSP algorithm," *IEEE Transactions on Biomedical Engineering*, vol. 60, no. 8, pp. 2123–2132, 2013.

[18] A. K. Aniyan, N. S. Philip, V. J. Samar, J. A. Desjardins, and S. J. Segalowitz, "A wavelet based algorithm for the identi-

fication of oscillatory event-related potential components," *Journal of Neuroscience Methods*, vol. 233, pp. 63–72, 2014.

[19] Z. Huang and H. Zheng, "Combining AR filter and sparse wavelet representation for P300 speller," in *Proceedings of 2015 IEEE International Conference on Bioinformatics and Biomedicine (BIBM)*, Washington, USA, November 2015.

[20] G. Schalk, D. J. McFarland, T. Hinterberger, N. Birbaumer, and J. R. Wolpaw, "BCI2000: a general-purpose brain-computer interface (BCI) system," *IEEE Transactions on Biomedical Engineering*, vol. 51, no. 6, pp. 1034–1043, 2004.

[21] R. O. Duda, P. E. Hart, and D. G. Stork, *Pattern Classification*, John Wiley and Sons, Hoboken, NJ, USA, 2nd edition, 2001.

[22] Z. Huang, "A MapReduce computation model for brain-computer interface," *Journal of Fuzhou University*, vol. 41, no. 6, pp. 981–985, 2013.

[23] A. Toshniwal, S. Taneja, A. Shukla et al., "Storm@twitter," in *Proceedings of 2014 ACM SIGMOD International Conference on Management of Data*, Snowbird, UT, USA, June 2014.

[24] C. Li, J. Zhang, and Y. Luo, "Real-time scheduling based on optimized topology and communication traffic in distributed real-time computation platform of storm," *Journal of Network and Computer Applications*, vol. 87, pp. 100–115, 2017.

[25] S. Guo, S. Lin, and Z. Huang, "Feature extraction of P300s in EEG signal with discrete wavelet transform and fisher criterion," in *Proceedings of 8th International Conference on Biomedical Engineering and Informatics(BMEI)*, Shenyang, China, October 2015.

[26] W. Huang and Z. Huang, "A real-time distributed computing mechanism for P300 speller BCI," in *Proceedings of 10th International Conference on Biomedical Engineering and Informatics(BMEI)*, Shanghai, China, October 2017.

[27] B. Rivet, A. Souloumiac, V. Attina, and G. Gibert, "xDAWN algorithm to enhance evoked potentials: application to brain–computer interface," *IEEE Transactions on Biomedical Engineering*, vol. 56, no. 8, pp. 2035–2043, 2009.

[28] F. Lotte, L. Bougrain, A. Cichocki et al., "A review of classification algorithms for EEG-based brain–computer interfaces: a 10 year update," *Journal of Neural Engineering*, vol. 15, no. 3, article 031005, 2018.

[29] T. Fawcett, "An introduction to ROC analysis," *Pattern Recognition Letters*, vol. 27, no. 8, pp. 861–874, 2006.

5

Sex Determination of 3D Skull based on a Novel Unsupervised Learning Method

Hongjuan Gao,[1,2] **Guohua Geng** ⓘ**,**[1] **and Wen Yang**[1]

[1]*College of Information Science and Technology, Northwest University, Xi'an, China*
[2]*College of Xinhua, Ningxia University, Yinchuan, China*

Correspondence should be addressed to Guohua Geng; ghgeng@nwu.edu.cn

Academic Editor: Reinoud Maex

In law enforcement investigation cases, sex determination from skull morphology is one of the important steps in establishing the identity of an individual from unidentified human skeleton. To our knowledge, existing studies of sex determination of the skull mostly utilize supervised learning methods to analyze and classify data and can have limitations when applied to actual cases with the absence of category labels in the skull samples or a large difference in the number of male and female samples of the skull. This paper proposes a novel approach which is based on an unsupervised classification technique in performing sex determination of the skull of Han Chinese ethnic group. The 78 landmarks on the outer surface of 3D skull models from computed tomography scans are marked, and a skull dataset of a total of 40 interlandmark measurements is constructed. A stable and efficient unsupervised algorithm which we abbreviated as MKDSIF-FCM is proposed to address the classification problem for the skull dataset. The experimental results of the adult skull suggest that the proposed MKDSIF-FCM algorithm warrants fairly high sex determination accuracy for females and males, which is 98.0% and 93.02%, respectively, and is superior to all the classification methods we attempted. As a result of its fairly high accuracy, extremely good stability, and the advantage of unsupervised learning, the proposed method is potentially applicable for forensic investigations and archaeological studies.

1. Introduction

Sex analysis and determination are indispensable and foremost steps in confirming the personal identification of an individual in forensic investigations. The best result is achieved when confirming an individual sex by accessing the entire skeleton, but most of the time the skeleton is incomplete. Thus, various local skeletons such as the patella [1], hip joint [2], pelvis [3], calcaneus [4], carpal [5], and skull and its parts have been utilized for sex determination in different populations worldwide. Among all parts of the skeleton, the skull is a small and distinctive collection of bones. The skull is composed of hard tissue and can be well preserved in most cases. Hence, the skull and its parts are most widely and commonly used in providing information about human origin, ancestry, stature, and sex in forensic anthropological analysis [6].

Sex determination of the skull involves two major techniques: the first one is the measurement of skull traits, which

reflects difference of skull morphology between males and females. The second one is the analysis and classification of skull measurements. Both will affect the classification accuracy in sex identification for the skull. The approach earlier used to measure skull traits is subjective visual method. Visual assessment depends heavily on the experience and knowledge of the forensic scientist or biological anthropologist. Thus, it is likely to be inaccurate when performed by an inexperienced observer due to its great subjectivity. To reduce subjectivity, efforts to physically quantify skull traits by using an ordinal scale or software are undertaken. With the development and success of medical imaging, skull traits measurement by means of images and computed tomography (CT) is established. For example, some studies used radiograph to provide morphological details of the skull, and some researchers utilized three-dimensional (3D) imaging of the skull from clinical scans of known individuals to discover metric variables. No matter what method is used to measure the morphological features of the skull, it is very important to employ a high-performance classification method. In existing studies, typically statistical and supervised classification methods are linear discriminant analysis (LDA), logistic regression, and support vector machines (SVM).

At present, many approaches in sex determination of the skull, which consist of skull measurement and data classification techniques, have been published and have achieved a high or higher accuracy of discrimination between the sexes. Walker obtained five cranial traits (glabella, mental, orbital, nuchal, and mastoid) by visual assessment and achieved the best classification results of 88% of the modern skulls with a negligible sex bias of 0.1% via the logistic regression model [7]. Robinson and Bidmos selected 230 skull samples from South Africa and extracted 12 measured skull characteristics and got 72.0–95.5 accuracy by establishing five discriminant function equations [8]. Ogawa et al. obtained anthropological measurements of 113 skulls of modern Japanese individuals from forensic anthropological test records. Ten skull measurements were used for statistical analysis, and nine discriminant functions were established. The classification accuracy is between 79% and 93% [9]. Franklin et al. used OsiriX 03 to mark 31 landmarks on 3D skulls of Australian individuals. They calculated a total of 18 linear interlandmark measurements, which were analyzed by discriminant function. The maximum classification accuracy was 90% [10]. Abdel Fatah et al. utilized 222 cranial CT images of White Americans to construct a statistical bone atlas. They obtained >95% accuracy (97.5% with 11 variables and 95.5% with 8 variables) by cross-validated linear discriminant analysis on metric variables [11]. Musilová et al. used coherent point drift-dense correspondence to analyze the entire cranial surface and used an SVM with a radial kernel to perform classification. The method provided a high level of classification accuracy (90.3%) in the sex determination of male and female skulls of Southern French population [12]. Li manually extracted the mid-sagittal frontal arc on dried skulls and adopted the Fourier transform to analyze the sex difference of adult skull in Northeast China. He obtained the results of 84.21% and 83.33% for male and female classification rates, respectively [13]. Li Ming et al. selected 67 skulls from Southwest China and measured 16 anthropometric characters. They established the equations of single-variable and multivariable analysis and obtained the highest accuracy of 89.2% for males and 90.0% for females [14]. Shui et al. chose 133 digital adult skull samples from Han ethnic group of North China and separately computed a total of 14 measurements (12 geometric measurements and 2 angle measurements). Then, they performed the Fisher step method to build the sex discriminant function and obtained the accuracy of 87.5% for male and 86.67% for female separately for the complete skull [15]. Luo et al. constructed a statistical shape model for 208 Chinese skulls by projecting the high-dimensional skull data into a low-dimensional shape space. Fisher discriminant analysis (FDA) was utilized to classify skulls in the shape space; the correct rates were 95.7% and 91.4% for females and males, respectively [16]. Liu et al. divided the skull into seven partitions and quantized immeasurable features by means of marking the feature points. Then, they used

the forward stepwise regression method based on maximum likelihood estimation to select the optimal feature subset of each partition. Experiments showed that any three partitions are enough to determine the sex of incomplete skulls with a high accuracy [17].

Although existing methods fully demonstrate their usefulness in sex identification of the skull, a notable problem is that these methods are not applicable in cases in which category labels in the skull samples are absent. Another situation is that when the distribution of the male and female skull samples is not balanced, the effect of using supervised learning for classification may not be better than unsupervised learning. LDA, logic regression, SVM, and other supervised learning methods need to use a training set with category labels to train the classification model. It is therefore the aim of this study to propose a stable and efficient sex determination approach for the skull that is based on unsupervised robust classification technology.

The contribution of our work is as follows: In terms of sex determination of the skull, the current works are mainly focused on the methods of skull measurement, while the methods of data analysis and data classification are less explored, especially the unsupervised learning method. In this study, we attempt to improve the classification accuracy of sex determination of the skull from the perspective of data mining. Inspired by the clustering theories, we extend the fuzzy C-means clustering (FCM) method and put forward an improved algorithm that is used to classify the skull dataset we have measured. We named it as MKDSIF-FCM. The proposed MKDSIF-FCM is based on an unsupervised learning theory where input is presented without desired output. Compared with existing supervised learning methods, the proposed MKDSIF-FCM can divide the skulls into two categories without known category labels and obtain fairly high accuracy for 3D adult skull from the Han Chinese ethnic group.

2. Materials and Methods

Our process of sex determination of the skull consists of three broad phases outlined in Figure 1. In the first stage, our approach relies on acquiring skull data and building a database of skull models (Section 2.1). In the second stage, feature points from 3D skull models are marked by utilizing a semi-automatic method, and skull characteristics are extracted that are required to identify a skull (Section 2.2). In the last stage, the extracted characteristics are passed to the classifier. The proposed MKDSIF-FCM algorithm is undertaken to distinguish the skull's sex (Section 2.3).

2.1. Skull Data Acquisition. This study is based on the specimens of 186 whole skulls from living adults representative of Han Chinese ethnic group, which were obtained by a clinical multislice CT scanner system at Xianyang Hospital located in Shaanxi province of China. The total database consisted of 100 female skulls with a mean age of 49.8 years (range: 18–75) and 86 male skulls with a mean age of 48.3 years (range: 18–76). Only intact, undamaged skulls were included in this study;

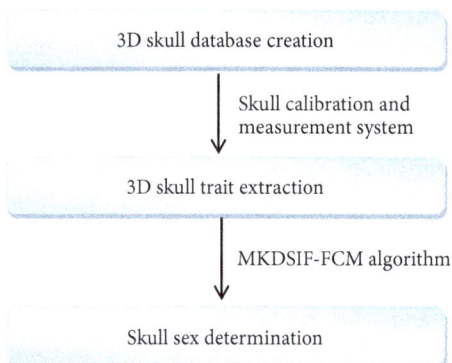

FIGURE 1: Depiction of the sex determination process.

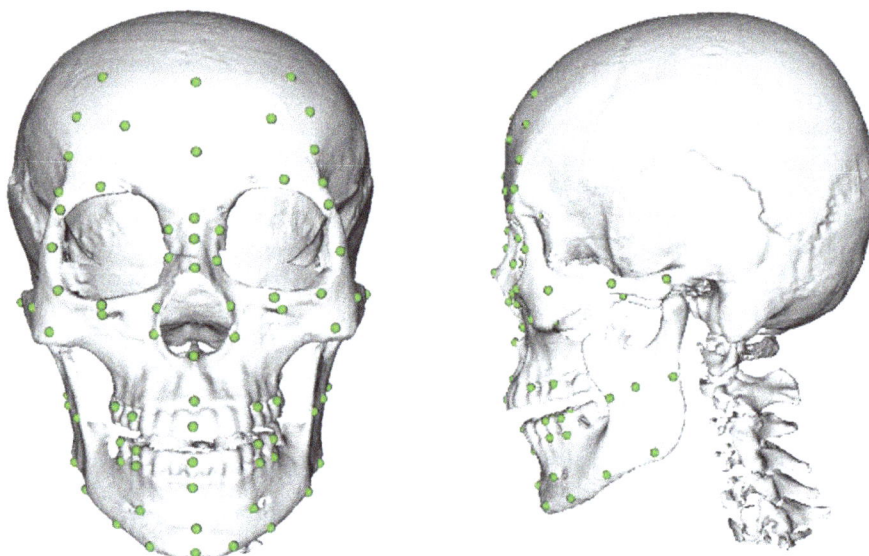

FIGURE 2: Seventy-eight landmarks on the outer surface of the skull.

each skull contains all the bones from calvaria to jaw with the full mouth of teeth.

2.2. Skull Characteristics Measurement.

In this study, in order to adequately illustrate the anatomy of the skull, we use the skull calibration and measurement system (with independent research and development by our research group) to extract the characteristics of the 3D skull.

According to the research achievements of forensic anthropology experts, 78 landmarks on the outer surface of the skull are marked, 12 of them are located in the midline, and the rest are symmetrically located about the midline sagittal line on both sides (Figure 2).

Distances and angles between different skull landmarks may be important components of skull sexual dimorphism. The size-related variables which reflect sex differences between male and female are obtained by calculating a total of 40 interlandmark measurements. Then, essential characteristic indexes for each skull were successfully constructed. Table 1 shows the characteristics and their brief descriptions; the data unit is mm.

2.3. Method.

FCM [19] is an unsupervised learning algorithm and a normal tool for data mining. Clustering is a process for grouping a set of data into classes so that the data within a cluster have high similarity but are very dissimilar to data in other clusters.

To classify our skull measurements via the unsupervised learning method, we propose an improved FCM algorithm that puts forward the concept of distance weighting coefficient with influence factor (IF) and incorporates the advantage of multiple kernel learning. We named it as MKDSIF-FCM.

2.3.1. Distance Weighting Coefficient with IF.

In the generic FCM algorithm, $u_{ik} \in U$ is a membership function value from k^{th} vector x_k to i^{th} cluster center v_i. It reflects to what degree the same sample belongs to each cluster center. In (1a)–(1d), there is an example of distance weighting coefficient with IF. (1a) X is a set of two-dimensional samples. (1b) V represents the initial cluster center in the FCM algorithm. (1c) U represents the initial membership function value in the FCM algorithm. (1d) W^{β}

TABLE 1: Description of the skull measurements.

Index	Descriptions	Index	Descriptions
I1	Maximum cranial length	I21	Maximum breadth of the frontal bone
I2	Basicranial length	I22	Upper facial width
I3	Maximum cranial breadth	I23	Orbital width
I4	First cranial height	I24	Width of the superior alveolar arch
I5	Bizygomatic breadth	I25	Length of the maxillary alveolar arch
I6	Bimaxillary width	I26	Palatal length
I7	Upper facial height	I27	Palatal width
I8	Minimum frontal breadth	I28	Palatal height
I9	First orbital width of the right eye	I29	Bigonial breadth
I10	Second orbital width of the right eye	I30	Height of the mandibular joint
I11	Distance between the outer corners of both eyes	I31	Height of the right mandibular ramus
I12	Height of right eye	I32	Mandibular condylar width
I13	Distance between the inner corners of the both eyes	I33	Coracoid width
I14	Nasal height	I34	Width of the mandibular notch
I15	Height of the nose forehead	I35	Depth of the mandibular notch
I16	Nasal width	I36	Height of the mandibular ramus
I17	Right mastoid length	I37	Thickness of the mandibular body
I18	Bimastoid width	I38	Mandibular angle
I19	Distance from the occipital to right mastoid point	I39	Second cranial height
I20	Frontal string	I40	Superciliary arch

represents the proposed distance weighting coefficient with IF.

In this example, three samples are a, b, and c; two cluster centers are v_1 and v_2. Suppose the membership function values of the sample a belonging to v_1 and v_2 are 0.7 and 0.3, respectively. It is obvious that sample a belongs to the v_1-centered class. The membership function values 0.7, 0.6, and 0.2 could not be compared in generic FCM. Nevertheless, this comparability is very important for classification or clustering analysis. It can reflect the distance of samples a, b, and c to the cluster center v_1.

$$X = \begin{bmatrix} a \\ b \\ c \end{bmatrix} = \begin{bmatrix} 1 & 1 \\ 1 & 2 \\ 4 & 4 \end{bmatrix} \tag{1a}$$

$$V = \begin{bmatrix} v_1 \\ v_2 \end{bmatrix} = \begin{bmatrix} 1 & 0 \\ 5 & 5 \end{bmatrix} \tag{1b}$$

$$U = \begin{matrix} & a & b & c & \\ \begin{bmatrix} 0.7 & 0.6 & 0.2 \\ 0.3 & 0.4 & 0.8 \end{bmatrix} & \begin{matrix} v_1 \\ v_2 \end{matrix} \end{matrix} \tag{1c}$$

$$W^\beta = \begin{bmatrix} \dfrac{7}{15} & \dfrac{6}{15} & \dfrac{2}{15} \\ \dfrac{3}{15} & \dfrac{4}{15} & \dfrac{8}{15} \end{bmatrix} \quad (\beta = 1) \tag{1d}$$

This paper puts forward a new concept of distance weighting coefficient with IF and provides a new approach of distance definition. Distance weighting coefficient is defined according to different contributions of sample to the same cluster center in data space. Distance weighting coefficient with IF is defined as follows:

$$w_i = \sum_{k=1}^{n} u_{ik} \quad k = 0, 1, 2, \cdots, n \tag{2}$$

$$w_{ik} = \frac{u_{ik}}{w_i} \tag{3}$$

$$w_{ik} = \left(\frac{1}{w_{ik}} \right)^\beta \tag{4}$$

Let w_{ik} be a fuzzy weighting coefficient from k^{th} vector x_k to i^{th} cluster center v_i. Moreover, w_{ik} plays an important role in measuring the distance between k^{th} vector x_k and i^{th} cluster center v_i. For different types of sample set, the influence on distance d_{ik} by w_{ik} is different. In order to be able to ensure the stable clustering performance of our improved algorithm in regard to different datasets, we introduce an IF for w_{ik}, denoted as β.

2.3.2. Euclidean Distance Based on Distance Weighting Coefficient with IF. In generic FCM, Euclidean distance is commonly used as distance d_{ik}. The notion of distance weighting coefficient with IF is introduced by the proposed MKDSIF-FCM algorithm, and the distance from k^{th} vector x_k to i^{th} cluster center v_i is defined in the form of square:

$$d_{ik} = \sqrt{\left(\frac{1}{w_{ik}} \right)^\beta \sum_{j=1}^{m} \left(x_{kj} - v_{ij} \right)^2} = \left\| \left(\frac{1}{w_{ik}} \right)^\beta \left(x_k - v_i \right) \right\|^2 \tag{5}$$

We can prove that (5) obeys with distance definition in Euclidean space. We shall discuss the significance of $(1/w_{ik})^{\beta}$. In (1a)–(1d), the Euclidean distances of three samples a, b, and c to cluster center v_1 are 1, 2, and 5, respectively. Suppose the value of β is 1. According to (2), (3), and (4), we can get w_{11}=7/15, w_{12}=6/15, and w_{13}=2/15. According to (5), we can obtain our defined distances of three samples a, b, and c to cluster center v_1: $d_{11} \approx 1.46$, $d_{12} \approx 2.24$, and $d_{13} \approx 13.69$.

From calculating the results, we introduce distance weighting coefficient with IF to distance in Euclidean space, which is equivalent to the function of a zoom lens. It enlarges ($\beta \geq 0$) or shortens ($\beta < 0$) all distances, but an enlarged or shortened yardstick is different. For long distances, the enlarged or shortened yardstick is slightly bigger, and for short distances the enlarged or shortened yardstick is slightly smaller. It leads to polarization, in which long distances become much longer, and short distances become much shorter. Thus, an appropriate assignment of distance weighting coefficient with IF can improve the performance of FCM.

2.3.3. Multiple Kernel Learning. In general, the reliability of the traditional clustering algorithms strictly depends on the feature difference of data. If the feature differences are large, it is easy to implement clustering. However, if the feature differences are small and even some features are crossed in the original space, it is difficult for traditional algorithms to cluster correctly. By using the traditional clustering methods and kernel technique, Wu et al. constructed the kernel clustering algorithm [20]. Kernel-based fuzzy clustering can map the data in the original space to a high-dimensional feature space in which it can produce a remarkable improvement over standard FCM. Then, Sonnenburg et al. put forward the concept of multicore learning [21].

The proposed MKDSIF-FCM algorithm incorporates the advantage of multiple kernel learning. Usually, multiple kernel methods consist of polynomial kernel, Gaussian kernel, and hyperbolic tangent kernel. According to different properties of samples, we can choose different parameters of different kernel functions to extend applicability of single kernel function, and we can choose different kernel functions to make the global kernel function and local complementary kernel function, further improving the categorization of different samples. Ultimately, good clustering effect is achieved, and generalization performance of the kernel is improved.

The form of Gaussian kernel function is as follows:

$$K(m,n) = \exp\left(-\frac{\|m-n\|^2}{2\sigma^2}\right) \qquad (6)$$

where n is the center of kernel function and σ is the width parameter and controls the radial range of the function.

The form of polynomial kernel function is as follows:

$$K(m,n) = (m \cdot n + c)^d, \quad c \geq 0, \ d \in N \qquad (7)$$

The form of hyperbolic tangent kernel function is as follows:

$$K(m,n) = \tanh(-b \cdot (m \cdot n) - c) \qquad (8)$$

Any function which satisfies the mercer condition [22] can be regarded as a kind of kernel function. The combination of k kernel functions according to different weight coefficients is still a kernel function, denoted as the following:

$$K^*(m,n) = \sum_{k=1}^{K} \beta_k K_k(m,n) \qquad \beta_k \geq 0, \ k = 1, 2, \cdots, K \qquad (9)$$

Under the constraint,

$$\sum_{k=1}^{K} \beta_k = 1 \qquad \beta_k \geq 0, \ k = 1, 2, \cdots, K \qquad (10)$$

By constraining to the Euclidean distance, the squared distance is computed in the kernel space using multiple kernel functions such that

$$\begin{aligned} d_{ki} &= \|\Phi(x_k) - \Phi(v_i)\|^2 \\ &= K^*(x_k, x_k) + K^*(v_i, v_i) - 2K^*(x_k, v_i) \end{aligned} \qquad (11)$$

If we select the Gaussian kernel which is used almost exclusively in the literature, then $k(x,x) = 1$ and

$$d_{ki} = \|\Phi(x_k) - \Phi(v_i)\|^2 = 2 - 2K^*(x_k, v_i) \qquad (12)$$

In this way, the objective function J_S will become the following:

$$J_S(U,V) = \sum_{i=1}^{c}\sum_{k=1}^{n} (u_{ik})^S \|\Phi(x_k) - \Phi(v_i)\|^2 \qquad (13)$$

where $\Phi(.)$ is the nonlinear map kernel function and $\Phi(x_k)$ and $\Phi(v_i)$ express sample x_k and clustering center v_i in feature space, respectively.

Minimizing (13), we then can obtain the update expressions of membership function u_{ik} and center of cluster v_i as follows:

$$u_{ik} = \frac{\left(1 - K^*(x_k, v_i)\right)^{-1/(s-1)}}{\sum_{j=1}^{c}\left(1 - K^*(x_k, v_j)\right)^{-1/(s-1)}} \qquad (14)$$

$$v_i = \frac{\sum_{k=1}^{n} u_{ik}^s K^*(x_k, v_i) x_k}{\sum_{k=1}^{n} u_{ik}^s K^*(x_k, v_i)} \qquad (15)$$

2.3.4. The Proposed MKDSIF-FCM Algorithm. Assume $X = \{x_1, x_2, \ldots, x_n\}$ is a set of m-dimensional samples, where $x_k = \{x_{k1}, x_{k2}, \ldots, x_{km}\}$ represents the kth sample for k=1,2,..,n and an integer $c(2 \leq c \leq n)$ is the number of clusters. The ith cluster is supposed to have the center vector $v_i = \{v_{i1}, v_{i2}, \ldots, v_{im}\}$ $(1 \leq i \leq c)$.

$U \in R_{c \times n}$ is an $c \times n$ matrix of fuzzy partition for given training data x_k=$\{x_{k1}, x_{k2}, \ldots, x_{km}\}$ (k=1,2,...,n), where $u_{ik} \in U$ is a membership function value from k^{th} vector x_k to i^{th} cluster center v_i and u_{ik} satisfies the following conditions:

$$\sum_{i=1}^{c} u_{ik} = 1, \quad \forall k \qquad (16)$$

$$0 < \sum_{k=1}^{n} u_{ik} < n, \quad \forall i \qquad (17)$$

$$0 \leq u_{ik} \leq 1, \quad \forall k, i \qquad (18)$$

The MKDSIF-FCM algorithm aims to determine cluster centers v_i ($i=1, 2, \ldots, c$) and the fuzzy partition matrix U by minimizing the objective function J_S defined as follows:

$$J_s(U, V) = \sum_{i=1}^{c} \sum_{k=1}^{n} (u_{ik})^s \left\| \left(\frac{1}{w_{ik}} \right)^\beta \right.$$

$$\left. \cdot \left(K^*(x_k, x_k) + K^*(v_i, v_i) - 2K^*(x_k, v_i) \right) \right\|^2 \tag{19}$$

where parameter s($1<s<\infty$) influences the fuzziness of the clusters. Large s will increase the fuzziness of the function. For most data, $1.5 \leq s \leq 3.0$ gives good results. The value of s is often set to 2. Moreover, d_{ki} is the Euclidean distance of the kernel space from sample x_k to cluster center v_i defined as (11).

The MKDSIF-FCM algorithm uses iterative optimization to approximate minima of an objective function J_S. In minimizing J_S, the basic step of MKDSIF-FCM algorithm is performed in the following procedures.

Step 1. Given a value of parameters c and commonly in the literature, we let $s=2$.

Step 2. Initialize the matrix U of fuzzy partition by generating $c \times n$ random numbers in the interval $[0, 1]$.

Step 3. For $t=0, 1, 2, \ldots$, adopt FCM algorithm to calculate cluster centers v_i ($i=1, 2, \ldots, c$) by using U as follows:

$$v_i = \frac{\sum_{k=1}^{n} (u_{ik})^S x_k}{\sum_{k=1}^{n} (u_{ik})^S} \tag{20}$$

Step 4. According to (2), (3), and (4), we can obtain w_{ik}.

Step 5. U and V are updated by minimizing objective function J_S. We can derive the calculating formula of u_{ik} and v_i as (14) and (15), respectively.

Step 6. Compute the objective function J_S by using (19); stop the MKDSIF-FCM process if the following condition holds:

$$|J_S(t+1) - J_S(t)| < \varepsilon \tag{21}$$

where it converges or the difference between two adjacent computed values of objective functions J_S is less than the given threshold ε.

Otherwise, go to Step 4.

The input of MKDSIF-FCM algorithm is a set of samples $X=\{x_1, x_2, \ldots, x_n\}$, and the number of clusters is required to be predefined. Further, two parameters (s and ε) need to be given in advance. The output of MKDSIF-FCM algorithm are the cluster centers v_i ($i=1, 2, \ldots, c$) and the fuzzy partition matrix U.

3. Results

We use a 3.40 GHZ Core(TM) I7-3770 CPU 4GB RAM desktop computer and MATLAB 2015a software in conducting all

TABLE 2: Comparative analysis of the proposed MKDSIF-FCM and original FCM algorithms on the skull dataset.

Result	FCM	MKDSIF-FCM
	$s=2$	$s=2$ $\beta=0.5$ $p_1=0.9$ $p_2=0.1$ $\sigma_1=30$ $\sigma_2=110$
TPR [%]	28.00	98.00
TNR [%]	100.0	93.02
ACC [%]	61.29	95.70
T[s]	0.0074	0.1281
Iterations	17	102

experiments. For all algorithms presented in this paper, the experiments were repeated 50 times, and the average results were obtained for comparison.

In MKDSIF-FCM algorithm, there is a parameter group $X = \{s, p_1, p_2, \sigma_1, \sigma_2, \beta\}$, where s represents the fuzziness index, p_1 and p_2 represent the probability, σ_1 and σ_2 represent the parameters of the Gaussian kernel function, and β represents the IF.

For all supervised classification methods presented in this paper, the skull dataset is split into a training set and testing set; 60 samples were randomly picked as the testing set and the numbers of positive and negative examples are kept the same in each sampling.

3.1. The Results of Sex Determination for 3D Skulls. The metrics used for evaluating the performance of the algorithm on the skull dataset are described below:

ACC: it is the number of skulls that are correctly classified as male or female skulls.

TPR: it is the proportion of the male skulls that are correctly identified.

TNR: it is the proportion of the female skulls that are correctly identified.

T: it represents running time.

From Table 2, it can be seen that when selecting a group of suitable parameter values ($s=2$, $\beta=0.5$, $p_1=0.9$, $p_2=0.1$, $\sigma_1=30$, and $\sigma_2=110$), the MKDSIF-FCM algorithm can obtain the best classification accuracy of sex determination of the skull. For 186 skulls of the Han Chinese ethnic group, we obtain the accuracy of 95.70% compared to 87.09%, 92.2%, and 93.55% found in the literature [15–17], respectively. There is a classification accuracy of 93.02% for males and 98% for females, respectively.

3.2. Comparison with Other Unsupervised Methods. It is clear from Table 2 that the accuracy had a significant and sharp improvement of nearly 34% for the MKDSIF-FCM algorithm over the original FCM algorithm for the skull dataset. The running time for MKDSIF-FCM is greater than that for FCM, because the number of iterations to convergence is greater.

It is also clear from Table 3 that the MKDSIF-FCM algorithm achieved better classification performance on the Iris dataset. There is an improvement of nearly 6% for MKDSIF-FCM over the original FCM algorithm with detecting a group

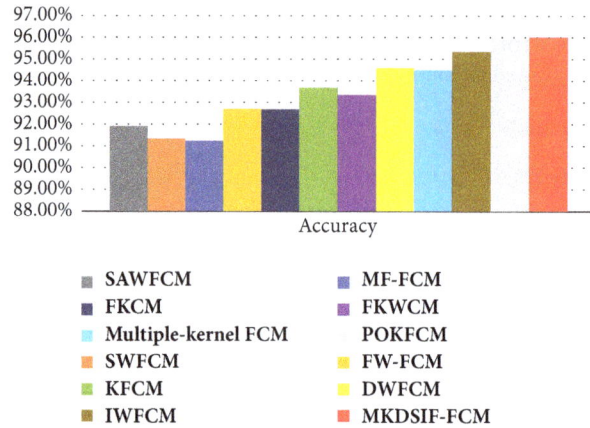

FIGURE 3: Accuracy analysis of the proposed MKDSIF-FCM and existing improved FCM algorithms on the Iris dataset.

TABLE 3: Comparative analysis of the proposed MKDSIF-FCM and original FCM algorithms on the Iris dataset.

Result	FCM	MKDSIF-FCM
	s=2	s=2 β=0.5 p_1=0.7 p_2=0.3 σ_1=3 σ_2=0.5
Accuracy [%]	89.33	96.00
T [s]	0.0042	0.0145
Iterations	16	11

of suitable parameters. The proposed algorithm appears to have the quite similar time complexity and iterations as the original FCM algorithm.

As shown in Figure 3, it is easily observed that the accuracy of MKDSIF-FCM algorithm is higher than that of SAWFCM [23], SWFCM [24], MF-FCM [25], FW-FCM [26], FKCM [27], KFCM [28], FKWCM [29], DWFCM [30], multiple kernel FCM [31], and IWFCM [32]. The accuracy of the MKDSIF-FCM algorithm is quite similar to that of POKFCM [33].

3.3. Comparison with Popular Supervised Classification Methods. Table 4 unfolds a clear comparison between the proposed MKDSIF-FCM algorithm and the other six supervised classification methods in three aspects, ACC, TPR, and TNR. All the results we have obtained are as follows (in order of increasing ACC): decision tree (80.47%), BP neural network (83%), H-ELM (88.2%), logistic regression (88.73), SVM (92.8%), FDA (92.87%), and MKDSIF-FCM (95.70%). It is obvious that the proposed MKDSIF-FCM algorithm obtained not only the highest classification accuracy of 95.7% but also the highest TPR and TNR of 93.02% and 98%, respectively. Both FDA (with the best feature) and SVM did a good job with higher accuracy. The classification accuracies of other methods are no more than 90%. The results reveal several similarities between TPR and TNR. And we can observe that the correct classification rate of females is uniformly higher than that of males.

3.4. Stability Analysis of the MKDSIF-FCM Algorithm. The experimental procedure is repeated 50 times for each

classification method; the maximum, minimum, and mean of the accuracy are represented via error-bar plots (Figure 4). The proposed MKDSIF-FCM algorithm presents an extremely stable performance on the skull dataset, and the classification accuracy of other methods fluctuates greatly. The difference between maximum and minimum accuracy ranged from 37% using BP neural network to 17% for SVM.

4. Discussion

FCM [19] is one of the best-known unsupervised algorithms. However, its performance has been limited to Euclidean distance. In recent years, various kinds of improved FCM algorithms have been reported [23–33]. This paper proposes an improved FCM algorithm to determine the sex of adult skulls from the Han Chinese ethnic group. In order to verify the effectiveness and generality of the proposed algorithm, we performed a comparative analysis among the original FCM, some improved FCM algorithms, and the proposed MKDSIF-FCM algorithm.

The MKDSIF-FCM algorithm achieved better classification performance on both publicly available Iris dataset and skull dataset. Especially in the skull database, the accuracy has been greatly improved. On the Iris dataset, our MKDSIF-FCM algorithm has little change in time complexity and iterations compared with FCM. On the skull dataset, the number of iterations of the MKDSIF-FCM algorithm is much larger than that of FCM. This finding implies that the proposed algorithm can tend to become very computationally demanding when the data has high dimensionality and large volume. Experimental results on the Iris datasets show that, for accuracy, our algorithm is almost better than all algorithms in the literature [23–33].

Our innovative algorithm introduces distance-weights with IF into the commonly used Euclidean distance and increases the difference degree of category between samples. The proposed algorithm incorporates the idea of multiple kernel learning that maps the data into a higher-dimensional space in which the nonlinearity fades away and the data become linearly separable. It is the reason that the proposed

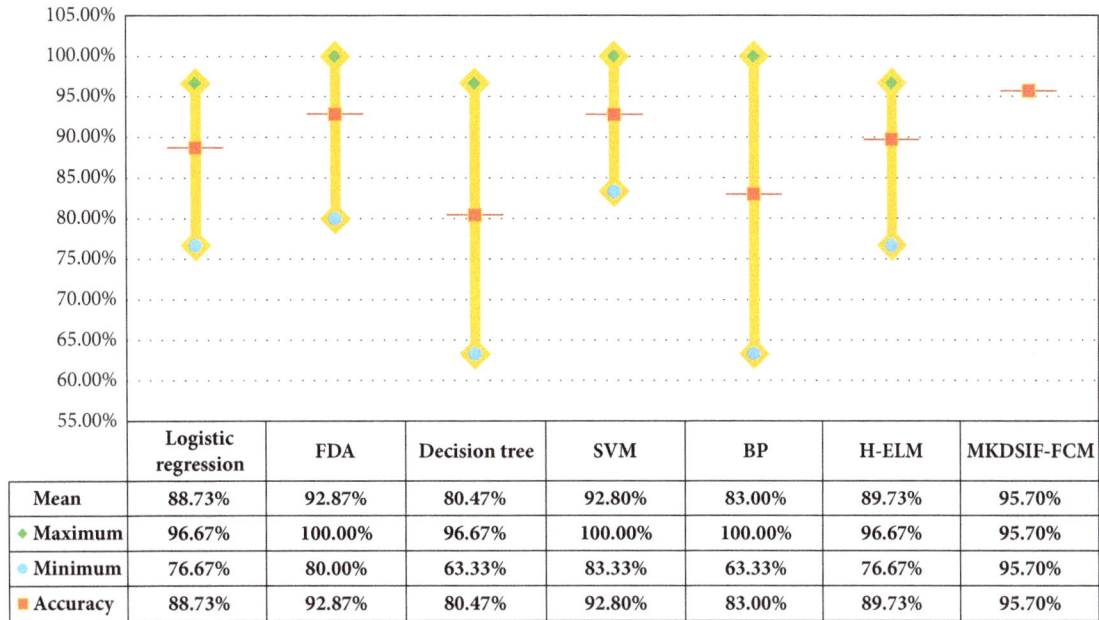

	Logistic regression	FDA	Decision tree	SVM	BP	H-ELM	MKDSIF-FCM
Mean	88.73%	92.87%	80.47%	92.80%	83.00%	89.73%	95.70%
◆ Maximum	96.67%	100.00%	96.67%	100.00%	100.00%	96.67%	95.70%
● Minimum	76.67%	80.00%	63.33%	83.33%	63.33%	76.67%	95.70%
■ Accuracy	88.73%	92.87%	80.47%	92.80%	83.00%	89.73%	95.70%

FIGURE 4: Comparative analysis of stability for the proposed MKDSIF-FCM and other classification methods on the skull dataset.

TABLE 4: Comparative analysis of the proposed MKDSIF-FCM and other popular classification methods on the skull dataset.

Classifier	TPR [%]	TNR [%]	ACC [%]
Decision tree	78.82	82.10	80.47
BP neural network	80.93	85.07	83.00
H-ELM [18]	88.27	88.13	88.20
Logistic regression	84.93	92.53	88.73
SVM	91.60	94.00	92.80
FDA	90.93	94.80	92.87
MKDSIF-FCM (proposed)	93.02	98.00	95.70

MKDSIF-FCM algorithm can improve the performance of clustering.

So far, to our knowledge, supervised learning remains the most widely employed method in sex determination of a skull. In particular, logistic regression and discriminant function analysis are the two most representative statistical learning methods. According to the method used in literature [17], we established the best model using logistic regression and stepwise variable selection. When selecting nine variables (I8, I11, I14, I16, I20, I29, I31, I38, I40), the model obtains 84.93% and 92.53% classification rates for males and females, respectively. In the same way, we select the best feature subset from skull measurements to establish the FDA model. With ten variables (I8, I11, I14, I16, I20, I23, I29, I31, I38, I40), the classification rates for males and females are 90.93% and 94.80%, respectively. In order to choose the most suitable classifier for the skull dataset, we also compared the results using other popular supervised classification methods, including decision tree, SVM, BP neural networks, and H-ELM [18]. In all the methods we attempted, the proposed MKDSIF-FCM algorithm gives the best classification performance for both male and female skulls.

When classifying the skull dataset, we hope that the results can be reproduced. Thus, it is very important that the classification algorithm is stable. In the 50 repeated experiments, our algorithm obtained the same result. It is obvious that the proposed MKDSIF-FCM algorithm presents extremely stable performance on the skull dataset.

In conclusion, by means of its fairly high accuracy, extremely good stability, and the advantage of unsupervised learning, we have the reason to believe that the MKDSIF-FCM algorithm is the most suitable classifier for our skull dataset. Of course, our experimental results also indicate that skull characteristics we extracted were very accurate and effective in sex determination of the skull.

5. Conclusions

In this paper, we propose a novel approach to sex determination of skulls of the Han Chinese ethnic group. The first step in our method is extraction of morphological features from the 3D skull. In the second step, the MKDSIF-FCM algorithm is employed to conduct sex determination of the skull of the Han Chinese ethnic group. A comparison with other popular classifiers, such as decision tree, BP neural network, logistic regression, FDA, SVM, and H-ELM [18], showed that our proposed MKDSIF-FCM algorithm worked better. The experimental results suggest that the use of the proposed MKDSIF-FCM algorithm in the classification of the skull dataset is an accurate, robust, and reproducible technique. For the Han Chinese ethnic group, there is an accuracy improvement of nearly 8.6%, 3.5%, and 2.2% for our sex determination approach over other methods in the literature [15–17].

It is worth noting that the proposed method achieves a better and stable performance for skull sex determination while maintaining its advantages of unsupervised learning. We believe that the methods described here are noteworthy, particularly for researchers who are attempting (or are considering attempting) to engage in skull sex determination by means of unsupervised learning methods.

Conflicts of Interest

The authors declare that they have no conflicts of interest regarding the publication of this paper.

Acknowledgments

This research was supported by the National Natural Science Foundation of China (nos. 61673319, 61731015, and 61602380), Institutions of Higher Learning Scientific Research Foundation in the Ningxia Hui Autonomous Region of China (no. NGY2016216), and Natural Science Fundamental Research Funds for Shaanxi Province of China (no. 2014JQ8315).

References

[1] M. R. Dayal and M. A. Bidmos, "Discriminating sex in South African blacks using patella dimensions," *Journal of Forensic Sciences*, vol. 50, no. 6, pp. 1294–1297, 2005.

[2] C. Papaloucas, A. Fiska, and T. Demetriou, "Sexual dimorphism of the hip joint in Greeks," *Forensic Science International*, vol. 179, no. 1, pp. 83–e1, 2008.

[3] S. J. Decker, S. L. Davy-Jow, J. M. Ford, and D. R. Hilbelink, "Virtual determination of sex: metric and nonmetric traits of the adult pelvis from 3d computed tomography models," *Journal of Forensic Sciences*, vol. 56, no. 5, pp. 1107–1114, 2011.

[4] T. R. Peckmann, K. Orr, S. Meek, and S. K. Manolis, "Sex determination from the calcaneus in a 20th century Greek population using discriminant function analysis," *Science & Justice*, vol. 55, no. 6, pp. 377–382, 2015.

[5] A. L. M Didi, R. R. Azman, and M. Nazri, "Sex determination from carpal bone volumes: A Multi Detector Computed Tomography (MDCT) study in a Malaysian population," *Legal Medicine*, vol. 20, pp. 49–52, 2016.

[6] M. Yoshino, H. Matsuda, S. Kubota, K. Imaizumi, S. Miyasaka, and S. Seta, "Computer-assisted skull identification system using video superimposition," *Forensic Science International*, vol. 90, no. 3, pp. 231–244, 1997.

[7] P. L. Walker, "Sexing skulls using discriminant function analysis of visually assessed traits," *American Journal of Physical Anthropology*, vol. 136, no. 1, pp. 39–50, 2008.

[8] M. S. Robinson and M. A. Bidmos, "The skull and humerus in the determination of sex: Reliability of discriminant function equations," *Forensic Science International*, vol. 186, no. 1-3, pp. 86–e5, 2009.

[9] Y. Ogawa, K. Imaizumi, S. Miyasaka, and M. Yoshino, "Discriminant functions for sex estimation of modern Japanese skulls," *Journal of Forensic and Legal Medicine*, vol. 20, no. 4, pp. 234–238, 2013.

[10] D. Franklin, A. Cardini, A. Flavel, and A. Kuliukas, "Erratum to 'Estimation of sex from cranial measurements in a Western Australian population' [Forensic Sci. Int. 229 (2013) 158.e1-158.e8]," *Forensic Science International*, vol. 232, no. 1-3, p. 153, 2013.

[11] E. E. Abdel Fatah, N. R. Shirley, R. L. Jantz, and M. R. Mahfouz, "Improving sex estimation from crania using a novel three-dimensional quantitative method," *Journal of Forensic Sciences*, vol. 59, no. 3, pp. 590–600, 2014.

[12] B. Musilová, J. Dupej, J. Velemínská, K. Chaumoitre, and J. Bruzek, "Exocranial surfaces for sex assessment of the human cranium," *Forensic Science International*, vol. 269, pp. 70–77, 2016.

[13] C. Li, "A study on sex difference of adult skull of the northeast china by fourier transform," *Acta Anthropologica Sinica*, 1992.

[14] M. Li, Y. Fan, Y. Yu, P. Xia, H. Li, and G. Dai, "Sex assessment of adult from southwest area of China by bones of facial cranium," *Chinese Journal of Forensic Medicine*, vol. 27, no. 2, pp. 132–134, 2012.

[15] W. Shui, R. Yin, M. Zhou, and Y. Ji, "Sex determination from digital skull model for the Han people in China," *Chinese Journal of Forensic Medicine*, vol. 28, no. 6, pp. 461–468, 2013.

[16] L. Luo, M. Wang, and Y. Tian, "Automatic sex determination of skulls based on a statistical shape model," in *Computational & Mathematical Methods in Medicine*, vol. 2013, 1 edition, 2013.

[17] X. Liu, L. Zhu et al., "Sex determination of incomplete skull of han ethnic in China," in *nternational Conference on Intelligent Computing*, pp. 574–585, Springer, 2017.

[18] J. Tang, C. Deng, and G. B. Huang, "Extreme learning machine for multilayer perceptron," *IEEE Transactions on Neural Networks & Learning Systems*, vol. 27, no. 4, pp. 809–821, 2016.

[19] J. C. Bezdek, R. Ehrlich, and W. Full, "FCM: the fuzzy c-means clustering algorithm," *Computers & Geosciences*, vol. 10, no. 2-3, pp. 191–203, 1984.

[20] Z. Wu, W. Xie, and J. Yu, "Fuzzy C-Means Clustering Algorithm Based on Kernel Method," in *Proceedings of the International Conference on Computational Intelligence and Multimedia Applications*, 54, 49 pages, 2003.

[21] S. Sonnenburg, G. Rätsch, C. Schäfer, and B. Schölkopf, "Large scale multiple kernel learning," *Journal of Machine Learning Research*, vol. 7, pp. 1531–1565, 2006.

[22] C. J. C. Burges, "A tutorial on support vector machines for pattern recognition," *Data Mining & Knowledge Discovery*, vol. 2, no. 2, pp. 121–167, 1998.

[23] Ren L.-n., Y.-b. Qin, and D.-y. Xu, "Fuzzy C-means clustering based on self-adaptive weight," *Application Research of Computers*, vol. 29, no. 8, pp. 2849–2851, 2012.

[24] M. Qi and H.-x. Zhang, "Research on modified fuzzy C -means clustering algorithm," *Computer Engineering and Applications*, vol. 45, no. 20, pp. 133–135, 2009.

[25] J. Cai and F. Xie, "New fuzzy clustering algorithm based on feature weighted mahalanobis distances," *Computer Engineering & Applications*, 2012.

[26] Y. Yue, D. Zeng, and L. Hong, "Improving fuzzy C-means clustering by a novel feature-weight learning," *Computational Intelligence and Industrial Application*, pp. 173–177, 2008.

[27] Z.-D. Wu, X.-B. Gao, and W.-X. Xie, "Study of a new fuzzy clustering algorithm based on the kernel method," *Xi'an Dianzi Keji Daxue Xuebao/Journal of Xidian University*, vol. 31, no. 4, pp. 533–537, 2004.

[28] A. Yang, L. Jiang, and Y. Zhou, "A KFCM-based fuzzy classifier," in *Proceedings of the 4th International Conference on Fuzzy Systems and Knowledge Discovery, FSKD 2007*, pp. 80–84, August 2007.

[29] C. Zhao and B. Qi, "Hyperspectral image classification based on fuzzy kernel weighted C-means clustering," *Yi Qi Yi Biao Xue Bao/Chinese Journal of Scientific Instrument*, vol. 33, no. 9, pp. 2016–2021, 2012.

[30] F. X. Wang, Y. Cheng, and Q. X. Qin, "Improved Density Weighted Fuzzy C Means Algorithm," *Computer Systems & Applications*, 2012.

[31] F. L. Zhao, I. L. Xin, and W. Dong, *Clustering Algorithm Based on Multiple Kernel SVM*, vol. 5, Periodical of Ocean University of China, 2009.

[32] Q. Liu, X. S. Xia, Y. Zhou et al., "Fuzzy clustering algorithm using two weighting methods," *Application Research of Computers*, vol. 28, no. 12, pp. 4437–4439, 2011.

[33] Y. Liu, F. Liu, T. Hou et al., "Kernel-based fuzzy C-means clustering method based on parameter optimization," *Jilin Daxue Xuebao*, vol. 46, no. 1, pp. 246–251, 2016.

6

DINOSARC: Color Features based on Selective Aggregation of Chromatic Image Components for Wireless Capsule Endoscopy

Michael D. Vasilakakis,[1] **Dimitris K. Iakovidis** [iD],[1] **Evaggelos Spyrou** [iD],[1,2] **and Anastasios Koulaouzidis** [iD][3]

[1]*Department of Computer Science and Biomedical Informatics, University of Thessaly, Lamia, Greece*
[2]*Institute of Informatics and Telecommunications, National Center for Scientific Research "Demokritos", Athens, Greece*
[3]*Endoscopy Unit, The Royal Infirmary of Edinburgh, Edinburgh, UK*

Correspondence should be addressed to Dimitris K. Iakovidis; dimitris.iakovidis@ieee.org

Academic Editor: Chuangyin Dang

Wireless Capsule Endoscopy (WCE) is a noninvasive diagnostic technique enabling the inspection of the whole gastrointestinal (GI) tract by capturing and wirelessly transmitting thousands of color images. Proprietary software "stitches" the images into videos for examination by accredited readers. However, the videos produced are of large length and consequently the reading task becomes harder and more prone to human errors. Automating the WCE reading process could contribute in both the reduction of the examination time and the improvement of its diagnostic accuracy. In this paper, we present a novel feature extraction methodology for automated WCE image analysis. It aims at discriminating various kinds of abnormalities from the normal contents of WCE images, in a machine learning-based classification framework. The extraction of the proposed features involves an unsupervised color-based saliency detection scheme which, unlike current approaches, combines both point and region-level saliency information and the estimation of local and global image color descriptors. The salient point detection process involves estimation of DIstaNces On Selective Aggregation of chRomatic image Components (DINOSARC). The descriptors are extracted from superpixels by coevaluating both point and region-level information. The main conclusions of the experiments performed on a publicly available dataset of WCE images are (a) the proposed salient point detection scheme results in significantly less and more relevant salient points; (b) the proposed descriptors are more discriminative than relevant state-of-the-art descriptors, promising a wider adoption of the proposed approach for computer-aided diagnosis in WCE.

1. Introduction

Wireless Capsule Endoscopy (WCE) has now been established as a first-line diagnostic tool for small bowel diseases [1]. It makes use of a capsule endoscope (CE) which is a miniaturized, swallowable device, equipped with a miniaturized color video camera. Current CEs travel along the whole gastrointestinal tract (GI) by exploiting both gravity and its peristaltic movements. CEs are also equipped with a light source and transmit the captured images to an external recording device. Typically, a commercially available CE is able to capture approximately 100 K images during its journey allowing therefore collection of rich information

about the GI tract in a minimally invasive manner. Since this amount of visual content is substantial, WCE video reading is a time-consuming process, prone to human errors, and it has been shown that detection rate of lesions is approximately 40% [2]. To overcome this, many research efforts have turned towards fully automatic analysis of WCE videos [3] and have been successfully applied on the problem of diagnosis of GI lesions, aiming to recognize several kinds of abnormalities, such as ulcers, polyps, and bleeding.

The majority of research works in WCE and in the broader field of endoscopic image analysis focuses on the interpretation of their visual content by either classifying them to normal/abnormal or further characterizing the abnormal ones according to the pathology of the depicted abnormality [4]. Image classification methodologies proposed in the context of automatic WCE image analysis include mainly supervised approaches addressing the detection of only a single or a few kinds of abnormalities [5], for example, polyps, ulcer, and bleeding, whereas fewer have addressed the detection of various kinds of abnormalities [6–8].

Many WCE image analysis approaches begin by detecting salient points to possible regions of abnormalities. Iakovidis and Koulaouzidis [6] proposed the use of the Speeded Up Robust Features (SURF) [9] algorithm on the chromatic component a of CIE-Lab to detect such salient points. From each salient point, color descriptors were extracted to characterize it along with its local neighborhood. These include the CIE-Lab values of the salient point and the minimum and maximum values of a square window centered at this point. This approach was very effective in the detection of a total of 9 different kinds of abnormalities. The success of this method was attributed in the physical meaning of these features which encodes more robustly the differences between normal and abnormal tissues.

Most of the current WCE image analysis methods aim to detect bleeding. In this context, the method proposed in [9] was applied for the detection of salient superpixels corresponding to bleeding regions. Following a Correlation-based Feature Selection (CFS), best discrimination of the superpixels containing blood was achieved using a three-dimensional vector of central moments estimated from a and saturation. In a later study [10], another bleeding detection method was based on saliency maps generated by fusing color component a of the CIE-Lab color space, component M of the $CMYK$ color space, and the similarity to the red color values, that is, if a pixel has a greater R value and smaller G and B values, it would seem reddish and should be assigned higher saliency value. Other saliency detection methods exploiting saliency at a regional level for bleeding detection include the works of Fu et al. [11] and Shi et al. [12].

Fewer methods have been proposed for the detection of other kinds of abnormalities. Most challenging ones are those addressing polypoid lesion detection. Polypoid lesions are visible tissue masses protruding from the mucosal surface. They are characterized according to their color, appearance of their mucosal surface, presence of ulceration (s), their bleeding tendency, and the presence of pedunculus. In the context of polypoid lesions detection, most previous studies have been performed on images of flexible (conventional) endoscopy [13]. In a relevant study, Bernal et al. [14] proposed the Window Median Depth of Valleys Accumulation (WM-DOVA) energy maps, which were related with the likelihood of polyp presence and used them for polyp detection. Li and Meng [15] proposed a tumor detection system for WCE images, which exploited textural features based on Uniform Local Binary Pattern (ULBP) and wavelet transform. Recently, Yuan et al. [16] proposed a polyp detection approach for WCE. It was based on the Scale Invariant Feature Transform (SIFT) algorithm for the detection of salient points and the extraction of features using the SIFT descriptor and Complete Local Binary Pattern (CLBP). Several other relevant applications have been proposed for other kinds of abnormalities. For example, in [17] our earlier approach [6] was applied for weakly-supervised inflammatory lesion detection. The machine-learning approach used is called weakly-supervised because the images used for the training of the classifier need not be annotated in detail (pixel-by-pixel); instead, only keywords semantically describing their content are sufficient. In that study, weak supervision was achieved by the Bag of Visual Words (BoVW) model [18]. This model enables the representation of entire WCE images using histograms of visual words.

In this paper, we consider the saliency of a WCE image as the main component that can improve the discrimination of abnormal from normal WCE images, and we propose a novel feature extraction methodology that extends our previous approaches [6, 7, 19] for the detection of various kinds of abnormalities in WCE images. This methodology includes an unsupervised salient point and region detection algorithm and the estimation of local and global image descriptors enabling the characterization of various abnormalities both at a regional and at an image level. It consists of several novel components, including a color-based salient point detector, a salient region detector defining salient superpixels, and a method to derive a vectorial representation of the color of the salient superpixels by taking into account both point and region-level information. This enables more accurate localization and characterization of even very small abnormalities. Besides the local image descriptors derived, global image descriptors are derived for weakly-supervised abnormality detection based on a BoVW model.

The rest of this paper is organized in four sections. In Section 2, we describe the materials of this study, and in Section 3, we present the methodology proposed in this study. In Section 4, we evaluate the proposed methodology in comparison to relevant state-of-the-art approaches and discuss the obtained results. In the last section, we summarize the conclusions that can be derived from this study.

2. Materials

The research performed in this study was based on a rich and diverse collection of WCE images that include a variety of abnormalities and normal images from various parts of the GI tract. We provide this collection through an online database, called KID [20]. KID is composed of thousands of WCE images obtained from the whole GI tract using a MiroCam capsule endoscope with a resolution of 360×360 pixels. Abnormalities depicted within this dataset include 303 vascular (small bowel angiectasias and blood in the lumen), 44 polypoid (lymphoid nodular hyperplasia, lymphoma, Peutz–Jeghers polyps) and 227 inflammatory (ulcers, aphthae, mucosal breaks with surrounding erythema, cobblestone mucosa, luminal stenoses and/or fibrotic strictures, and mucosal/villous oedema) lesion images and 1,778 normal images obtained from the esophagus, the stomach, the small bowel, and the colon.

3. DINOSARC Feature Extraction

The proposed feature extraction methodology involves the detection of salient points based on image color, and these points are subsequently used for the definition of salient regions based on superpixel segmentation. From each detected salient point and region, a feature vector is calculated to describe the local color properties of the image that differentiate the abnormal from the normal tissues.

3.1. Salient Point Detection.

A novel algorithm is proposed for the detection of salient points, specifically in WCE images. Unlike previous approaches, saliency is defined with respect to *color differences*. The proposed approach is based on the observation that within WCE images, the appearance of abnormalities may be described within a relatively small color range that is usually located on the margins of the overall color range of an image. In many cases, this range is nonoverlapping with the color range of the normal image content. By examining each WCE image separately, one may observe that the color ranges are different for each image, even for the same kind of abnormalities (Figure 1). Also, given a diverse set of WCE images, the color ranges of both the normal and abnormal content are completely overlapping. Therefore, it is not straightforward to specify a standard color range discriminating the abnormalities from normal content.

The rationale of the proposed saliency detection algorithm can be explained by the respective color histograms of WCE images. We consider that WCE images are represented in the CIE-*Lab* color space, which describes color with approximately decorrelated components [6]. The components of this space represent lightness (L), the quantity of red ($a > 0$) or the quantity of green ($-a > 0$), and the quantity of yellow ($b > 0$) or the quantity of blue ($-b > 0$) of a pixel. This way, color can be examined separately from lightness, which in our case varies significantly depending on the distance and the angle of the endoscope from the tissue surface. Thus, by only using the chromatic components a and b, the color information can be isolated, and an approximately illumination-invariant description of the image content may be obtained.

Let H^A and H^N be the normalized histograms (probability distributions) of a WCE image for abnormal and normal regions, respectively. For the images of Figure 1, the respective histograms are illustrated in Figure 2. H^A is represented by a red line, and H^N is represented by a green line. We provide the histograms for the chromatic components, that is, a or b, of the images where a nonoverlapping range between the two histograms can be observed. For example, in Figure 2(a), a nonoverlapping region between H^A and H^N can be observed only in component a (in the chromatic region $a \in [-9, -1]$); the respective histograms of component b are omitted. Similarly, Figures 2(b)–2(d) present the nonoverlapping histograms of the images illustrated in Figures 1(b)–1(d). In Figure 3, the normalized histograms estimated over all images of KID dataset (Section 2) are provided, where a total overlap

between the abnormal and normal chromatic ranges can be observed.

We propose a novel algorithm named SARC (Algorithm 1), which performs a Selective Aggregation of chRomatic image Components after an automatic segmentation process. This is based on the observation that abnormal image regions are usually characterized by higher positive or negative values of the a and b chromatic components. SARC produces saliency maps which emphasize on the regions that correspond to possible abnormalities.

Let I_{Lab} be a $M \times N$-pixel CIE-*Lab* input image, and I_a and I_b be the grayscale images representing a and b components of I_{Lab}. This algorithm uses the histogram H_c of image I_c, $c = a$, b, to determine optimal thresholds maintaining the image regions that have a higher probability to include an abnormality. It calculates the first (r_c) and second derivatives (R_c) of the positive (+) and negative (−) axes of H_c and determines the maximum of each of the second derivatives as an optimal image threshold for maintaining as much as discriminating information about the possible abnormal regions within the chromatic components of the image as possible. This process determines the value of the chromatic component (a or b) where the rate of the first derivative changes. Considering that the chromatic ranges of the abnormal regions are located at the margins of the histograms, this value will be the most probable one for the abnormality. Figure 4 illustrates this concept. It can be noticed that the maximum of the second derivative corresponds approximately to the value of the chromatic component a with the maximum probability of the abnormality.

By applying the determined thresholds on the respective chromatic image components, four images are obtained. Indicative examples of such images for the cases of Figures 1(a) and 1(b) are illustrated in the first and in the second row of Figure 5, respectively. These images are subsequently filtered using a sliding window of $n \times n$ pixels, which aims to discard local nonmaxima. The final step of SARC algorithm is the aggregation of the four filtered images using the sum operator.

Algorithm 2 uses I_{SARC} to detect regions with significant changes in the chromatic components of CIE-Lab color space. Initially, I_{SARC} is sampled using concentric square windows of $s \times s$ and $s/2 \times s/2$ pixels, respectively, at each pixel of I_{SARC} with nonzero value. These pixels are more considered as points of more interest, since they have a maximum value within their neighborhood. From these points, we define as salient ones those that are characterized by a significant change in the chromatic values of their local neighborhood. This change is calculated by the distance between the maxima and the minima extracted from the concentric square windows. This definition of saliency is inspired by the fact that such chromatic changes are usual in the neighborhoods of most abnormalities.

3.2. Salient Region Detection.

The salient point detection process is followed by sampling image regions from their neighborhoods in order to estimate relevant descriptors. Instead of sampling square-shaped neighborhoods, as in

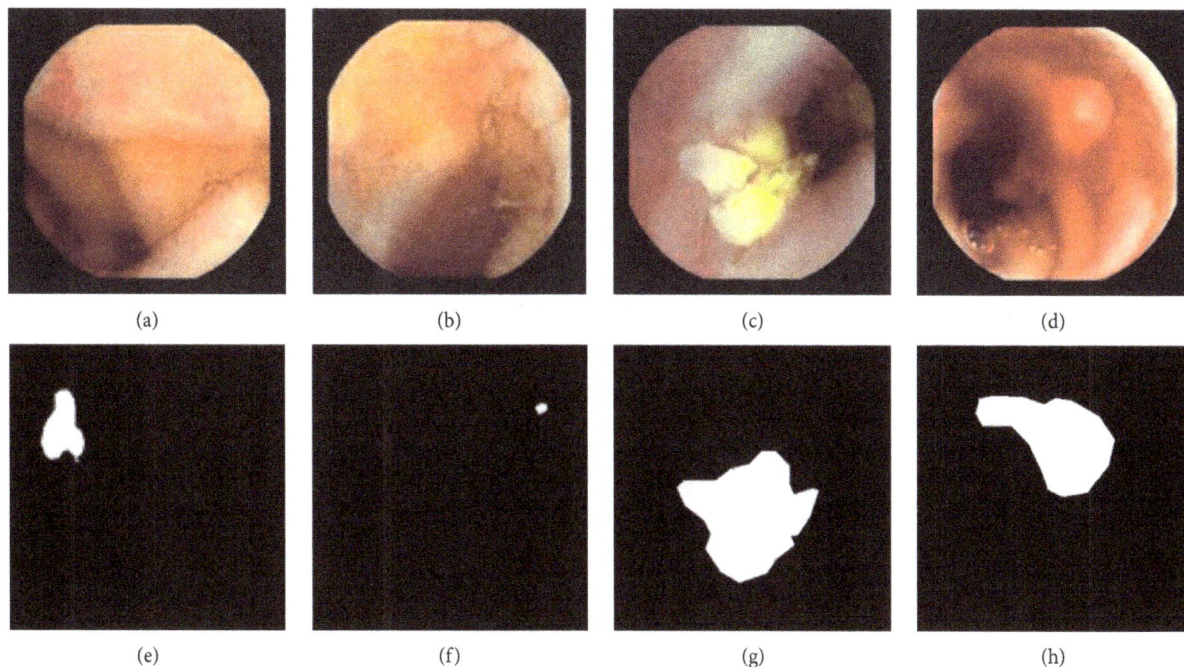

FIGURE 1: Representative images from KID dataset [20]. (a) Vascular lesion. (b) Small inflammatory lesion. (c) Large inflammatory lesion. (d) Polypoid lesion. (e–h) Detailed graphic annotations indicating the locations of the abnormalities within the respective WCE images (a–d).

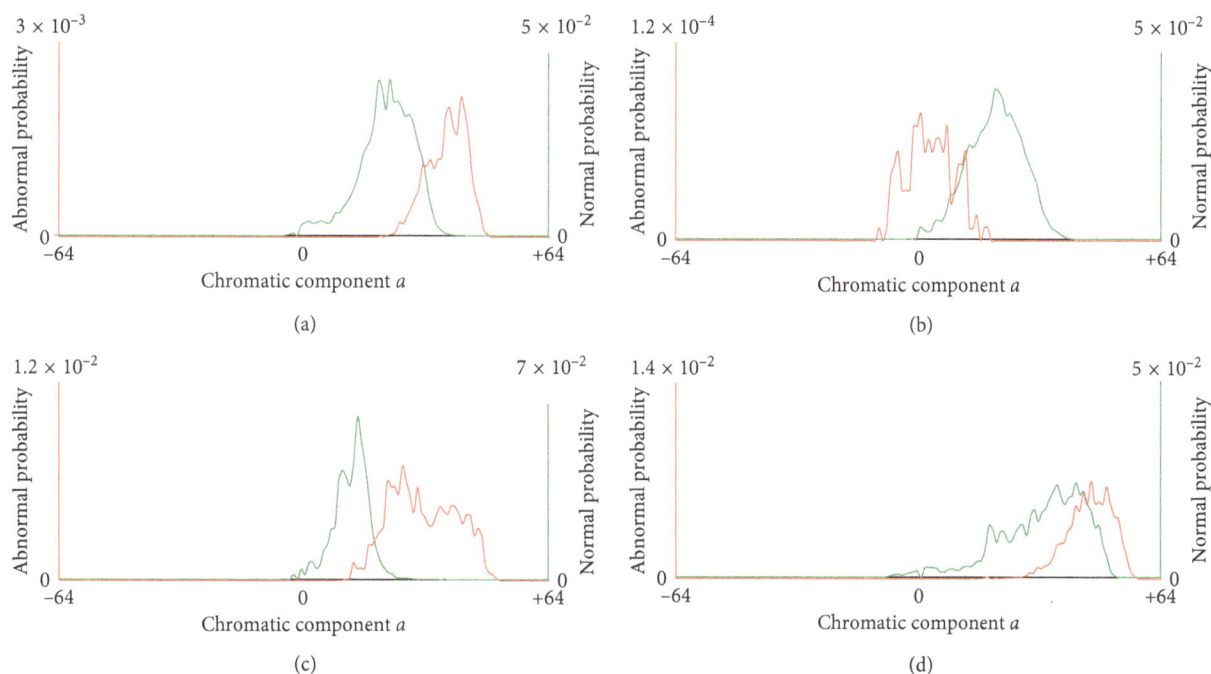

FIGURE 2: Normalized chromatic histograms of WCE images of Figure 1 (for chromatic components that have nonoverlapping regions). Histogram H^A which is estimated from abnormal image regions is represented with a solid red line, and H^N which is estimated from normal image regions is represented with a dashed green line. (a) Vascular lesion. (b) Small inflammatory lesion. (c) Large inflammatory lesion. (d) Polypoid lesion.

[5, 6], the DINOSARC descriptors are extracted from arbitrary-shaped neighborhoods. To this end, the input images are segmented using the simple iterative linear clustering (SLIC) algorithm [21]. SLIC creates clusters of pixels defining regions of homogeneous color properties, called superpixels (Figure 6). Considering the approach we

(a)

(b)

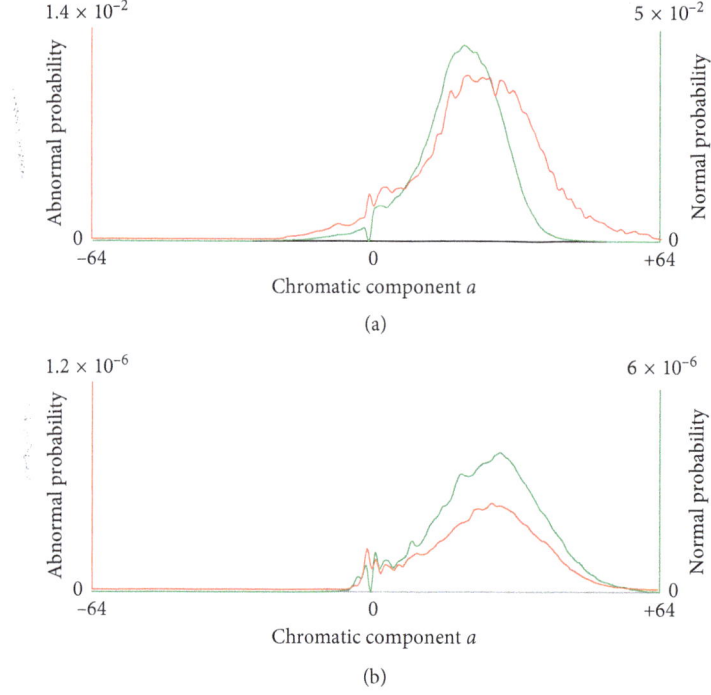

FIGURE 3: Normalized chromatic histograms estimated from all WCE images in KID dataset [20]. Histogram H^A which is estimated from abnormal image regions is represented with a solid red line, and H^N which is estimated from normal image regions is represented with a dashed green line. (a) Chromatic component a. (b) Chromatic component b.

Input: Images I_c $(M \times N)$, $c = a, b$
Output: Image I_{SARC}
(1) **Compute** histogram H_c of images I_c,
(2) $L = $ **length** (H_c);
(3) //Calculate the first and second derivatives of H_c
(4) //r_c^+ first rate
(5) $r_c^+ \longleftarrow dH_c(i)/di, \quad i = L/2 - 1, \ L/2 - 2, \ \ldots, \ 0;$
(6) $r_c^- \longleftarrow dH_c(i)/di, \quad i = -L/2 + 1, \ -L/2 + 2, \ \ldots, \ 0;$
(7) $R_c^+(i) \longleftarrow r_c^+(i)/di, \quad i = L/2 - 2, \ L/2 - 3, \ \ldots, \ 0;$
(8) $R_c^-(i) \longleftarrow r_c^-(i)/di, \quad i = -L/2 + 2, \ -L/2 + 3, \ \ldots, \ 0;$
(9) //denote the max values of value field
(10) $T_c^{+/-} \longleftarrow \arg\max(R_c^{+/-});$
(11) **For each** $(x, \ y) \in [M, \ N]$ **do**
(12)   **If** $I_c^+(x, \ y) < T_c^+$ **then** $I_c^+(x, \ y) \longleftarrow 0;$
(13)   **If** $I_c^-(x, \ y) > T_c^-$ **then** $I_c^-(x, \ y) \longleftarrow 0;$
(14) **End For**
(15) $I_c^{+/-} \longleftarrow$ Normalize $|I_c^{+/-}|;$ //Enhance contrast
(16) //Non-maxima filtering
(17) **For each** $(x, \ y) \in [M, \ N]$ in $I_c^{+,-}$ **do**
(18)   temp[] $\longleftarrow n \times n$ neighborhood centered at $I_c^{+,-}(x, \ y)$
(19)   **For** $i = 0$ to $n \times n$ **do**
(20)   **If** temp$[i] < p(x, \ y)$ **then** temp$[i] = 0;$
(21)   **End For**
(22)   //Temp is matrix with odd number of rows and columns
(23)   **If** $\sum_{i \in [0, n \times n]}$temp $[i] > 0$ **then** temp$\lceil (n \times n/2) + n/2 \rceil = 0; \ I_c^{+,-}(x, \ y) \longleftarrow$ temp$[];$
(24) **End For**
(25) $I_{\text{SARC}} = \sum_{c=a,b} I_c^+ + \sum_{c=a,b} I_c^-$

ALGORITHM 1: Selective aggregation of chromatic image components (SARC).

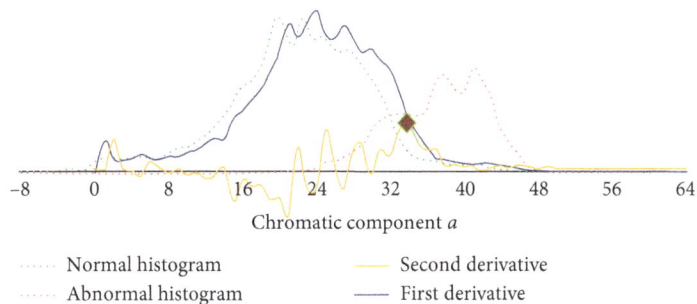

FIGURE 4: Determination of the optimal threshold T_a^+ (black point) based on the second derivative R_a^+ of the histogram estimated from chromatic component a of the WCE image of Figure 1(a). The application of this threshold results in Figure 5(a).

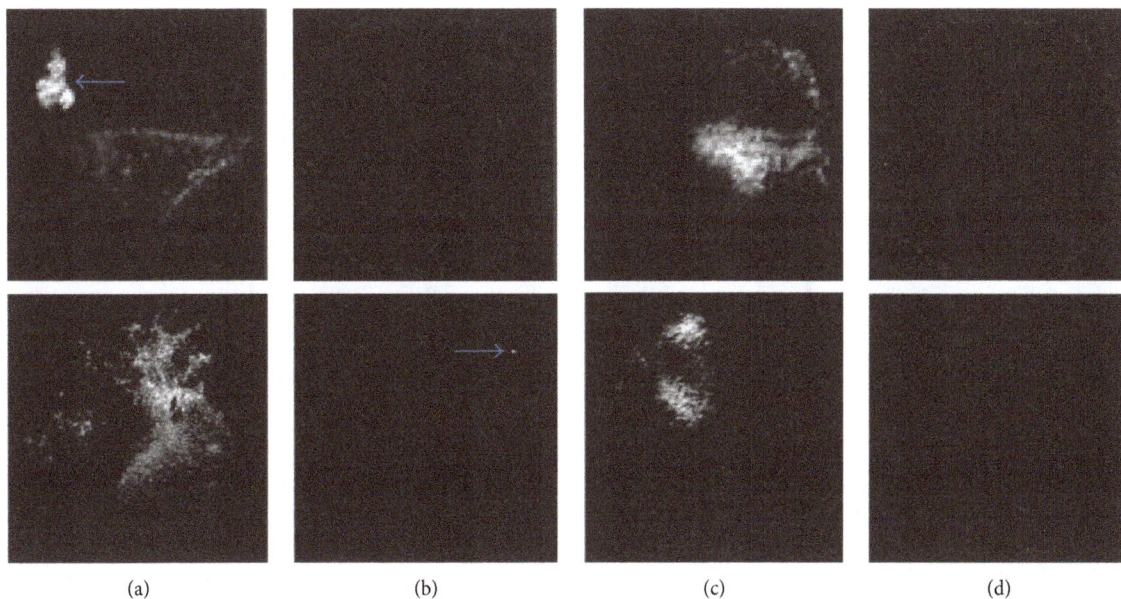

FIGURE 5: Representative output images obtained from the application of Algorithm 1 on the WCE images illustrated in Figure 1(a) (first row) and Figure 1(b) (second row) respectively. (a) I_a positive. (b) I_a negative. (c) I_b positive. (d) I_b negative. The arrows indicate the locations of the lesions. The vascular lesion of Figure 1(a) is clearly discriminated in the respective I_a positive image. Also the small inflammatory lesion of Figure 1(b) is clearly discriminated in the respective I_a negative image.

proposed in [19], the superpixels that contain at least one salient point are also characterized as salient. However, in that study, the pixel-level saliency was disregarded and the localization of abnormalities smaller than a superpixel was impossible. In this study, the pixel-level saliency defined by DINOSARC algorithm is not superseded by the region-level saliency defined by the superpixels. Each DINOSARC salient region is defined by a superpixel that includes only a single, representative salient point. If the superpixel contains a cluster of salient points, then the cluster centroid is regarded as its corresponding salient point.

3.3. Local and Global Color Image Descriptors. Another novel contribution of this work is that both DINOSARC salient regions and points are represented by a local color feature vector. The local feature vectors are subsequently used for the formation of feature vectors globally representing the WCE images. The feature extraction process presented in

this paper is an extension of the approach we originally proposed in [6] for only local representation of square WCE image patches along with their central point.

The proposed, extended approach forms a 9-dimensional feature vector from the color components (L, a, b) of the CIE-*Lab* representation of a salient point, as well as the minimum and maximum values of each of the L, a, and b components within the DINOSARC salient region, that is, min (L), max (L); min (a), max (a); and min (b), max (b). This is inspired by the way the WCE video reviewers empirically assess the image regions for the detection of abnormalities, which, takes into account regional color differentiations [7]. By only including the minimum and maximum values from the salient regions (which are also determined by salient points derived from color differences), such differentiations can be captured.

The local image representation approach is extended by adopting the BoVW model [18] for the extraction of global features from the WCE images. This model considers that an

---

Input: Images I_c $(M \times N)$, $c = a$, b; I_{SARC} $(M \times N)$
Output: List of salient points $I[]$
(1) //Initialize
(2) $i \longleftarrow 0$;
(3) $d[] \longleftarrow$ **null**;
(4) $I[] \longleftarrow$ **null**;
(5) //Sample I_{SARC} and evaluate saliency
(6) **For each** $I_{SARC}(x, y) \neq 0$, $(x, y) \in [M, N]$ **do**
(7) $temp^{large}[] \longleftarrow s \times s$ neighborhood centered at $I_c(x, y)$;
(8) $temp^{small}[] \longleftarrow s/2 \times s/2$ neighborhood centered at $I_c(x, y)$;
(9) $M^{large} \longleftarrow \max(temp^{large}[])$;
(10) $m^{large} \longleftarrow \min(temp^{large}[])$;
(11) $M^{small} \longleftarrow \max(temp^{small}[])$;
(12) $m^{small} \longleftarrow \min(temp^{small}[])$;
(13) $i \longleftarrow i + 1$;
(14) $d[i] \longleftarrow \sqrt{(M^{large} - M^{small})^2 + (m^{large} - m^{small})^2}$
(15) $I[i] \longleftarrow I_c(x, y)$;
(16) **End For**
(17) //Filter salient points upon their proximity
(18) **For** $i = 1$ **to** length $(d[])$ **do**
(19)   **If** $d[i] \leq$ average $(d[])$ **then**
(20)   remove$(d[i])$;
(21)   remove$(I[i])$;
(22)   **End If**
(23) **End For**

ALGORITHM 2: Distances on SARC (DINOSARC) salient point detection.

entire image can be represented by a visual vocabulary. Such a vocabulary may be seen as a set of "exemplar" image patches (visual words), in terms of which any given image may be described. The vocabulary may be seen as a means of quantization of the feature space derived from the local feature vectors. Then, any previously unseen descriptor may be easily quantized to its nearest visual word. Thus, the DINOSARC feature vectors are used to form histograms of visual words for the representation of entire WCE images.

4. Results and Discussion

Experiments on the WCE images were performed to evaluate the proposed DINOSARC feature extraction methodology in comparison to the state-of-the-art using the publicly available data described in Section 2. The results obtained are organized as follows: (a) evaluation of the proposed salient point detector with respect to its capability to detect abnormalities; (b) evaluation of the proposed local descriptor for the discrimination of abnormal from normal salient regions; (c) evaluation of the proposed global descriptor for the detection of abnormal images.

4.1. Salient Point Detection. Prior to the application of DINOSARC algorithm, we performed a series of experiments to determine its optimal parameters. The criterion considered for this tuning process was the number of false negative images, that is, the number of images that were actually containing abnormalities, but no salient points were

detected on these abnormalities. Since the salient point detection process is considered as the first step in the analysis of the WCE images, it is important to be able to detect points on abnormalities, in as many as possible (ideally in all) abnormal images.

To this end, the salient point detection performance of DINOSARC algorithm was investigated using various window sizes $s \times s$ between 4×4 and 20×20 pixels in each component of CIE-*Lab* color space. The results are illustrated in Figure 7. By using window sizes of 6×6 and 10×10 pixels in component a, at least one salient point was detected within the abnormalities. Among these choices, the 10×10 pixel window is considered preferable because it results in less salient points per image (Figure 7(b)).

The DINOSARC salient point detector was compared with the standard SIFT [22] (SIFT-*L*) and SURF [9] (SURF-*L*) algorithms, as they are typically applied on the luminance component (L) of images. Also, it was compared with the SURF-*a* color salient point detection method proposed in [6], where SURF was applied on component a of CIE-*Lab* color space. For completeness, SIFT was also tested on that color component (SIFT-*a*). The evaluation criterion for every detector was the minimum number of salient points needed in order to have the zero false negative images (Figure 8).

Further reduction of the DINOSARC salient points is achieved by the salient region detection process (Section 3.2), which results in only a single salient point per salient region. In the evaluation of DINOSARC detection algorithm, we also computed the percentage of the salient points

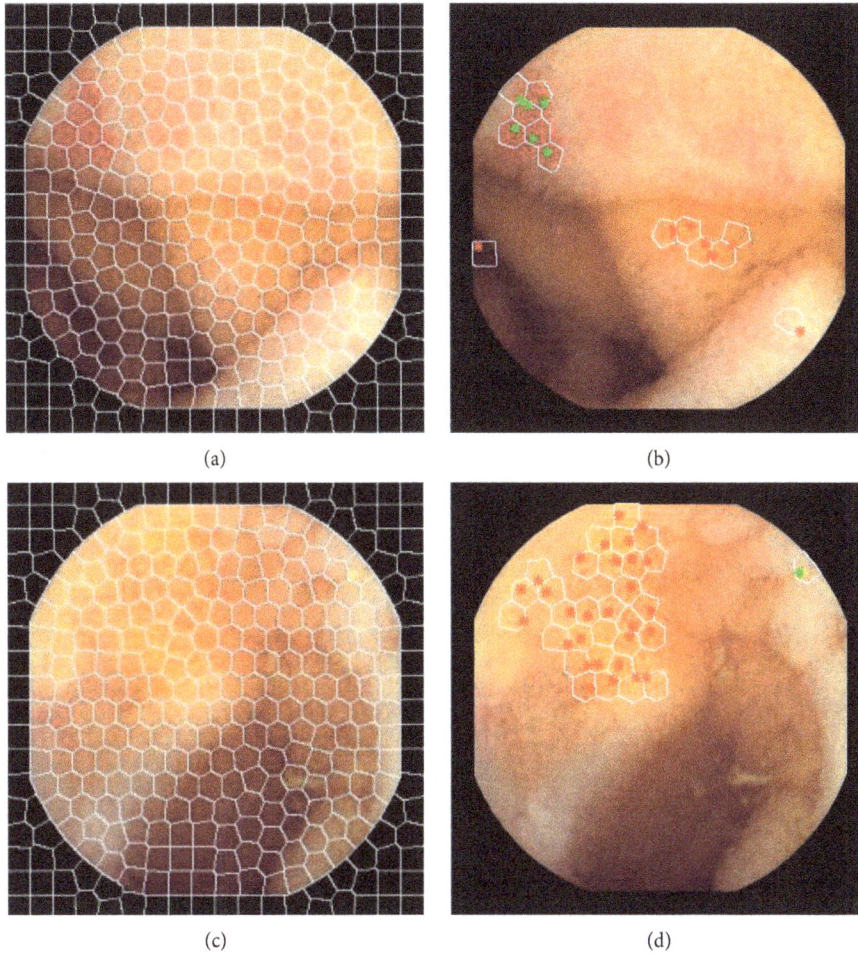

FIGURE 6: Result of SLIC algorithm on an endoscopy image (a) and superpixels with DINOSARC points (b). The images (c) and (d) show the effectiveness of saliency detection for small lesions.

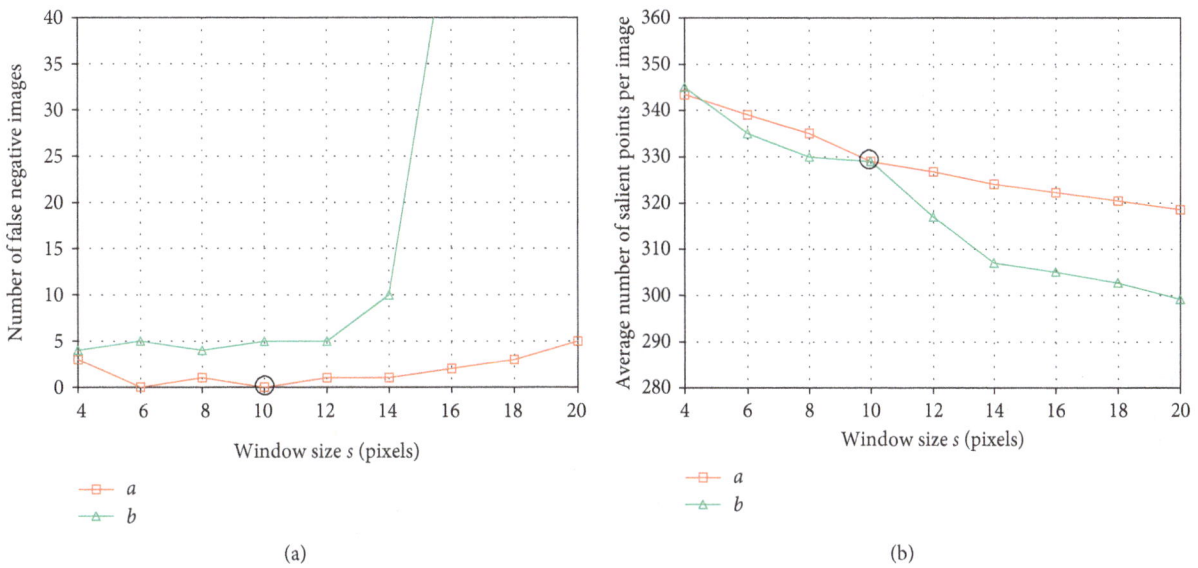

FIGURE 7: Salient point detection results for different (square) window sizes $s \times s$. (a) Average number of salient points detected per image. (b) Number of images in which salient points have not been detected within abnormal regions (false negative).

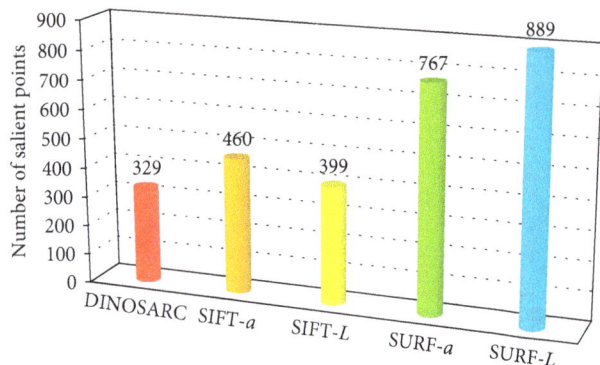

FIGURE 8: Number of salient points detected within abnormal regions over abnormal images using different methods.

TABLE 1: True positive points for each image.

Algorithm	Salient points (%)
DINOSARC	20
SIFT-L	14
SURF-L	11
SIFT-a	15
SURF-a	12

TABLE 2: Classification results of salient regions using local image descriptors.

	Hue histogram	Iakovidis and Koulaouzidis [6]	Yuan et al. [16]	Li and Meng [15]	DINOSARC
AUC	0.584	0.774	0.606	0.718	**0.813**
Accuracy	0.671	0.772	**0.874**	0.698	0.809
Sensitivity	0.833	0.699	0.142	0.432	0.680
Specificity	0.232	0.782	**0.974**	0.829	0.814

falling on the abnormal regions of the images. The percentages of these true positive points over the total number of detected points in the image are presented in Table 1. It can be noticed that the proposed salient point detection algorithm results in more true positive points in every abnormal image than the other algorithms.

4.2. Salient Region Discrimination Using Local Descriptors. For the discrimination of abnormal from normal salient regions, classification experiments were performed using various local image descriptors. As a baseline to compare our DINOSARC descriptor, we considered the hue histogram of the area around each salient point. Since this descriptor is not associated with a particular salient point detection algorithm, the DINOSARC salient point detector was used. The hue histogram was quantized into 15 bins, which was the best performing one among histograms of 15 i, $i = 1, \ldots, 24$ bins. Also, for comparison purposes, we selected three state-of-the-art methodologies. The methodology of Yuan et al. [16], which is very recent, the methodology of Li and Meng [15], and the methodology of Iakovidis and Koulaouzidis[6], which is a predecessor of the proposed approach. The experiments were performed using the 10-fold cross validation evaluation scheme, and a Support Vector Machine (SVM) with Radial Basis Function (RBF) kernel, as a standard classifier. The classification performance was thoroughly investigated using Receiver Operating Characteristic (ROC) analysis [23]. These curves illustrate the trade-off between sensitivity and specificity for various decision thresholds. The Area Under the ROC (AUC) was estimated to be able to compare the classification performances using a single measure. The classification accuracy, the sensitivity, and the specificity are provided as additional measures facilitating comparisons.

The results are presented in Table 2. The best AUC was obtained with the proposed methodology. The respective ROCs are illustrated in Figure 9. It can be noticed that methodology of Yuan et al. provides a higher accuracy; however, this is due to the high specificity, whereas the sensitivity is very low, that is, its capability to detect positive image regions is low. Also low was the performance of the

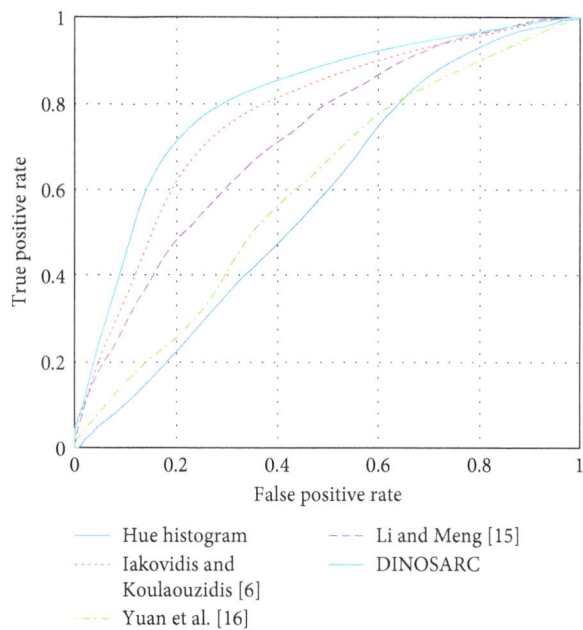

FIGURE 9: The ROCs corresponding to the AUCs reported in Table 2 for the classification of salient regions using local image descriptors.

hue histogram descriptor. The second best performance was obtained by the method of Iakovidis et al.

An interpretation of these results can be based on the physical meaning of the respective descriptors. The descriptors proposed by Yuan et al. [16] and Li and Meng [15] encode the texture of an image area (both SIFT/CLBP and ULBP/wavelet transform are textural descriptors), and hue histograms encode its colors as they are perceived by humans [24]. The best performing approaches are also based on color; however, the regional minima and maxima of the opponent color components tend to provide more discriminative information about the abnormalities. The approach of Yuan et al. [16] was originally proposed for the detection of polyps, and the approach of Li and Meng [15] was proposed for the detection of tumors, including adenomas and adenocarcinomas. Texture has been a discriminative feature of polyps and tumors in several studies with flexible endoscopy images [13, 25]. However, the significantly lower resolution of WCE images limits the visibility of texture, and consequently, texture becomes less discriminative. More importantly, the database used in our experiments not only contains polyps but also several other kinds of abnormalities, for which texture may not be as discriminative as color, for example, vascular lesions.

4.3. Abnormal Image Detection Using Global Descriptors. Experiments were performed for the investigation of the classification performance of entire WCE images using the DINOSARC features. For image representation, global features were extracted using the BoVW model. The BoVW model was constructed with a range of visual vocabulary sizes in the range from 500 to 700 words. The experiments were performed using the 10-fold cross validation evaluation scheme and an RBF-SVM classifier. Table 3 summarizes the results obtained. The proposed DINOSARC features achieved better results from the other methods. The respective ROCs are illustrated in Figure 10. As in Section 4.2, considering the AUCs, the method of Iakovidis and Koulaouzidis was ranked second, the method of Li and Meng [15] was ranked third, the method of Yuan et al. was ranked fourth, and the lowest classification performance was obtained by the hue histograms.

5. Conclusions

We presented DINOSARC, a color feature extraction methodology for WCE image analysis. The proposed methodology aims to the discrimination of various abnormal tissues from normal image contents. Major contributions of this study include the following:

(i) A novel salient point detection method, which considers saliency with respect to color differences observed in abnormality regions.

(ii) A novel definition of regional saliency based on superpixel segmentation that extends the approach we previously proposed for bleeding detection [19]. The extension relies on the fact that region-level saliency is defined based on DINOSARC salient points and that point-level saliency is preserved to enable the localization of smaller abnormalities.

(iii) A novel descriptor, which extends the descriptor we proposed in [6] by applying the calculations on an arbitrarily shaped local region defined by a salient superpixel.

(iv) The proposed methodology was applied for both supervised and weakly-supervised detection of abnormalities in a rich publicly available dataset. The supervised approach was based on the proposed local descriptors, and the weakly-supervised

TABLE 3: Classification results of WCE images using global image descriptors.

	Hue histogram	Iakovidis and Koulaouzidis [6]	Yuan et al. [16]	Li and Meng [15]	DINOSARC
AUC	0.684	0.774	0.701	0.754	**0.815**
Accuracy	0.730	0.786	0.746	0.751	**0.818**
Sensitivity	0.391	0.496	0.406	0.358	**0.512**
Specificity	0.871	0.890	0.884	0.870	**0.908**

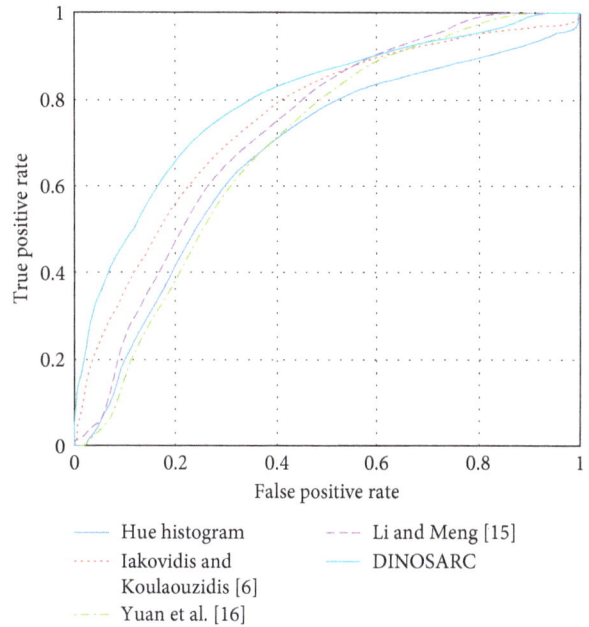

FIGURE 10: The ROCs corresponding to the AUCs reported in Table 3 for the classification of WCE images using global image descriptors.

approach was based on global image descriptors derived from the local ones by application of the BoWV model.

The results showed that the proposed methodology can be more efficient and more effective than relevant state-of-the-art methods for the detection of abnormal images. More, specifically:

(i) The proposed salient point detection approach results in a smaller number of salient points, which are more likely to fall within regions of abnormality than other current approaches

(ii) The proposed local image descriptors result in better discrimination of the abnormalities from the normal image contents

(iii) The global image descriptors enable more accurate detection of the abnormal images in the WCE dataset

Future research directions include investigation of methods towards further decreasing the total number of salient points, further improvement of the discrimination capability of the image descriptors, and the extension of the experimentation to entire video sequences.

Conflicts of Interest

The authors declare that there are no conflicts of interest regarding the publication of this paper.

Acknowledgments

This project was supported in part by the project "Klearchos Koulaouzidis," Grant no. 5151, Special Account of Research Grants of the University of Thessaly, Greece.

References

[1] A. Koulaouzidis, D. K. Iakovidis, A. Karargyris, and E. Rondonotti, "Wireless endoscopy in 2020: will it still be a capsule?," *World Journal of Gastroenterology*, vol. 21, no. 17, pp. 5119–5130, 2015.

[2] A. Riphaus, S. Richter, M. Vonderach, and T. Wehrmann, "Capsule endoscopy interpretation by an endoscopy nurse—a comparative trial," *Zeitschrift für Gastroenterologie*, vol. 47, no. 3, pp. 273–276, 2009.

[3] D. K. Iakovidis, R. Sarmiento, J. S. Silva et al., "Towards intelligent capsules for robust wireless endoscopic imaging of the gut," in *Proceedings of IEEE International Conference on Imaging Systems and Techniques (IST)*, Macau, China, September 2014.

[4] I. N. Figueiredo, C. Leal, L. Pinto, P. N. Figueiredo, and R. Tsai, "Hybrid multiscale affine and elastic image registration approach towards wireless capsule endoscope localization," *Biomedical Signal Processing and Control*, vol. 39, pp. 486–502, 2018.

[5] D. K. Iakovidis and A. Koulaouzidis, "Software for enhanced video capsule endoscopy: challenges for essential progress," *Nature Reviews Gastroenterology and Hepatology*, vol. 12, no. 3, pp. 172–186, 2015.

[6] D. K. Iakovidis and A. Koulaouzidis, "Automatic lesion detection in wireless capsule endoscopy—a simple solution for a complex problem," in *Proceedings of IEEE International Conference on Image Processing (ICIP)*, pp. 2236–2240, Paris, France, October 2014.

[7] D. K. Iakovidis and A. Koulaouzidis, "Automatic lesion detection in capsule endoscopy based on color saliency: closer to an essential adjunct for reviewing software," *Gastrointestinal Endoscopy*, vol. 80, no. 5, pp. 877–883, 2014.

[8] A. Karargyris and N. Bourbakis, "Detection of small bowel polyps and ulcers in wireless capsule endoscopy videos," *IEEE Transactions on Biomedical Engineering*, vol. 58, no. 10, pp. 2777–2786, 2011.

[9] H. Bay, A. Ess, T. Tuytelaars, and L. Van Gool, "Speeded-up robust features (SURF)," *Computer Vision and Image Understanding*, vol. 110, no. 3, pp. 346–359, 2008.

[10] Y. Yuan, B. Li, and M. Q.-H. Meng, "Bleeding frame and region detection in the wireless capsule endoscopy video," *IEEE Journal of Biomedical and Health Informatics*, vol. 20, no. 2, pp. 624–630, 2016.

[11] Y. Fu, W. Zhang, M. Mandal, and M. Q.-H. Meng, "Computer-aided bleeding detection in WCE video," *IEEE Journal of Biomedical and Health Informatics*, vol. 18, no. 2, pp. 636–642, 2014.

[12] W. Shi, J. Chen, H. Chen, Q. Peng, and T. Gan, "Bleeding fragment localization using time domain information for WCE videos," in *Proceedings of 8th International Conference on BioMedical Engineering and Informatics (BMEI)*, pp. 73–78, Shenyang, China, October 2016.

[13] M. Liedlgruber and A. Uhl, "Computer-aided decision support systems for endoscopy in the gastrointestinal tract: a review," *IEEE reviews in Biomedical Engineering*, vol. 4, pp. 73–88, 2011.

[14] J. Bernal, F. J. Sánchez, G. Fernández-Esparrach, D. Gil, C. Rodríguez, and F. Vilariño, "WM-DOVA maps for accurate polyp highlighting in colonoscopy: validation vs. saliency maps from physicians," *Computerized Medical Imaging and Graphics*, vol. 43, pp. 99–111, 2015.

[15] B. Li and M. Q.-H. Meng, "Tumor recognition in wireless capsule endoscopy images using textural features and SVM-based feature selection," *IEEE Transactions on Information Technology in Biomedicine*, vol. 16, no. 3, pp. 323–329, 2012.

[16] Y. Yuan, B. Li, and M. Q.-H. Meng, "Improved bag of feature for automatic polyp detection in wireless capsule endoscopy images," *IEEE Transactions on Automation Science and Engineering*, vol. 13, no. 2, pp. 529–535, 2016.

[17] M. Vasilakakis, D. K. Iakovidis, E. Spyrou, and A. Koulaouzidis, "Weakly-supervised lesion detection in video capsule endoscopy based on a bag-of-colour features model," in *Lecture Notes in Computer Science*, T. Peters, G. Yang, N. Navab et al., Eds., pp. 1–8, Springer, Berlin, Germany, 2017.

[18] G. Csurka, C. Dance, L. Fan, J. Willamowski, and C. Bray, "Visual categorization with bags of keypoints," in *Proceedings of Workshop on Statistical Learning in Computer Vision, ECCV*, vol. 1, pp. 1–2, Prague, Czech Republic, May 2004.

[19] D. K. Iakovidis, D. Chatzis, P. Chrysanthopoulos, and A. Koulaouzidis, "Blood detection in wireless capsule endoscope images based on salient superpixels," in *Proceedings of Annual International Conference on IEEE Engineering in Medicine and Biology Society, EMBS*, pp. 731–734, Milano, Italy, August 2015.

[20] A. Koulaouzidis, D. K. Iakovidis, D. E. Yung et al., "KID Project: an internet-based digital video atlas of capsule endoscopy for research purposes," *Endoscopy International Open*, vol. 5, no. 6, pp. E477–E483, 2017.

[21] R. Achanta, A. Shaji, K. Smith, A. Lucchi, P. Fua, and S. Süsstrunk, "SLIC superpixels compared to state-of-the-art superpixel methods," *IEEE Transactions on Pattern Analysis and Machine Intelligence*, vol. 34, no. 11, pp. 2274–2282, 2012.

[22] D. G. Lowe, "Distinctive image features from scale-invariant keypoints," *International Journal of Computer Vision*, vol. 60, no. 2, pp. 91–110, 2004.

[23] T. Fawcett, "An introduction to ROC analysis," *Pattern Recognition Letters*, vol. 27, no. 8, pp. 861–874, 2006.

[24] G. Wyszecki and W. S. Stiles, *Color Science*, Wiley, Vol. 8, Wiley, New York, NY, USA, 1982.

[25] S. A. Karkanis, D. K. Iakovidis, D. E. Maroulis, D. A. Karras, and M. Tzivras, "Computer-aided tumor detection in endoscopic video using color wavelet features," *IEEE Transactions on Information Technology in Biomedicine*, vol. 7, no. 3, pp. 141–152, 2003.

7

Stimulation Strategies for Tinnitus Suppression in a Neuron Model

Alessandra Paffi ⓘ**, Francesca Camera** ⓘ**, Chiara Carocci,**
Francesca Apollonio ⓘ**, and Micaela Liberti** ⓘ

Sapienza University of Rome, Via Eudossiana 18, 00184 Rome, Italy

Correspondence should be addressed to Micaela Liberti; liberti@diet.uniroma1.it

Academic Editor: György Thuróczy

Tinnitus is a debilitating perception of sound in the absence of external auditory stimuli. It may have either a central or a peripheral origin in the cochlea. Experimental studies evidenced that an electrical stimulation of peripheral auditory fibers may alleviate symptoms but the underlying mechanisms are still unknown. In this work, a stochastic neuron model is used, that mimics an auditory fiber affected by tinnitus, to check the effects, in terms of firing reduction, of different kinds of electric stimulations, i.e., continuous wave signals and white Gaussian noise. Results show that both white Gaussian noise and continuous waves at tens of kHz induce a neuronal firing reduction; however, for the same amplitude of fluctuations, Gaussian noise is more efficient than continuous waves. When contemporary applied, signal and noise exhibit a cooperative effect in retrieving neuronal firing to physiological values. These results are a proof of concept that a combination of signal and noise could be delivered through cochlear prosthesis for tinnitus suppression.

1. Introduction

Tinnitus is a debilitating perception of sound in the absence of external auditory stimuli that affects more than 10% of the world population [1–3] and tends to increase with the age [2, 3].

The origin of this debilitating disorder may be central or peripheral; i.e., it can originate in the cochlea, in the primary hearing cortex or in any other point of the auditory pathway [4].

Based on frequency and permanence of sound perception, tinnitus is classified in continuous low frequency tinnitus (CLFT) for frequencies below 100 Hz, continuous high frequency tinnitus (CHFT) for frequencies above 3 kHz, and transient spontaneous tinnitus (TST) [5]. Several studies [6, 7] confirm that the CHFT is the most widespread tinnitus typology, generally associated with a reduction of cochlear functionality at high frequency, due to a damage of the basal section of the cochlea. In the tonotopic organization of sound perception [8], the cochlea basal section encodes for high frequency stimuli, above 3 kHz.

This close association between tinnitus and hearing loss suggests that, in many cases, it is due to an impairment of the outer hair cells (OHC) of the cochlear basal section that, in turn, induces a pathologic state of depolarization of the inner hair cells (IHC) [9].

In 1995 Le Page [9] proposed a cochlear model to explain tinnitus origin. The OHCs determine the hair deflection of the IHCs that, in turn, depolarize the acoustic fibers. In physiologic conditions, in the absence of an external stimulus, the OHCs fix the operating point on the IHC transfer function (acoustic neuron depolarization versus IHC hair deflection) to a position that brain recognizes as absence of sound. When the OHCs are damaged, the control input to the IHCs gets lost with a consequent shift of the operating IHC point and a permanent firing rate of the acoustic fiber interpreted by the brain as a real acoustic pattern [9].

This modification of the nerve fiber firing pattern due to OHC impairment was experimentally observed in different animal models [10–13].

Several experimental studies [14–16] revealed that an electric stimulation of the cochlea, delivered through cochlear prosthesis or transtympanic electrode, could alleviate tinnitus perception in a significant percentage of treated patients. McKerrow and colleagues [14] used continuous wave (CW) high frequency signals (2-6 MHz) superposed to a Gaussian white noise (GWN), whereas other authors used pulse trains with repetition frequency up to 5 kHz [15, 17]. Recently, Tyler and colleagues [18] efficiently used pulsed modulated signals delivered to the Vagus nerve on human volunteers.

However, the electric signals delivered in stimulation, in terms of type (CW, pulse train, white noise), frequency content, amplitude, and modulation, were empirically chosen and their mechanisms of action on the auditory fibers were not defined.

Moving from a recent study by the authors [19] showing an inhibitory effect of an electric exogenous stimulation on a hyperexcited neuronal network model, it was hypothesized that an electric stimulation may interfere with the neuron firing pattern of a pathologically polarized acoustic neuron by reducing its firing rate to the physiologic one.

Aim of this work is to verify such a hypothesis and to study the efficacy of a combination of signal and noise in tinnitus inhibition, using a simple model of a hyperexcited auditory fiber.

In a biomedical perspective, the final aim is to deliver this stimulation to the auditory nerve using cochlear prosthesis to suppress tinnitus in patients with acoustic impairment.

2. Models and Methods

2.1. Neuron Model. To describe the single Ranvier node of an auditory fiber, a stochastic Hodgkin-Huxley (HH) model was used [20–22]. In this model, the neuronal membrane patch is represented by an electrical equivalent, in which the balance of the currents per unit area is given by

$$C_m \frac{dV}{dt} = -g_l (V - E_l) - g_K (V - E_K)$$
$$- g_{Na} (V - E_{Na}) + I_0 \tag{1}$$

where C_m is the unit area capacitance that takes into account the dielectric properties of the membrane phospholipidic bilayer, V is the transmembrane potential, g_{Na}, g_K, g_l are sodium, potassium and leakage conductances per unit area, respectively, and E_{Na}, E_K, E_l are the reversal potentials of the corresponding current densities. Finally, I_0 is the bias current density that controls the transition between the resting state and the firing activity of the neuron [23]. For the deterministic HH model at 6.3°C, the threshold value above which the neuron starts its firing activity is equal to 6.3 μA/cm^2 [23].

Despite the model limitation concerning the operating temperature equal to 6.3°C, it is simple, very well characterized in terms of neuronal response as a function of model parameters, and the most used in different applications, with more than 10000 citations in the Scopus database [24], so that it can be considered as a golden standard when a new hypothesis has to be tested. Moreover, the possibility of including channel gating stochasticity allowed us to realistically model

channel noise which is particularly relevant in the auditory fibers, due to their small size [25, 26].

To account for the random gating of sodium and potassium channels, the ionic current densities $I_{Na} = g_{Na}(V - E_{Na})$ and $I_K = g_K(V - E_K)$ were calculated using a channel-state-tracking algorithm [27, 28] where Markov chains [27, 29] modeled independent gating particles belonging to each ionic channel.

The magnitude of fluctuations in current densities (channel noise) depends on the number of ionic channels and, thus, for fixed channel densities (ρ_{Na}=60 channels/μm^2, ρ_K=18 channels/μm^2), on the area of the considered membrane patch. Specifically, channel noise is inversely proportional to the square root of the number of ionic channels in the membrane patch [21, 30]. Acoustic fibers are characterized by small Ranvier nodes, whose size may vary from 2.2 [25] to 15.7 μm^2 [26] and thus by high levels of intrinsic channel noise. In this work, three patch areas were considered: 2.2, 11.0, and 15.7 μm^2, corresponding to the maximum, the minimum, and an intermediate fiber size.

Besides Na, K, and leakage current densities, I_0 represents here the background level of stimulation coming from the OHCs. This current density determines the firing rate of the neuron, i.e., the operating point on the IHC transfer function.

To simulate different states of pathologic neuron depolarization, I_0 was set to a value close to the threshold: 6 μA/cm^2 and to suprathreshold values: 7 and 10 μA/cm^2 [23]. Conversely, physiological spontaneous firing of the auditory fiber was modeled by using a subthreshold bias current density I_0 equal to 2 μA/cm^2. With respect to this physiological condition, the other conditions increased the background firing activity from 30 to 80%, as suggested by experimental recordings in animals with induced tinnitus [12, 13].

In this paper, for each patch area, four bias currents densities were used: 2, 6, 7, and 10 μA/cm^2. The first value was used to model a healthy acoustic fiber; the other ones modeled paroxysmal excitation underlying tinnitus.

The model was run in the C++ environment using the forward Euler integration method with time step 10 μs.

In principle, the HH model extends its validity up to frequencies that short-circuit the membrane capacitance. According to [31], this occurs above the beta relaxation frequency of the cell membrane, at about 100 MHz. Moreover, the ionic channel modeling using Markov chains [32] is valid if the sampling time is much longer than the channel protein transition time (order of ps) [33]. The used time step of 10 μs imposes a practical limitation of 50 kHz to the maximum frequencies that can be studied with the model. This is well below the theoretical frequency limitations of the model previously discussed.

For each studied condition, 300 independent runs of the model, 1 s in duration, were considered. The number of runs was approximately the number of afferent fibers contemporary stimulated by a single electrode of the cochlear prosthesis; this number was calculated by considering the size of the electrode (0.3 mm), the diameter of a IHC ($\approx$10 μm), and the number of auditory fibers ($\approx$10) contacting a single IHC.

TABLE 1: Mean firing rate (spikes/s) exhibited by the neuron model for different bias current densities I_0 and patch areas in the absence of external electric stimulation.

Patch area (μm^2)	Sub-threshold (physiologic) $I_0=2\ \mu A/cm^2$	Close to threshold (pathologic) $I_0=6\ \mu A/cm^2$	Supra-threshold (pathologic)	
			$I_0=7\ \mu A/cm^2$	$I_0=10\ \mu A/cm^2$
2.2	53.7	64.9	66.8	72.2
11.0	44.5	57.8	60.7	67.2
15.7	42.1	56.5	59.3	66.2

2.2. Stimulation. The exogenous stimulation was introduced in the model as an additional voltage over the membrane potential [34–36]. In terms of equivalent HH electric circuit, the electric stimulus was represented as a voltage generator in series with the membrane capacitor and the ionic conductances per unit area [37–40].

The applied electric stimulation was either a CW or a zero-mean GWN or a combination of both.

It should be noticed that the CW is a deterministic signal completely characterized by amplitude (A) and frequency (f), whereas the GWN, being a stochastic process, is described by its statistic moments, namely, average value, variance (σ_N^2), and autocorrelation function.

The GWN had zero-mean value, flat spectrum, and variance values: $\sigma_N^2 = 3, 25, 100\ mV^2$. The variance can be associated with the average power that the process dissipates on a 1 Ω resistance. The CW signal was chosen to have amplitude values: A=1.73, 5, 10 mV, equal to the standard deviations (σ_N) of the considered GWN processes, where σ_N was taken as a measure of the amplitude of noise fluctuations. The CW frequencies were chosen to be equal to 25, 35, 50 kHz

because they are above the upper perception threshold of human hearing (20 kHz). Due to the time step of 10 μs chosen for the model solution, 50 kHz is the maximum frequency allowed for an input signal. For the same reason, even the GWN spectrum is practically limited to that upper frequency.

After separately studying the two kinds of stimulation, all combinations of the CW signals and the GWN were applied to the model to check possible cooperative effects.

2.3. Quantification of Firing Reduction. As already mentioned in Introduction, a pathologic acoustic fiber exhibits a spontaneous firing rate higher than that of a healthy neuron [12, 13]. The mean firing rate, i.e., the number of spikes per second, is due to the operating point fixed by the OHC and to the endogenous noise related to the number of ionic channels. To quantify the level of firing inhibition, and thus of tinnitus suppression, induced by the electric stimulation, it is necessary to introduce a sensitive technique.

In this work, the inactivation function (IA) was defined as follows:

$$IA = \frac{\#spike\left(\sigma_N = 0; A = 0; f = 0; I_0 = 6,7,10\right) - \#spike\left(\sigma_N \neq 0; A \neq 0; f \neq 0; I_0 = 6,7,10\right)}{\#spike\left(\sigma_N = 0; A = 0; f = 0; I_0 = 6,7,10\right) - \#spike\left(\sigma_N = 0; A = 0; f = 0; I_0 = 2\right)} \times 100 \tag{2}$$

where $\#spike(\sigma_N=0; A=0; f=0; I_0=6,7,10)$ is the number of spikes per second of a pathologic neuron ($I_0=6,7, 10\ \mu A/cm^2$) in the absence of exogenous electric stimulation ($\sigma_N=0$ mV; A=0 mV; f=0 Hz); $\#spike(\sigma_N\neq0; A\neq0; f\neq0; I_0=6,7,10)$ is the number of spikes per second of a pathologic neuron during the exogenous electric stimulation ($\sigma_N\neq0$ mV; A$\neq$0 mV; f$\neq$0 Hz); $\#spike(\sigma_N=0; A=0; f=0; I_0=2)$ is the number of spikes per second of a healthy neuron ($I_0=2\ \mu A/cm^2$) in the absence of exogenous electric stimulation ($\sigma_N=0$ mV; A=0 mV; f=0 Hz).

This quantity furnishes the percentage of firing reduction obtained using the stimulation in the pathologic neuron with respect to the difference, in terms of firing activity, between a pathologic and a physiologic neuron. The inactivation function will be 0% if the stimulation does not change the number of spikes of pathologic neuron and 100% if the neuron activity is turned back to the physiologic one. In this latter case, tinnitus is considered completely suppressed. Inactivation could be also higher than 100% if the firing activity is reduced

below the physiologic condition or negative if the effect of electric stimulation is excitatory instead of inhibitory.

3. Results

3.1. Spontaneous Firing. The used stochastic neuron model exhibits a firing activity, quantified by the mean firing rate (spikes per second), that increases with the bias current density I_0 injected in the model, as shown in Table 1. Even in subthreshold conditions (see second column of Table 1) a not null firing rate is observed, due to the energy injected into the system by channel noise, that increases as the Ranvier node area becomes smaller (Table 1).

The neuron firing rate is due to the contemporary presence of channel noise and bias current density; the first one is determined by the typical sizes of the acoustic Ranvier nodes, the second one accounts for the operating point set by the OHC on the IHC transfer function, according to [9].

As shown in Table 1, for the same patch area, the three bias current densities, used to mimic the neuron with tinnitus (pathologic condition), increase the firing activity with respect to the physiologic condition, here modeled using the subthreshold bias current density I_0=2 μA/cm^2. These increases range from 21% (I_0=6 μA/cm^2) to 35% (I_0=10 μA/cm^2), for the 2.2 μm^2 patch area, from 25% (I_0=6 μA/cm^2) to 40% (I_0=10 μA/cm^2), for the 11.0 μm^2 patch area, and from 35% (I_0=6 μA/cm^2) to 57% (I_0=10 μA/cm^2), for the 15.7 μm^2 patch area (Table 1). This shows that when channel noise decreases, in correspondence of larger patch areas, bias current densities assume a stronger influence on neuron firing.

The increased firing activity obtained by using the close to threshold and the suprathreshold current densities reported in Table 1 agrees with the experimental recordings on animals with induced tinnitus, reporting an increase from 35 to 83% [12, 13].

In the next sections, it will be examined the efficacy of different exogenous electric stimulations (see Section 2.2) in reducing the firing activity of pathologic neurons down to physiologic conditions.

3.2. Effect of Different Electric Stimulations.
The effects of a GWN on the mean firing rate of the neuron model, in each operating condition, have been quantified by the inactivation function IA, defined in Section 2.3, and summarized in Figure 1. For each pathologic condition, Figure 1 shows inactivation versus patch area for three standard deviations σ_N of noise fluctuations: 1.73 mV (panel (a)), 5 mV (panel (b)), and 10 mV (panel (c)).

For the lowest σ_N (Figure 1(a)), the inactivation does not exceed 2% and, in some cases, assumes negative values, indicating an increase of the mean firing frequency instead of a reduction. For σ_N of 5 mV (Figure 1(b)) it is possible to observe higher inactivation values that increase with the patch area and decrease with the bias current density, reaching a value of about 10% for patch size 15.7 μm^2 and bias current density 6 μA/cm^2. However, such values are too low to induce considerable tinnitus alleviation. Further increasing σ_N up to 10 mV (Figure 1(c)), the inactivation could become considerable, reaching 53% for the highest patch area and the smallest bias current density. However, the inactivation is just some percent points for the smallest patch area, where the endogenous channel noise dominates on the exogenous stimulation in determining the neuron firing rate.

Therefore, a standard deviation of 10 mV is necessary for the GWN to induce an inactivation from 26 to 53% in acoustic fibers whose Ranvier nodes are larger than 11 μm^2.

However, a broadband stimulation with a quite high power, related to the variance of noise fluctuations, may in principle induce unwanted acoustic perceptions coming from neighboring healthy hear cells.

Thus, it is worth evaluating the effect of using a stimulation with comparable amplitude of noise at a single frequency (CW) above 20 kHz, the upper perception limit of the human hearing. In fact, this stimulation cannot be directly interpreted as a sound by the human auditory system.

Figure 2(a) shows the inactivation versus the bias current density for the larger patch area (best case) and an applied CW at 25 kHz and amplitude equal to 1.73, 5, or 10 mV. As discussed in Section 2.2, these amplitudes have been chosen to have the same standard deviation of the used GWNs.

Even in this case, the signal with 1.73 mV of amplitude is not efficient in inhibiting firing and that of 5 mV inactivates the neuron up to 10%. The effect becomes considerable for the 10 mV signal, when the inactivation is equal to 18% for I_0=10 μA/cm^2 and reaches a maximum of 35% for I_0=6 μA/cm^2. As already noticed for the GWN stimulation, the inactivation decreases with the bias current density, i.e., with the background firing activity of the pathologic neuron.

To evaluate the sensitivity to different stimulation frequencies, also 35 and 50 kHz CW signals have been considered. Figure 2(b) shows the inactivation induced by 25 kHz, 35 kHz and 50 kHz CW signals with the amplitude set to 10 mV.

It is worth noticing that the CW is almost ineffective at 50 kHz, being the inactivation always less than 20%, whereas 25 kHz and 35 kHz signals behave in a similar way, with a slightly better performance of the 25 kHz CW. This evidences a frequency sensitivity of the neuron already observed also in a lower frequency range (50-500 Hz) [41, 42].

Results of simulations show that the GWN, having the standard deviation equal to the sinusoidal amplitude, is always more efficient than the 25 kHz CW in inducing firing reduction. Figure 3 compares the inactivations induced by these two exogenous stimulations in the best case (I_0=6 μA/cm^2; patch area=15.7 μm^2). Although the inactivation values are very similar when both the noise standard deviation (σ_N) and the signal amplitude (A) are equal to 1.73 and 5 mV, for σ_N=10 mV the inactivation induced by GWN is 52% versus 35% obtained by using the 25 kHz CW signal with the same amplitude. In fact, while the CW inactivation trend versus the amplitude (purple line in Figure 3) is accurately approximated (R=0.99976) by a quadratic curve with the second-order coefficient equal to 0.35, in the case of GWN (orange line in Figure 3), the quadratic function which best fits the inactivation trend (R=0.99964) has a second-order coefficient equal to 0.64.

To obtain 100 % inactivation, too high amplitude values for the CW signal would be necessary; conversely GWN has the disadvantage of having a spectrum segment in the auditory frequency band.

For these reasons, it would be useful to combine in a suitable way these two kinds of stimulation.

3.3. Effects of Combined Stimulation.
The question arises on what happens if monochromatic and white stimulations are combined.

Results of the combined stimulation have been compared to the superposition of the effects induced by the two stimulations applied individually. Figure 4 shows a comparison of inactivation obtained by combining the two kinds of stimulation IA(CW+GWN) with the sum of the inactivations obtained by using the two single stimulations

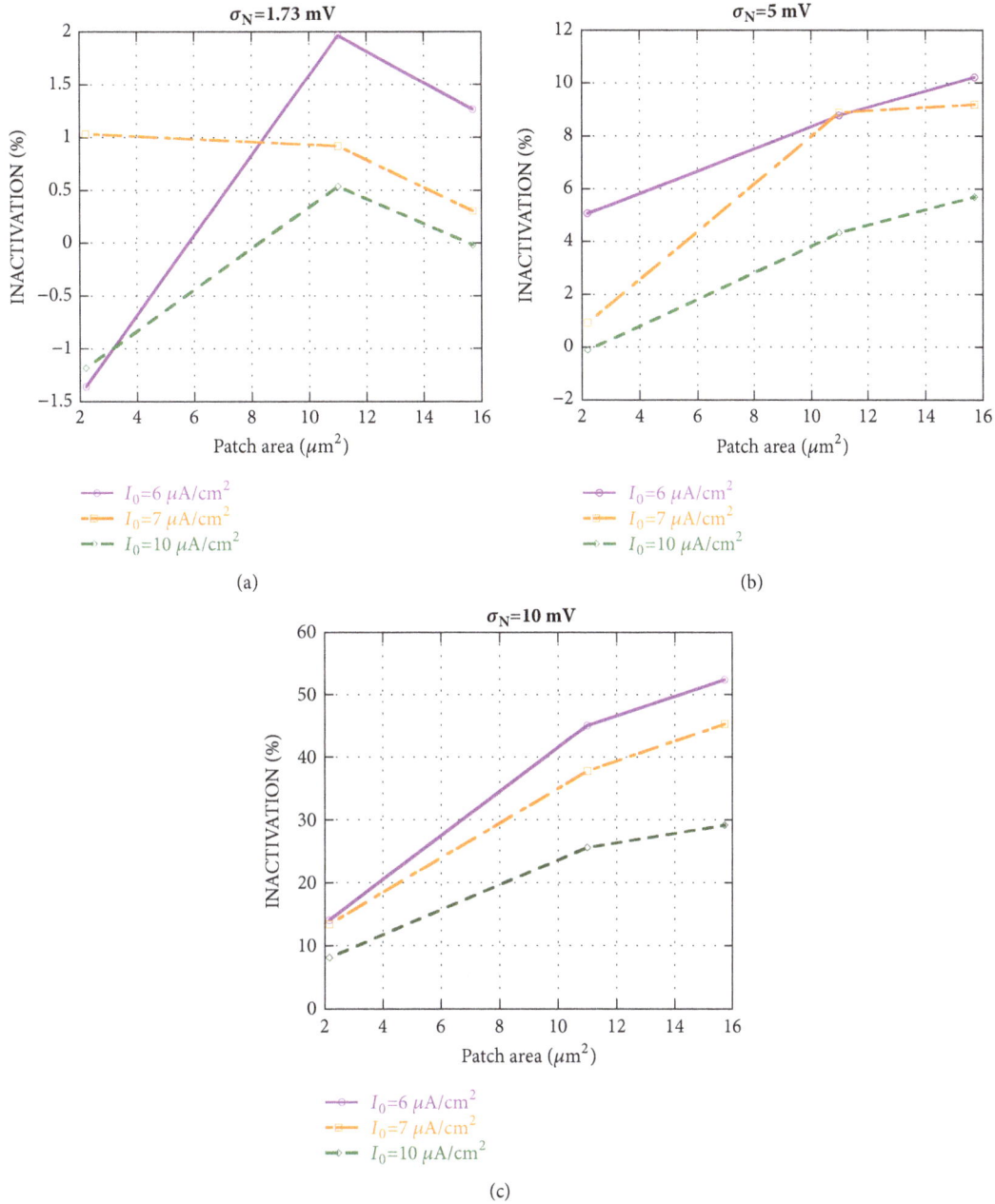

FIGURE 1: Inactivation versus patch area for different bias current densities I_0. The exogenous stimulation is given by a Gaussian white noise GWN with different standard deviations: σ_N=1.73 mV (panel (a)), σ_N=5 mV (panel (b)), and σ_N=10 mV (panel (c)).

IA(CW)+IA(GWN), in the best case: CW at 25 kHz with amplitude 10 mV, and GWN with σ_N=10 mV.

As evident from Figure 4, except for the lowest patch area and I_0=6 μA/cm^2, IA(CW+GWN) is always higher than IA(CW)+IA(GWN) and, for I_0=6 μA/cm^2 and patch area 15.7 μm^2, it reaches 100%. This means that the firing rate of the stimulated neuron is reduced to physiologic conditions.

These results, due to the nonlinear neuronal behavior, show a cooperative effect of the applied signal and noise that can be usefully exploited in applications. So, a good stimulation solution could be a combination of CW and

GWN to maximize tinnitus suppression while reducing possible side effects.

4. Discussion

Results of this work furnish a proof of concept that a suitable exogenous electrical stimulation, consisting of a high frequency (25-35 kHz) CW and/or Gaussian noise, can alleviate tinnitus through a mechanism of firing inhibition. This finding is coherent with studies on human volunteers, where the electrical stimulation was delivered to the cochlea [14–16], and suggests a possible interaction mechanism based on

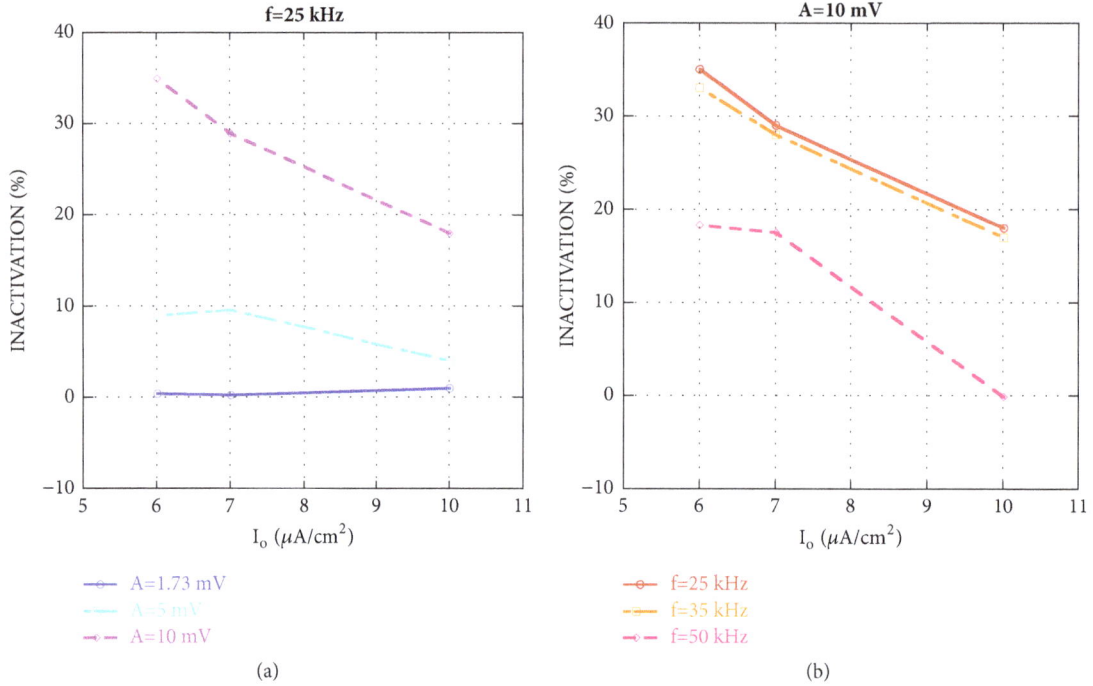

FIGURE 2: Inactivation versus bias current density I_0 for a patch area equal to 15.7 μm^2. The exogenous stimulation is given by a CW at 25 kHz and amplitudes 1.73 mV, 5 mV, and 10 mV (panel (a)) or a CW of amplitude 10 mV and frequencies 25 kHz, 35 kHz, and 50 kHz (panel (b)).

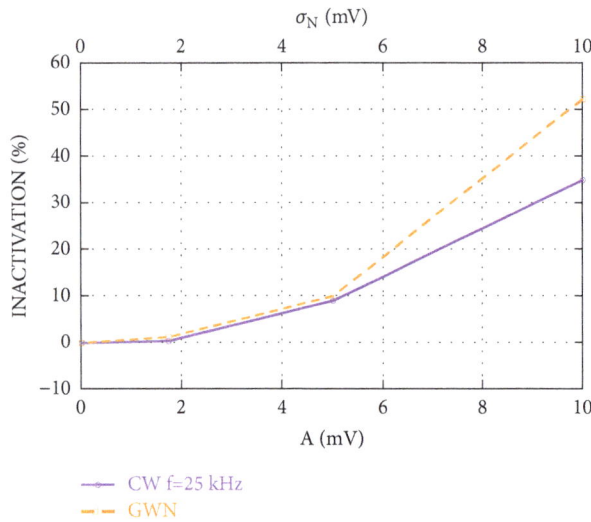

FIGURE 3: Inactivation induced by the CW stimulation versus the amplitude A of the CW at 25 kHz (purple solid line) and inactivation induced by the GWN stimulation versus its standard deviation σ_N (orange dashed line); A and σ_N assume the same values; $I_0 = 6$ $\mu A/cm^2$; patch area = 15.7 μm^2.

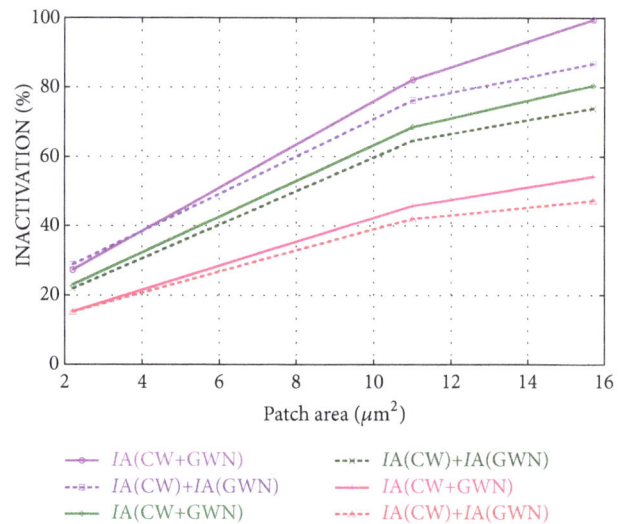

FIGURE 4: Inactivation IA versus patch area for $I_0 = 6$ $\mu A/cm^2$ (purple lines), $I_0 = 7$ $\mu A/cm^2$ (green lines), and $I_0 = 10$ $\mu A/cm^2$ (magenta lines), obtained by combining the CW at 25 kHz 10 mV and the GWN, $\sigma_N = 10$ mV (solid lines), compared with the superposition of the inactivations induced by the two stimulations applied individually (dashed lines).

the reduction of the pathologic firing rate to the spontaneous activity of a healthy auditory fiber.

To simulate the single Ranvier node of an auditory fiber, a stochastic HH neuron model was used, since it is well characterized and considered as a reference model in the literature for a lot of different applications with more than

10000 citations in the Scopus database [24]. The authors themselves already used it to study neuronal encoding [37, 38, 42, 43] and to explain the analgesic effect of the Complex Neuroelectromagnetic Pulse [44] by means of a silencing mechanism [19].

A limitation of the used model is that, even if a temperature correction factor is used [45], it cannot work at the mammalian temperature of 37°C. In the HH model, a temperature increase causes the threshold current density to shift towards higher values, and the firing rate to change depending on the patch size [45]. So, different operating conditions, in terms of bias current densities, would mimic healthy and pathologic neuronal activities. Similar mechanisms of relative firing reduction are expected to occur for a suitable combination of signal and noise since the model anyway presents two attraction basins for firing ad resting states and the exogenous stimulation can push the system from one state to the other. However, since the temperature adjustment in neuronal models is still an open question, here it was preferred to use the well-assessed reference temperature for the HH model.

Due to the generality of the used model and the high number of degrees of freedom, a complete evaluation of the uncertainty budget is not practicable but, besides the temperature, the other main variables that may influence results are examined in the following.

An aspect that could contribute to the uncertainty of results is that, for frequencies above 10 kHz, the membrane capacitance per unit area (C_m) is not constant, differently from what was assumed in our model. In fact, the permittivity of the cell membrane decreases with frequency due to the relaxation of the alpha polarization phenomenon [46]. Nevertheless, our simplification is largely acceptable since the frequency dependence of C_m was shown to have a negligible effect on the stimulation threshold of a HH model (median = 1.4%) [47].

Other model parameters that induce a great variability of results are the bias current density I_0 and the patch area. When applying a combination of the CW (f=25 kHz, A=10 mV) and the GWN (σ_N=10 mV) to the neuronal patch of 15.7 μm^2, the inactivation ranges from 54% (I_0=10 $\mu A/cm^2$) to 100% (I_0=6 $\mu A/cm^2$). Conversely, for I_0=6 $\mu A/cm^2$, the inactivation passes from 28% to 100% if the patch size increases from 2.2 to 15.7 μm^2. Such variations could explain the great variability of results on human volunteers [16] that could be attributed to the individual variability of auditory fiber size (patch area in the model) and tinnitus severity (bias current density in the model).

This study suggests a plausible mechanism of tinnitus suppression using exogenous electrical excitation and is a first step towards the characterization of kind and parameters of stimulation that maximize the efficacy while reducing possible short-term or long-term side effects, such as unwanted sound perception or adaptation.

To control side effects, charge-balanced signals should be used and the induced currents should not exceed typical currents used in cochlear prostheses. A recent dosimetric study [48] revealed that a typical cochlear implant delivered, at the location of the afferent fibers of the auditory nerve, a peak voltage of several tens of mVs, higher than the signal amplitudes used in this work ($\leq$ 10 mV). This suggests that the stimulation signals used in this work are plausible to be released from cochlear implants without severe side effects, even though it will be necessary to conduct a careful risk analysis to assess the safety of the proposed technique.

5. Conclusions

A stochastic HH neuron model was used to evaluate the efficacy of different electric stimulation strategies in tinnitus suppression. The used stimulations were CW signals at different frequencies in the range of tens of kHz and GWN.

Results of simulations show that both a CW and a white noise, applied individually to the neuron model, may induce a firing inhibition. The inactivation level is shown to depend on many parameters, such as patch area, bias current density, CW frequency and amplitude, and noise standard deviation. The more the background activity is low (larger patch size and lower bias currents), the more the inactivation is high. Considerable inactivation values are obtained by using either CW at 25 or 35 kHz or GWN with 10 mV of standard deviation, but GWN is shown to be more efficient than CW (IA=53% versus IA=35% in the best condition) for a comparable amplitude of fluctuations.

Moreover, the inactivation induced by a combination of signal and noise is almost always higher than the sum of the inactivations induced by the two stimulations applied individually and it reaches 100% for the lowest I_0 and the highest patch area.

These results are a proof of concept that signal and noise act on the neuron in a cooperative way and could be suitably delivered in combination through cochlear prosthesis to alleviate tinnitus while reducing possible side effects due to a broadband stimulation.

Future works will concern the validation of the presented results on a mammalian neuronal model at 37°C, such as the Spatially Extended Nonlinear Node (SENN) [49] and the McIntyre-Richardson-Grill (MRG) [50] models and the identification of a colored stimulating noise suitably filtered considering the typical frequency selectivity of the used model.

Disclosure

This work was partially performed within the context of the European COST EMF-MED Action BM1309. Preliminary results were presented at the Joint Annual Meeting of the Bioelectromagnetics Society and the European BioElectromagnetics Association, Ghent, Belgium, 2016.

Conflicts of Interest

The authors report no conflicts of interest. The authors alone are responsible for the content and writing of the paper.

References

[1] K. Brunger, "Managing tinnitus," *The Journal of Family Health Care*, vol. 18, no. 2, pp. 47-48, 2008.

[2] J. Shargorodsky, G. C. Curhan, and W. R. Farwell, "Prevalence and characteristics of tinnitus among US adults," *American Journal of Medicine*, vol. 123, no. 8, pp. 711–718, 2010.

[3] B. Scott and P. Lindberg, "Psychological profile and somatic complaints between help-seeking and non-help-seeking tinnitus subjects," *Psychosomatics*, vol. 41, no. 4, pp. 347–352, 2000.

[4] H. P. Zenner, M. Pfister, and N. Birbaumer, "Tinnitus sensitization: Sensory and psychophysiological aspects of a new pathway of acquired centralization of chronic tinnitus," *Otology & Neurotology*, vol. 27, no. 8, pp. 1054–1063, 2006.

[5] G. Baracca, L. Del Bo, and U. Ambrosetti, "Tinnitus and hearing loss," in *Textbook of Tinnitus*, A. R. Møller, B. Langguth, D. De Ridder, and T. Kleinjung, Eds., pp. 285–291, Springer, New York, NY, USA, 2011.

[6] C. Nicolas-Puel, T. Akbaraly, R. Lloyd et al., "Characteristics of tinnitus in a population of 555 patients: Specificities of tinnitus induced by noise trauma," *International Tinnitus Journal*, vol. 12, no. 1, pp. 64–70, 2006.

[7] F. Martines, D. Bentivegna, E. Martines, V. Sciacca, and G. Martinciglio, "Characteristics of tinnitus with or without hearing loss: Clinical observations in Sicilian tinnitus patients," *Auris Nasus Larynx*, vol. 37, no. 6, pp. 685–693, 2010.

[8] G. Ehret, "Tonotopic organization (maps)," in *Encyclopedia of Neuroscience*, pp. 4083–4088, 2009.

[9] E. L. Le Page, "A model for cochlear origin of subjective tinnitus: excitatory drift in the operating point of inner hair cells," in *Mechanisms of Tinnitus*, J. A. Vernon and A. R. Moller, Eds., pp. 115–148, Allyn and Bacon, London, 1995.

[10] A. J. Noreña, M. Tomita, and J. J. Eggermont, "Neural changes in cat auditory cortex after a transient pure-tone trauma," *Journal of Neurophysiology*, vol. 90, no. 4, pp. 2387–2401, 2003.

[11] A. J. Noreña and J. J. Eggermont, "Changes in spontaneous neural activity immediately after an acoustic trauma: implications for neural correlates of tinnitus," *Hearing Research*, vol. 183, no. 1-2, pp. 137–153, 2003.

[12] J. A. Kaltenbach, "Tinnitus: models and mechanisms," *Hearing Research*, vol. 276, no. 1-2, pp. 52–60, 2011.

[13] P. G. Finlayson and J. A. Kaltenbach, "Alterations in the spontaneous discharge patterns of single units in the dorsal cochlear nucleus following intense sound exposure," *Hearing Research*, vol. 256, no. 1-2, pp. 104–117, 2009.

[14] W. S. Mckerrow, C. E. Schreiner, M. M. Merzenich, R. L. Snyder, and J. G. Toner, "Tinnitus suppression by cochlear implants," *Annals of Otology, Rhinology & Laryngology*, vol. 100, no. 7, pp. 552–558, 1991.

[15] J. T. Rubinstein, R. S. Tyler, A. Johnson, and C. J. Brown, "Electrical suppression of tinnitus with high-rate pulse trains," *Otology & Neurotology*, vol. 24, no. 3, pp. 478–485, 2003.

[16] J. E. Chang and F. Zeng, "Tinnitus suppression by electric stimulation of the auditory nerve," *Frontiers in Systems Neuroscience*, vol. 6, article 19, 2012.

[17] F.-G. Zeng, Q. Tang, A. Dimitrijevic, A. Starr, J. Larky, and N. H. Blevins, "Tinnitus suppression by low-rate electric stimulation and its electrophysiological mechanisms," *Hearing Research*, vol. 277, no. 1-2, pp. 61–66, 2011.

[18] R. Tyler, A. Cacace, C. Stocking et al., "Vagus Nerve Stimulation Paired with Tones for the Treatment of Tinnitus: A Prospective Randomized Double-blind Controlled Pilot Study in Humans," *Scientific Reports*, vol. 7, no. 1, 2017.

[19] F. Camera, A. Paffi, A. W. Thomas et al., "The CNP signal is able to silence a supra threshold neuronal model," *Frontiers in Computational Neuroscience*, vol. 9, Article 44, pp. 1–11, 2015.

[20] A. L. Hodgkin and A. F. Huxley, "A quantitative description of membrane current and its application to conduction and excitation in nerve.," *The Journal of Physiology*, vol. 117, no. 4, pp. 500–544, 1952.

[21] E. Schneidman, B. Freedman, and I. Segev, "Ion Channel Stochasticity May be Critical in Determining the Reliability and Precision of Spike Timing," *Neural Computation*, vol. 10, no. 7, pp. 1679–1703, 1998.

[22] J. R. Clay and L. J. DeFelice, "Relationship between membrane excitability and single channel open-close kinetics," *Biophysical Journal*, vol. 42, no. 2, pp. 151–157, 1983.

[23] E. M. Izhikevich, *Dynamical Systems in Neuroscience: The Geometry of Excit- ability and Bursting*, MIT Press, Cambridge, UK, 2006.

[24] Scopus database, (https://www.scopus.com).

[25] F. Rattay, "Basics of hearing theory and noise in cochlear implants," *Chaos, Solitons & Fractals*, vol. 11, no. 12, pp. 1875–1884, 2000.

[26] H. Mino and W. M. Grill Jr., "Effects of stochastic sodium channels on extracellular excitation of myelinated nerve fibers," *IEEE Transactions on Biomedical Engineering*, vol. 49, no. 6, pp. 527–532, 2002.

[27] H. Mino, J. T. Rubinstein, and J. A. White, "Comparison of algorithms for the simulation of action potentials with stochastic sodium channels," *Annals of Biomedical Engineering*, vol. 30, no. 4, pp. 578–587, 2002.

[28] J. H. Goldwyn, N. S. Imennov, M. Famulare, and E. Shea-Brown, "Stochastic differential equation models for ion channel noise in Hodgkin-Huxley neurons," *Physical Review E: Statistical, Nonlinear, and Soft Matter Physics*, vol. 83, no. 4, 2011.

[29] J. T. Rubinstein, "Threshold fluctuations in an N sodium channel model of the node of Ranvier," *Biophysical Journal*, vol. 68, no. 3, pp. 779–785, 1995.

[30] J. A. White, J. T. Rubinstein, and A. R. Kay, "Channel noise in neurons," *Trends in Neurosciences*, vol. 23, no. 3, pp. 131–137, 2000.

[31] C. Merla, M. Liberti, F. Apollonio, and G. D'inzeo, "Quantitative assessment of dielectric parameters for membrane lipid bilayers from rf permittivity measurements," *Bioelectromagnetics*, vol. 30, no. 4, pp. 286–298, 2009.

[32] E. Neher and B. Sakmann, "Single-channel currents recorded from membrane of denervated frog muscle fibers," in *A Century of Nature: Twenty-One Discoveries that Changed Science and the World*, L. Garwin and T. Lincoln, Eds., 2003.

[33] P. Marracino, M. Liberti, E. Trapani et al., "Human aquaporin 4 gating dynamics under perpendicularly-oriented electric-field impulses: A molecular dynamics study," *International Journal of Molecular Sciences*, vol. 17, no. 7, article no. 1133, 2016.

[34] C. Merla, A. Denzi, A. Paffi et al., "Novel passive element circuits for microdosimetry of nanosecond pulsed electric fields," *IEEE Transactions on Biomedical Engineering*, vol. 59, no. 8, pp. 2302–2311, 2012.

[35] F. Apollonio, M. Liberti, A. Paffi et al., "Feasibility for microwaves energy to affect biological systems via nonthermal mechanisms: a systematic approach," *IEEE Transactions on Microwave Theory and Techniques*, vol. 61, no. 5, pp. 2031–2045, 2013.

[36] A. Denzi, C. Merla, P. Camilleri et al., "Microdosimetric study for nanosecond pulsed electric fields on a cell circuit model with nucleus," *Journal of Membrane Biology*, vol. 246, no. 10, pp. 761–767, 2013.

[37] A. Paffi, F. Apollonio, G. d'Inzeo, and M. Liberti, "Stochastic resonance induced by exogenous noise in a model of a neuronal

network," *Network: Computation in Neural Systems*, vol. 24, no. 3, pp. 99–113, 2013.

[38] A. Paffi, F. Camera, F. Apollonio, G. D'Inzeo, and M. Liberti, "Restoring the encoding properties of a stochastic neuron model by an exogenous noise," *Frontiers in Computational Neuroscience*, vol. 9, Article 42, pp. 1–11, 2015.

[39] T. Y. Tsong and R. D. Astumian, "Electroconformational coupling and membrane protein function," *Progress in Biophysics and Molecular Biology*, vol. 50, no. 1, pp. 1–45, 1987.

[40] H. Mino, J. T. Rubinstein, C. A. Miller, and P. J. Abbas, "Effects of electrode-to-fiber distance on temporal neural response with electrical stimulation," *IEEE Transactions on Biomedical Engineering*, vol. 51, no. 1, pp. 13–20, 2004.

[41] F. Liu, J. Wang, and W. Wang, "Frequency sensitivity in weak signal detection," *Physical Review E: Statistical, Nonlinear, and Soft Matter Physics*, vol. 59, no. 3, pp. 3453–3460, 1999.

[42] S. Orcioni, A. Paffi, F. Camera, F. Apollonio, and M. Liberti, "Automatic decoding of input sinusoidal signal in a neuron model: Improved SNR spectrum by low-pass homomorphic filtering," *Neurocomputing*, vol. 267, pp. 605–614, 2017.

[43] S. Orcioni, A. Paffi, F. Camera, F. Apollonio, and M. Liberti, "Automatic decoding of input sinusoidal signal in a neuron model: high pass homomorphic filtering," *Neurocomputing*, vol. 292, pp. 165–173, 2018.

[44] A. W. Thomas, M. Kavaliers, F. S. Prato, and K.-P. Ossenkopp, "Antinociceptive effects of a pulsed magnetic field in the land snail, Cepaea nemoralis," *Neuroscience Letters*, vol. 222, no. 2, pp. 107–110, 1997.

[45] L. Yang and Y. Jia, "Effects of patch temperature on spontaneous action potential train due to channel fluctuations: Coherence resonance," *BioSystems*, vol. 81, no. 3, pp. 267–280, 2005.

[46] K. R. Foster and H. P. Schwan, "Dielectric properties of tissues and biological materials: a critical review," *Critical Reviews in Biomedical Engineering*, vol. 17, pp. 25–104, 1989.

[47] B. Howell, L. E. Medina, and W. M. Grill, "Effects of frequency-dependent membrane capacitance on neural excitability," *Journal of Neural Engineering*, vol. 12, no. 5, Article ID 056015, 2015.

[48] G. Tognola, A. Pesatori, M. Norgia et al., "Numerical modeling and experimental measurements of the electric potential generated by cochlear implants in physiological tissues," *IEEE Transactions on Instrumentation and Measurement*, vol. 56, no. 1, pp. 187–193, 2007.

[49] J. P. Reilly and A. M. Diamant, *Electrostimulation Theory, Applications, and Computational Models*, 2011, http://www.artechhouse.com.

[50] C. C. McIntyre, A. G. Richardson, and W. M. Grill, "Modeling the excitability of mammalian nerve fibers: Influence of afterpotentials on the recovery cycle," *Journal of Neurophysiology*, vol. 87, no. 2, pp. 995–1006, 2002.

8

Method for Calculating the Bending Angle of Puncture Needle in Preoperative Planning for Transjugular Intrahepatic Portal Systemic Shunt (TIPS)

Xiaoli Zhu,[1] **Zhao Ran,**[2] **Wanci Li,**[1] **Wansheng Wang,**[1] **Kangshun Zhu** [iD],[3] **Wensou Huang,**[3] **and Xin Gao** [iD][2]

[1]*Invasive Technology Department, The First Affiliated Hospital of Soochow University, No. 899, Pinghai Road, Suzhou, Jiangsu 215006, China*
[2]*Department of Medical Imaging, Suzhou Institute of Biomedical Engineering and Technology, Chinese Academy of Sciences, No. 88, Keling Road, Suzhou, Jiangsu 215163, China*
[3]*Department of Minimally Invasive Interventional Radiology, The Second Affiliated Hospital of Guangzhou Medical University, No. 250, Changgang East Road, Guangzhou, Guangdong 510260, China*

Correspondence should be addressed to Xin Gao; xingaosam@yahoo.com

Academic Editor: Hiro Yoshida

Transjugular Intrahepatic Portal Systemic Shunt is a comprehensive interventional therapy for portal hypertension. During this intervention, puncturing from hepatic vein into portal vein is a difficult step. Selecting puncture needle with a proper bending angle is vital to accurate puncture. Thus, this prospective study provides a method to calculate the angle of the puncture needle using preinterventional contrast-enhanced CT imaging. According to the geometrical characteristics of puncture needle, Bezier curve equation was adopted to describe its bending part. By testing whether each point in a specific region satisfied the equation set of Bezier curves, the possible position of needle tip was obtained. Then, the bending angle of puncture needle was obtained by calculating curvature. The method was evaluated in 13 patients from 2 centers showing now a success rate of 100% and a duration of the procedure of 141 and 161 minutes. The method based on Bezier curve equation for calculating a proper bending angle of puncture needle was proven to be effective. And the clinical study is preliminary and additional work for clinical evaluation is necessary.

1. Introduction

Portal hypertension (PH) refers to a group of clinical syndromes characterized by abnormal changes of hemodynamics in portal vein system. It is also a major complication of cirrhosis and can even lead to death. Transjugular Intrahepatic Portal Systemic Shunt (TIPS) is a kind of comprehensive interventional therapy for PH [1, 2]. TIPS adopts radiation technology and uses special equipment (puncture needle with an bending angle, stent, etc.) to build a shunt between inferior vena cava and the branch of portal vein, so part of the bloodstream in portal vein can flow into inferior vena cava. Finally, portal vein pressure is decreased and severe complications caused by PH can be controlled and even prevented [3, 4].

Currently, the frequently used puncture tools are RUPS100 or RTPS100 puncture kits manufactured by Cook Company (USA). In the puncture kits, the puncture needle has only one type of bending angle. However, the causes of PH vary with patients, and the structure of intrahepatic vascular system, especially the spatial relationship between hepatic vein and portal vein, also varies with patients. Thus, the puncture needle currently used cannot meet the requirement of personalized treatment. Clinical practice indicates that choosing a puncture needle with a proper bending angle is necessary for accurate puncture of the portal vein [5]. Currently, the bending angle of puncture needle is adjusted by doctors according to their experiences. This process lacks accuracy. Once an improper bending angle is chosen, puncture cannot be performed according to the preplanned path and there is even a high risk of abdominal bleeding, resulting in intervention failure.

Therefore, the aim of this preliminary study was to provide a method that enables calculating the bending angle of the puncture needle on the basis of a previous CT imaging. The method was then evaluated in a small pilot study including 13 patients receiving a TIPS. The clinical study is preliminary and additional work for clinical evaluation is necessary.

2. Methods

2.1. Subjects. Between July 2016 and December 2016, clinical image data of 4 subjects from the First Affiliated Hospital of Soochow University (SU hospital) and 9 subjects from the Second Affiliated Hospital of Guangzhou Medical University were collected. These 13 subjects were supposed to undergo TIPS. This study was approved by the local Institutional Review Board. Among the subjects, eight patients were male and five were female. Their average age was 45 ± 4 years. Inclusion criteria include the following: (1) endoscopy confirmed esophageal or gastric varices bleeding, and the medical treatment cannot control bleeding effectively; (2) a history of portal hypertension in upper gastrointestinal bleeding and endoscopic or CT examination showed that esophageal or gastric fundus is still significantly varicose and not suitable for endoscopic therapy. Exclusion criteria included the following: (1) suffering from hepatic vein or intrahepatic portal vein or inferior vena cava occlusion; (2) patients with absolute contraindications to TIPS; (3) unwilling to accept the TIPS intervention patients

2.2. Path Planning. Iterative threshold segmentation combined with morphological operation was adopted to segment liver. Then, double threshold method was used to extract hepatic veins and portal veins in the segmented liver. Subsequently, 3D visualization was performed by using a surface-rendering method. Finally, the visualized image was put into 3D Slicer and an interventional physician was asked to designate two puncture points according to the anatomical spatial relationship between hepatic vein and portal vein. The point at which the needle punctured outside the hepatic vein was denoted as the Initial Point (IP). The point at which the needle punctured into the portal vein was denoted as the Terminal Point (TP). The preferred IP location was on the right hepatic veins, about 2 cm from the IVC. The preferred TP position was on the right branch of portal or on the left branch of portal, about 2 cm from the portal vein bifurcation. According to IP and TP, the puncture path was constructed (Figure 1).

2.3. Calculation of Bending Angle. In the plane where the puncture path was, puncture needle moved forward from IP to TP. Puncturing into portal vein (branch) was a critical step, after which guide wire was induced into the portal vein (trunk) for subsequent stent implantation. The whole puncture process depended on the bending angle of puncture needle. Only a proper bending angle can ensure the needle

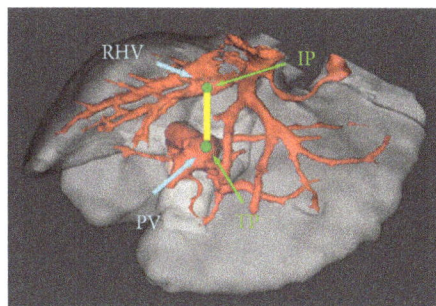

FIGURE 1: Schematic illustration of puncture path planning.

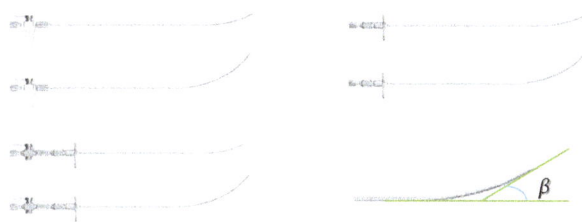

FIGURE 2: Puncture needle and its bending angle.

to move toward portal vein after puncturing outside hepatic vein and then puncture into the branch of portal vein. Otherwise, puncture process might be performed several times before success, and the risk of liver bleeding might be increased, resulting in intervention failure. As shown in Figure 2, the angle between the tangent of needle body and the tangent of needle tip was defined as the bending angle.

2.3.1. Construction of Puncture Plane. CT imaging system had self-defined coordinate system, which was denoted as S_{CT}. According to parameters (voxel position, voxel size, and layer distance) in DICOM file of CT image, the coordinates of voxel in S_{CT} can be determined. The coordinates of preplanned puncture points IP and TP in S_{CT} can also be obtained, which were (x_I, y_I, z_I) and (x_T, y_T, z_T), respectively. A successful puncture operation meant that the puncture needle passed through IP and TP as well as a random point (RP) (x_R, y_R, z_R) on the puncture path. These three points determined a puncture plane. According to equation of a plane passing through three points, that is,

$$\begin{vmatrix} x - x_R & y - y_R & z - z_R \\ x_I - x_R & y_I - y_R & z_I - z_R \\ x_T - x_R & y_T - y_R & z_T - z_R \end{vmatrix} = 0, \quad (1)$$

we could obtain the equation of the puncture plane:

$$Ax + By + Cz + D = 0 \quad (2)$$

where A, B, C, and D were coefficients. Then, the unit normal vector of the puncture plane was $\overrightarrow{n} = (A/\sqrt{A^2 + B^2 + C^2}, B/\sqrt{A^2 + B^2 + C^2}, C/\sqrt{A^2 + B^2 + C^2})$, which was denoted as $\overrightarrow{n} = (n_x, n_y, n_z)$.

To conveniently use equations of curves for calculation, the 3D coordinate system was projected into a 2D coordinate

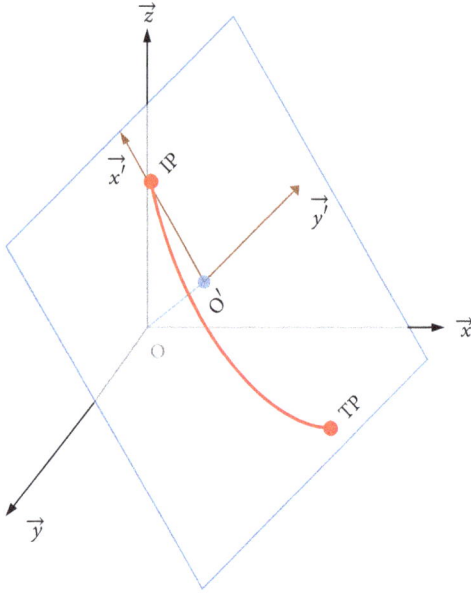

FIGURE 3: Projecting the 3D coordinate system into a 2D coordinate system. The gray plane was the puncture plane.

system. As shown in Figure 3, the origin O of S_{CT} was projected onto the puncture plane and O' was the projection of O. Then, O' was taken as the origin of the new 2D coordinate system, called S_{PUNC}. x-axis of the 2D coordinate system was the line passing through O' and IP. y-axis was perpendicular to x-axis and also in the puncture plane. Thus, the 2D coordinate system S_{PUNC} was built for the puncture plane:

(a) Origin O': $O' = -D(n_x, n_y, n_z)$. Because $\overrightarrow{OO'} // \vec{n}$, $O' = \partial \vec{n} = \partial(n_x, n_y, n_z)$. Since O' was on the puncture plane, it should satisfy the equation of the plane (see (2)). Thus, we had $\partial = -D/|\vec{n}|^2 = -D$ (length of unit vector was 1).

(b) Unit vector of x-axis: $\overrightarrow{N_{x'}} = \overrightarrow{O'I}/|\overrightarrow{O'I}|$. $\overrightarrow{O'I}$ was the vector passing through O' and IP. Coordinates of O' were obtained in (a) and coordinates of IP were obtained during above-mentioned preplanning process.

(c) Unit vector of y-axis: $\overrightarrow{N_{y'}} = \overrightarrow{O'I} \times \overrightarrow{O'O}$. Unit vector of y-axis was the cross product of $\overrightarrow{O'I}$ and $\overrightarrow{O'O}$, which was perpendicular to the puncture plane.

According to (b) and (c), the basis of S_{PUNC} was $(\overrightarrow{O'I}/|\overrightarrow{O'I}|, N_{y'})$. Any point $Q(x_q, y_q, z_q)$ inside a patient's body in the original 3D coordinate system projected onto the puncture plane had coordinates $Q'(\overrightarrow{O'Q} \cdot \overrightarrow{O'I}/|\overrightarrow{O'I}|, \overrightarrow{N_{y'}})$ in the 2D coordinate system S_{PUNC}. This projection process was denoted as $f: S_{CT} \rightarrow S_{PUNC}$.

2.3.2. Curve Fitting. Bezier curve was an important parametric curve in computer graphics. It can use mathematical language to precisely describe any complicated graphs. Bezier curve was developed by Paul de Casteljau in 1959 using de Casteljau algorithm and was published by Pierre Bezier,

a French engineer, in 1962 [6]. It had wide application in industrial design. Bezier curve had multiorder expressions. The second-order expression was defined as follows. As shown in Figure 4(a), three points including endpoints P_0 and P_2 and control points P_1 were given. Point Q_0 moved along line segment $P_0 P_1$ and divided this line segment into two parts with a ratio t:1-t (first-order Bezier curve). Another point Q_1 on line segment $P_1 P_2$ was chosen and it divided the line segment $P_1 P_2$ into two parts also with the ratio t:1-t. Finally, a point B on line segment $Q_0 Q_1$ was chosen and it also divided the line segment $P_1 P_2$ into two parts with the ratio t:1-t. When t changed from 0 to 1, Q_0 moved from P_0 to P_1 and Q_1 moved from P_1 to P_2. During this process, the movement trajectory of B was a second-order Bezier curve and had the following equation:

$$B(t) = (1-t)^2 \mathbf{p}_0 + 2t(1-t)\mathbf{p}_1 + t^2 \mathbf{p}_2, \quad t \in [0,1] \quad (3)$$

where $\mathbf{p}_0$, $\mathbf{p}_1$, and $\mathbf{p}_2$ are the coordinates of P_0, P_1, and P_2.

It was found that Bezier curve tool in vector mapping software can well fit the bending part of the needle (Figure 4(b)). It was thus assumed that the bending part of needle can be described by the Bezier curve. In Figure 4(b), the point at which the needle began to bend (bending point) was the starting point P_0 of Bezier curve, and the needle tip was the endpoint P_2 of Bezier curve.

Before intervention, the bending angle of puncture needle should be adjusted manually to meet the requirement of the preplanned path. When the bending point of puncture needle reached IP, the needle could hardly move forward. It was expected that the needle tip can reach TP. However, the currently used puncture needle had only one type of bending angle and length of the bending part was fixed. Moreover, the spatial relationship between IP and TP varied with patients. Therefore, the needle tip might not be able to reach TP. In fact, if the extension line of needle tip passed through TP, accurate puncture can also be achieved. As shown in Figure 5(a), it was assumed that the bending part of puncture needle can always be described by the equation of second-order Bezier curve when the bending angle was manually adjusted. In addition, the position of bending point and tangent at the bending point were assumed not to change, whereas the position of needle tip and tangent at the needle tip changed with the bending angle. The needle was rigid, so the length of its bending part was not supposed to change when the bending angle was adjusted. In the Bezier curve, this assumption conformed to the calculation rules. As shown in Figure 5(b), the change of the Bezier curve for puncture needle was simulated in Mathematica.

According to above assumptions, two conditions were always satisfied when the bending angle was adjusted.

(1) The Extension Line of Needle Tip Must Pass through Puncture Point TP. When the bending angle was proper, puncture can be successfully performed according to the preplanned path. In that case, bending point must be where IP was, and needle tip or its extension line must be able to reach TP. Bending point or IP was the starting point P_0 of Bezier curve, and needle tip was the endpoint P_2 of Bezier curve. The position of the needle tip changed with bending

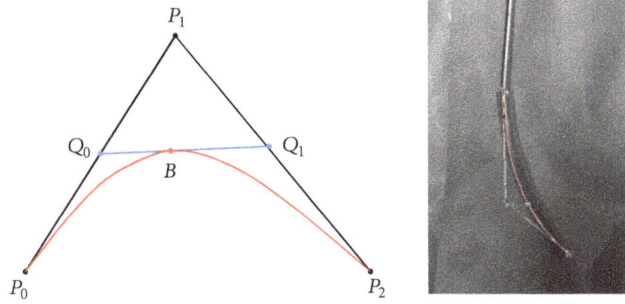

FIGURE 4: (a) Two-order Bezier curve. (b) Bezier curve matching puncture needle.

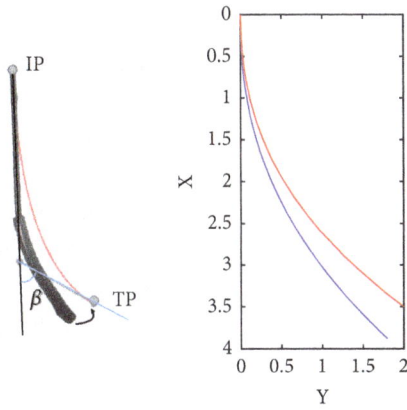

FIGURE 5: (a) Change of the bending part of puncture needle. (b) Change of corresponding Bezier curve in Mathematica.

where (x_0, y_0), (x_1, y_1), and (x_2, y_2) were coordinates of P_0, P_1, and P_2, respectively, of Bezier curve in 2D coordinate system. When the bending angle was adjusted, (x_0, y_0) (i.e., coordinates of IP in S_{PUNC}) remained the same, but (x_1, y_1) and (x_2, y_2) changed with bending angle. The slope at needle tip (t = 1, P2) was $k|_{t=1} = (-y_1 + y_2)/(-x_1 + x_2)$, where (x_1, y_1) and (x_2, y_2) were unknown. The slope of line segment TP P_2 was $k|_{TP,P_2} = (y_2 - y_T')/(x_2 - x_T')$, where (x_T', y_T') were coordinates of TP in S_{PUNC}.

(2) The Length of Bending Part of the Needle Remained the Same. First, we measured the length of bending part of the needle by using a soft thread. The bending part was found to have a length of 4.35 cm.

The bending part can be described by the equation of Bezier curve, so we had

$$x'(t) = -2(1 - t) x_0 + 2t (1 - 2t) x_1 + 2tx_2,$$
$$t \in [0, 1]$$
$$y'(t) = -2(1 - t) y_0 + 2t (1 - 2t) y_1 + 2ty_2,$$
$$t \in [0, 1] \tag{5}$$

According to integral formula

$$L = \int_\alpha^\beta 1 \cdot \sqrt{x'(t)^2 + y'(t)^2} dt, \quad t \in [0, 1] \tag{6}$$

we can obtain the length of bending part of the needle. The calculation formula was

angle, but its extension line always passed through puncture point TP. Thus, the movement pattern of the needle tip can be obtained. On this basis, we could obtain the slope of tangent at needle tip according to Bezier curve and further obtain the bending angle.

The slope at any point on the Bezier curve was

$$k = \frac{dy/dt}{dx/dt} = \frac{-(1 - t) y_0 + (1 - 2t) y_1 + ty_2}{-(1 - t) x_0 + (1 - 2t) x_1 + tx_2},$$
$$t \in [0, 1] \tag{4}$$

$$L$$
$$= \int_0^1 \sqrt{4(1 - t)^2 (x_0{}^2 + y_0{}^2) + 4(1 - 2t)^2 (x_1{}^2 + y_1{}^2) + 4t^2 (x_2{}^2 + y_2{}^2) + 8t(1 - 2t)(x_1 x_2 + y_1 y_2) - 8(1 - t)(1 - 2t)(x_0 x_1 + y_0 y_1) - 8t(1 - t)(x_0 x_2 + y_0 y_2)} dt \tag{7}$$

where (x_0, y_0), (x_1, y_1), and (x_2, y_2) were coordinates of P_0, P_1, and P_2, respectively, in 2D coordinate system.

According to the above two conditions, the following equations were obtained:

$$\int_0^1 \sqrt{4(1 - t)^2 (x_0{}^2 + y_0{}^2) + 4(1 - 2t)^2 (x_1{}^2 + y_1{}^2) + 4t^2 (x_2{}^2 + y_2{}^2) + 8t(1 - 2t)(x_1 x_2 + y_1 y_2) - 8(1 - t)(1 - 2t)(x_0 x_1 + y_0 y_1) - 8t(1 - t)(x_0 x_2 + y_0 y_2)} dt$$
$$= 4.35 \tag{8}$$
$$\frac{-y_1 + y_2}{-x_1 + x_2} = \frac{y_2 - y_T'}{x_2 - x_T'}$$

TABLE 1: Coordinates of puncture points in S_{CT} chosen by interventional physician for each subject.

Subject number	IP (x_I, y_I, z_I)	TP (x_T, y_T, z_T)
1	$(218, 263, 34)$	$(190, 230, 24)$
2	$(188, 243, 34)$	$(172, 240, 25)$
3	$(170, 275, 35)$	$(172, 258, 27)$
4	$(202, 258, 27)$	$(201, 251, 21)$
5	$(192, 241, 31)$	$(172, 228, 21)$
6	$(225, 285, 34)$	$(210, 263, 23)$
7	$(204, 258, 37)$	$(201, 248, 30)$
8	$(201, 255, 72)$	$(197, 236, 65)$
9	$(201, 332, 27)$	$(175, 317, 21)$
10	$(202, 262, 37)$	$(188, 257, 29)$
11	$(210, 265, 36)$	$(197, 248, 30)$
12	$(201, 264, 33)$	$(189, 257, 27)$
13	$(210, 283, 33)$	$(189, 257, 27)$

TABLE 2: Calculated bending angle of puncture needle for each subject.

Subject number	Bending angle (degree)
1	30.7
2	41.0
3	37.5
4	36.2
5	39.5
6	40.2
7	66.7
8	52.5
9	54.2
10	36.0
11	36.2
12	45.1
13	41.0

When the bending angle was adjusted, the position of starting point P_0 did not change, whereas the positions of control point P_1 and endpoint P_2 changed. There were four unknown parameters but only two equations, so we cannot obtain the exact solutions of the equations. Even obtaining the movement trajectory of P_2 (i.e., the equation that (x_2, y_2) satisfied) was difficult. In actual case, the range within which the bending angle changed would not be very large, since the needle was made of rigid material. Thus, we could use all the points in the circle whose center was at the initial position of the needle tip and radius was 2 cm to solve the problem. According to the resolution of the voxel space, all the points in the circle whose center was at the initial position of the needle tip and radius was 4 were tested if they satisfied (5). The step was set at 1. By doing so, we can obtain the position of P_2. The calculation was performed in Matlab and Mathematica.

According to the definition of the bending angle, we had

$$\beta = \arctan\ k|_{P_2} - \arctan\ k|_{P_0} \tag{9}$$

With the obtained position of P_2 (x_2, y_2), we could obtain β.

3. Results

13 patients with portal hypertension underwent TIPS placement in two centers from July 2016 to December 2016. CECT was performed on each subject before TIPS. The CECT data were then used for preoperative planning.

After the original DICOM data were obtained, liver and blood vessels were segmented and were three-dimensionally visualized. Then an interventional physician was asked to designate puncture points for each subject. The coordinates of puncture points in S_{CT} for each subject were shown in Table 1.

After calculation, the bending angle of puncture needle for each subject was obtained (Table 2).

Because of a lack of intraoperative real-time imaging, the positions of actual puncture points IP and TP were a little different from those of the preplanned puncture points. Thus, the actual path was also different from the preplanned one. To evaluate the effect of bending angle

on puncture efficiency, we adopted subjective and objective evaluations. The indicators were average puncture times, whether puncture needle deviated from the targeted point even punctured outside liver during intervention, whether there were puncture-related complications after intervention, and so forth. The clinical results were in Table 3.

Here, the procedure time referred to the time it took to perform the standard operations of TIPS. There were only two subjects whose results were not very good; the procedure time and puncture times of these two subjects were not as good as other patients. One was because the contrast time for CECT was improper, leading to the fact that the hepatic veins cannot be well segmented. Position of IP selected by interventional physician might be very inaccurate. The other was because the patient had undergone hepatectomy; hepatic tissue reconstruction led to difficulty in puncture.

4. Discussion

The bending angle of puncture needle is only one of the parameters determining the success of TIPS. Some parameters associated with the morphology of hepatic and portal venous systems as well as the positional relationship between them may also influence the accuracy and efficiency of puncture from hepatic vein to liver parenchyma and then into portal vein. However, the morphological structure of hepatic vascular system in patients with portal hypertension of cirrhosis is abnormal. This is caused by the atrophy of liver parenchyma and liver ascites after hepatic fibrosis. Thus, the puncture needle bending angle that we calculated is a reference value. Applying our method, probably many punctures will still not be successful because the needle bending may change during advancing the needle and the liver may move and twist during the puncture. Moreover, the procedure does not provide real-time guidance. Therefore, this does not replace sonographic real-time 3D guidance. It is definitely the gold standard. However, our method can be used as an adjunct, which may always improve the technique irrespective of other guiding attempts.

TABLE 3: Clinical results of subjects in two research centers.

Research center	Average puncture times	Average procedure time (min)	Puncture outside liver	Puncture-related complications
SU[1] (n=4)	3	161	1	0
SYSU[2] (n=9)	2	142	0	0

[1] SU refers to SU Hospital.
[2] SYSU refers to SYSU Hospital.

TIPS is a very difficult and highly risky intervention. In fact, it is thought to be one of the most complicated interventions by *Peripheral Vascular Interventional Diagnosis and Surgery Hierarchical Directory*. The process of puncture needle puncturing outside hepatic vein in a specific region and then precisely puncturing into portal vein branch is a difficult step of TIPS. To solve this problem, Image-guided TIPS intervention [7–9] and path planning method [10–13] have been developed. However, none of them performed calculation of the bending angle of puncture needle. In fact, the bending angle of puncture needle was often subjectively adjusted because of the lack of precise calculation, which might lead to the deviation of puncture needle from the targeted point and the damage to other tissues. In that case, the puncture needle needed to be taken out and reinserted in again, resulting in more puncture times. This paper proposed a method based on Bezier curve equation to precisely calculate a proper bending angle of puncture needle for TIPS. Bezier curve was used to describe the bending part of puncture needle, and Bezier curve equation was used to solve the problem of bending angle. Adjusting puncture needle to obtain a proper bending angle was a critical step during preoperative planning.

A path planning method based on numerical calculation model was proposed, where the critical puncture points can be selected according to preoperative 3D CECT. In addition, a proper bending angle of puncture needle can be calculated based on Bezier curve equation.

Clinical results showed that our method for adjusting the bending angle of puncture needle can well guide the puncture of the portal vein. In this case, the preplanned puncture path and the precisely calculated bending angle of puncture needle can improve puncture accuracy and reduce puncture times, ensuring an effective puncture operation. Knowledge of the bending angle has its own advantage whatever additional guidance is used.

The clinical study is preliminary; the method should be further evaluated intraoperatively and postoperatively on more cases. In the future, we will evaluate the performance of this method by using it in more clinical trials from multiple centers and will propose methods for calculating other parameters related to 3D puncture path.

Conflicts of Interest

The authors declare that there are no conflicts of interest regarding the publication of this article.

Authors' Contributions

Xiaoli Zhu and Zhao Ran are primary authors and contributed equally to this work.

Acknowledgments

This work was partially supported by Science and Technology Plan Projects of Jiangsu-Society Development Project (BE2017671), Science and Technology Plan Projects of Suzhou Health and Family Planning Commission (LCZX201704), and the National Natural Science Foundation of China (81571772).

References

[1] R. S. Rahimi and D. C. Rockey, "Complications of cirrhosis," *Current Opinion in Gastroenterology*, vol. 28, no. 3, pp. 223–229, 2012.

[2] J. Rösch, B. T. Uchida, J. S. Putnam, R. W. Buschman, R. D. Law, and A. L. Hershey, "Experimental intrahepatic portacaval anastomosis: Use of expandable Gianturco stents," *Radiology*, vol. 162, no. 2, pp. 481–485, 1987.

[3] G. M. Richter, G. Noeldge, J. C. Palmaz et al., "Transjugular intrahepatic portacaval stent shunt: Preliminary clinical results," *Radiology*, vol. 174, no. 3, pp. 1027–1030, 1990.

[4] D. Bettinger, E. Knüppel, W. Euringer et al., "Efficacy and safety of transjugular intrahepatic portosystemic shunt (TIPSS) in 40 patients with hepatocellular carcinoma," *Alimentary Pharmacology and Therapeutics*, vol. 41, no. 1, pp. 126–136, 2015.

[5] C. F. Cuijpers, Tips for TIPS [D]; TU Delft, Delft University of Technology, 2015.

[6] Y. Y. Xiong, "Collection of expressions of Bezier curve and their application," in *Proceedings of The Proceedings of The Sixth Geometric Design and Computing Academic Conference*, China Society for Industrial and Mathematics: Geometric Design and Computing Committee, p. 4, 2013.

[7] M. Darcy, "Transjugular intrahepatic portosystemic shunt: Techniques for portal localization," *Techniques in Vascular and Interventional Radiology*, vol. 3, no. 3, pp. 147–157, 2000.

[8] K. Farsad and J. A. Kaufman, "Novel image guidance techniques for portal vein targeting during transjugular intrahepatic portosystemic shunt creation," *Techniques in Vascular and Interventional Radiology*, vol. 19, no. 1, pp. 10–20, 2016.

[9] S.-H. Tang, J.-P. Qin, Q.-F. Shu, and M.-D. Jiang, "The imaging guidance for the portal vein branch puncturing in performing TIPS: recent progress in research," *Journal of Interventional Radiology*, vol. 23, no. 7, pp. 640–643, 2014.

[10] R. Adamus, M. Pfister, and R. W. R. Loose, "Enhancing transjugular intrahepatic portosystemic shunt puncture by using

three-dimensional path planning based on the back projection of two two-dimensional portographs," *Radiology*, vol. 251, no. 2, pp. 543–547, 2009.

[11] J. Tsauo, X. Luo, L. Ye, and X. Li, "Three-dimensional path planning software-assisted transjugular intrahepatic portosystemic shunt: a technical modification," *CardioVascular and Interventional Radiology*, vol. 38, no. 3, pp. 742–746, 2015.

[12] J.-P. Qin, S.-H. Tang, M.-D. Jiang et al., "Contrast enhanced computed tomography and reconstruction of hepatic vascular system for transjugular intrahepatic portal systemic shunt puncture path planning," *World Journal of Gastroenterology*, vol. 21, no. 32, pp. 9623–9629, 2015.

[13] K. Li, Z. Tang, G.-J. Liu, and S.-X. Zhang, "Three-dimensional reconstruction of paracentesis approach in transjugular intrahepatic portosystemic shunt," *Anatomical Science International*, vol. 87, no. 2, pp. 71–79, 2012.

9

A New Approach towards Minimizing the Risk of Misdosing Warfarin Initiation Doses

Ashkan Sharabiani ,[1] **Edith A. Nutescu,**[2] **William L. Galanter,**[2,3] **and Houshang Darabi**[1]

[1]*Department of Mechanical and Industrial Engineering, University of Illinois at Chicago, Chicago, IL, USA*
[2]*Department of Pharmacy Systems Outcomes and Policy and Center for Pharmacoepidemiology and Pharmacoeconomic Research, University of Illinois at Chicago, Chicago, IL, USA*
[3]*Department of Medicine, University of Illinois at Chicago, Chicago, IL, USA*

Correspondence should be addressed to Ashkan Sharabiani; ashara2@uic.edu

Academic Editor: Chen Yanover

It is a challenge to be able to prescribe the optimal initial dose of warfarin. There have been many studies focused on an efficient strategy to determine the optimal initial dose. Numerous clinical, genetic, and environmental factors affect the warfarin dose response. In practice, it is common that the initial warfarin dose is substantially different from the stable maintenance dose, which may increase the risk of bleeding or thrombosis prior to achieving the stable maintenance dose. In order to minimize the risk of misdosing, despite popular warfarin dose prediction models in the literature which create dose predictions solely based on patients' attributes, we have taken physicians' opinions towards the initial dose into consideration. The initial doses selected by clinicians, along with other standard clinical factors, are used to determine an estimate of the difference between the initial dose and estimated maintenance dose using shrinkage methods. The selected shrinkage method was LASSO (Least Absolute Shrinkage and Selection Operator). The estimated maintenance dose was more accurate than the original initial dose, the dose predicted by a linear model without involving the clinicians initial dose, and the values predicted by the most commonly used model in the literature, the Gage clinical model.

1. Introduction

Warfarin is a commonly used oral anticoagulant drug with over 30 million prescriptions written annually in the United States [1]. This drug is difficult to manage because of its narrow therapeutic index and wide interpatient variability in dose response. Warfarin is the leading cause of drug-related hospitalizations among adults in the United States [2]. There are numerous factors affecting the activity of warfarin. They vary from each individual patient's characteristics, such as height, weight, age, and race, to the patient's medical history, diet, genotype, such as VKORC1 and CYP2C9, and their concurrent medications. Since various factors impact warfarin's dose response, numerous mathematical prediction models have been proposed to assist clinicians in finding the optimal initial dose [3–18]. The models that only contain clinical variables are known as clinical models (CL); models which also contain the patients' genotype are known as pharmacogenetic models (PKG).

Gage et al. [3] proposed two linear multiple regression models (CL & PKG models) in 2008. The clinical factors that were incorporated in both models are body surface area, target INR (International Normalized Ratio), smoking status, age, race, amiodarone use, and indication of VTE (Venous Thromboembolism). The IWPC (International Warfarin Pharmacogenetics Consortium) research group [4] also proposed two linear regression models. The models' performances were satisfactory for the patients who required doses less than or equal to 21 mg/wk or more than or equal to 49 mg/wk. According to the "Clinical Pharmacogenetics Implementation Consortium Guidelines for CYP2C9 and VKORC1 Genotypes and Warfarin Dosing," the models proposed by Gage and IWPC are the most recommended models for predicting warfarin initiation doses [5]. Additionally, Grossi et al. [6] designed a novel model in Artificial Neural Networks (ANN) framework. After collecting the data of 377 patients, they derived the model and chose their variables using the TWIST system [7], which is designed in order to select the most relevant features for performing classification or prediction. They compared their model with IWPC and Gage's models, along with another model proposed by Zambon et al. [8] based on Mean Absolute Error (MAE) and model's fitness (R^2), which proved their model's outperformance.

In 2015, Sharabiani et al. [9, 10] developed a new methodology towards estimating the initial warfarin dose. The proposed methodology estimates the initial dose for warfarin in two stages. In the first stage, using relevance vector machines, the patients are classified into two classes: patients requiring high doses (>30 mg/wk) and patients who require low doses (≤30 mg/wk). In the second stage, the dose for each class is predicted using two clinical regression models, which are trained for each class. Their proposed model was examined against Gage, IWPC clinical models, the fixed-dose approach (35 mg/wk), and the model proposed by Sharabiani et al. [10, 18] for African American patients, and it outperformed all of them in terms of prediction accuracy.

Several prediction models have also been proposed which target patients of specific ethnicities. The general proposed models are much more accurate when they are applied to Caucasian and Asian patients and less accurate in African American patients [11–13].

Using machine learning techniques, Cosgun et al. [14] proposed three PKG prediction models for African American patients. The models that were investigated were Boosted Regression Tree (BRT), Random Forest Regression (RFR), and Support Vector Regression (SVR). They compared their models to the models proposed by Schelleman et al. [15, 16] and Limdi et al. [13, 17] and reported their outperformance based on R^2. Sharabiani et al. [10, 18] suggested a new clinical model for African American patients in 2013; the proposed model outperformed IWPC and Gage models in terms of prediction accuracy MAE and Root Mean Squared Error (RMSE). Hernandez et al. [19] also proposed a PKG model for African American patients. They used the data of 349 patients for training the model and 149 patients for validating it. They proved that their proposed model outperformed the PKG and CL models proposed by IWPC [4].

Clinicians are now faced with several alternative dosing approaches in order to determine the initiation dose of warfarin in clinical practice. They can use the loading dose method and the dose prediction models that are proposed in the literature or rely solely on their clinical knowledge and expertise.

The objective of this paper is to propose a method to minimize warfarin misdosing when the prescription of the initial dose is guided by clinical judgment alone.

The risk of misdosing is defined as a clinically significant percentage difference between the initial dose and the therapeutic dose. The therapeutic dose is defined as the dose leading to two consecutive INRs in the therapeutic INR range for at least 14 days apart. By prescribing an initial dose close to the therapeutic dose, the time to reach the target INR decreases and the risk of anticoagulant related complications such as bleeding and thrombosis can be reduced.

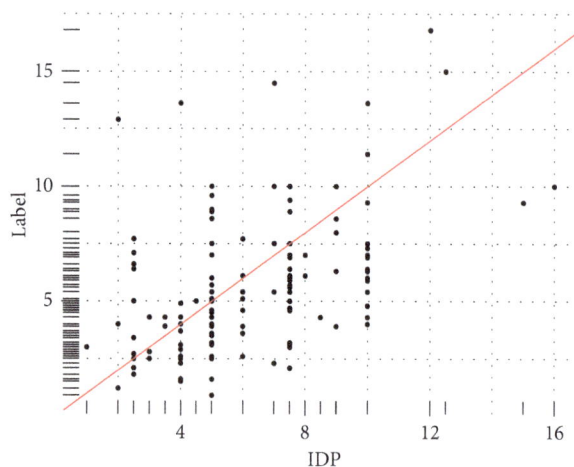

FIGURE 1: Distribution of the Initial Dose Prescribed by the Physician (IDP) Versus the Therapeutic Dose (Label).

Since the definition of a "clinically significant percentage difference" is subject to individual interpretation, we have examined our procedure based on different scenarios. The proposed model estimates the amount of percentage error which can be either positive (in case of overdose) or negative (in case of underdose). Once the amount of percentage error is estimated, the optimal initial dose can be determined by revising the prescribed initial dose accordingly. If the estimated percentage error is not considered significant, the prescribed dose will be used unaltered. It is shown that, by using the proposed method, the risk of misdosing decreases significantly.

2. Materials and Methods

The dataset, which was used for this project, contains the data of 150 warfarin-treated patients in the University of Illinois Hospital & Health Sciences System (UI-Health) who had reached the therapeutic warfarin dose in their course of treatment.

At the University of Illinois Hospital (UIH), the ordering clinicians select the initial dose of warfarin. If the resulting dose from the Gage clinical model [3] which is calculated using data in the electronic medical record (EMR) and the dose selected by the clinician are more than 20% different from the calculated dose, a warning is shown to the ordering clinician which includes the suggested dose. The ordering clinician is free to accept or reject this dose. If the ordering clinician chooses to order warfarin pharmacogenetic testing, a pharmacogenetics service pharmacist will assist with future doses of warfarin. Otherwise, the clinical team will manage the dosing of warfarin.

Numerous patient variables were recorded. The variables in the dataset and their frequencies are presented in Tables 1 and 2. As a small minority of our patient population, our model may not be appropriate in Asians. In Figure 1, the correlation between Initial Dose Prescribed by the Physician (IDP) and therapeutic dose is presented. The red line, in Figures 1, 3, and 4, indicates the ideal dosing scenario for each

TABLE 1: Categorical variables in the dataset.

Variable name	Values	Code	Frequency	Percentage
Race	African American	1	79	53%
	Hispanic	2	34	23%
	White	3	18	12%
	Asian	4	4	3%
	Others*	5	15	10%
Gender	Male	1	67	45%
	Female	2	83	55%
Liver disease	Yes	1	3	2%
	No	2	125	83%
	Missing	NA	22	15%
Warfarin Indication (WI)	A.fib	1	25	17%
	DVT	2	53	35%
	PE	3	34	23%
	TKA/THA	4	13	9%
	MVR	5	1	1%
	CVA	6	4	3%
	Others	7	20	13%
Goal INR	2-3	1	136	91%
	2.5–3.5	2	3	2%
	1.8–2.5	3	11	7%
Amiodarone	Yes	1	5	3%
	No	2	144	96%
	Missing	NA	1	1%
Bactrim	Yes	1	1	1%
	No	2	148	99%
	Missing	NA	1	1%
Azole	Yes	1	1	1%
	No	2	148	99%
	Missing	NA	1	1%
Which statin? (ST)	None	0	93	62%
	Simva	1	14	9%
	Atorva	2	23	15%
	Prava	3	7	5%
	Lova	4	8	5%
	Rosuva	5	4	3%
	Missing	NA	1	1%
Dialysis	Yes	1	8	5%
	No	2	142	95%
Rheumatoid arthritis	Yes	1	1	1%
	No	2	149	99%
Collagen vascular disease	Yes	1	2	1%
	No	2	148	99%
Deep Vein Thrombosis (DVT)	Yes	1	10	7%
	No	2	140	93%

TABLE 1: Continued.

Variable name	Values	Code	Frequency	Percentage
Smoking	Current smoker	1	13	9%
	Never smoker	2	107	71%
	Ex-smoker	3	30	20%
EtOH	Yes	1	24	16%
	No	2	119	79%
	Missing	NA	7	5%
Illicit	Yes	1	6	4%
	No	2	144	96%
Hypertension	Yes	1	86	57%
	No	2	64	43%
Angina	Yes	1	1	1%
	No	2	149	99%
Myocardial Infarction	Yes	1	3	2%
	No	2	147	98%
Percutaneous Coronary Intervention (PCI)	Yes	1	6	4%
	No	2	144	96%
Coronary Artery Bypass Graft (CABG)	Yes	1	5	3%
	No	2	145	97%
Atrial Fibrillation or Flutter	Yes	1	11	7%
	No	2	139	93%
Diabetes Mellitus (DM)	Yes	1	48	32%
	No	2	102	68%
Stroke	Yes	1	11	7%
	No	2	139	93%
Chronic Renal Insufficiency	Yes	1	15	10%
	No	2	135	90%
Chronic Obstructive Pulmonary Disease (COPD)	Yes	1	7	5%
	No	2	143	95%
Asthma	Yes	1	19	12%
	No	2	132	88%
Valvular heart disease	Yes	1	1	1%
	No	2	149	99%
Sickle cell	Yes	1	3	2%
	No	2	147	98%
Cancer history	Yes	1	12	8%
	No	2	138	92%
Pulmonary Embolism (PE)	Yes	1	5	3%
	No	2	144	96%
	Missing	NA	1	1%
Dyslipidemia	Yes	1	53	35%
	No	2	97	64%
Heart Failure (HF)	Yes	1	15	10%
	No	2	135	90%
Peripheral Vascular Disease (PVD)	Yes	1	7	4%
	No	2	143	95%

*These patients have predominantly unknown race.

TABLE 2: Continuous variables in the data set.

Continuous Variables	Unit	Number of missing instances	Mean	Median	Standard deviation	Min	Max
Therapeutic dose (Label)	mg/day	0	5.68	2.87	5.1	0.9	16.8
Initial Dose Prescribed By the Physician (IDP)	mg/day	2	6.12	2.59	5	1	16
Percentage error		2	0.26	0.7	0.12	−0.84	4.83
Age	Year	0	54.29	17.82	57	18	91
Height (Ht)	cm	0	168.28	10.35	169	142.2	195
Weight (Wt)	kg	0	89.9	31.12	83	40	220
Creatinine Clearance (CrCl)	ml/min	2	64.79	36.32	63.65	3.6	146.5
Albumin	g/dl	17	3.12	0.65	3.2	1.4	4.3
Aspartate Aminotransferase (AST)	u/L	22	33.56	41.04	22	9	379
Alanine Aminotransferase (ALT)	u/L	22	25.88	24.85	19	5	199
Baseline INR		1	1.18	0.14	1.2	1	1.8

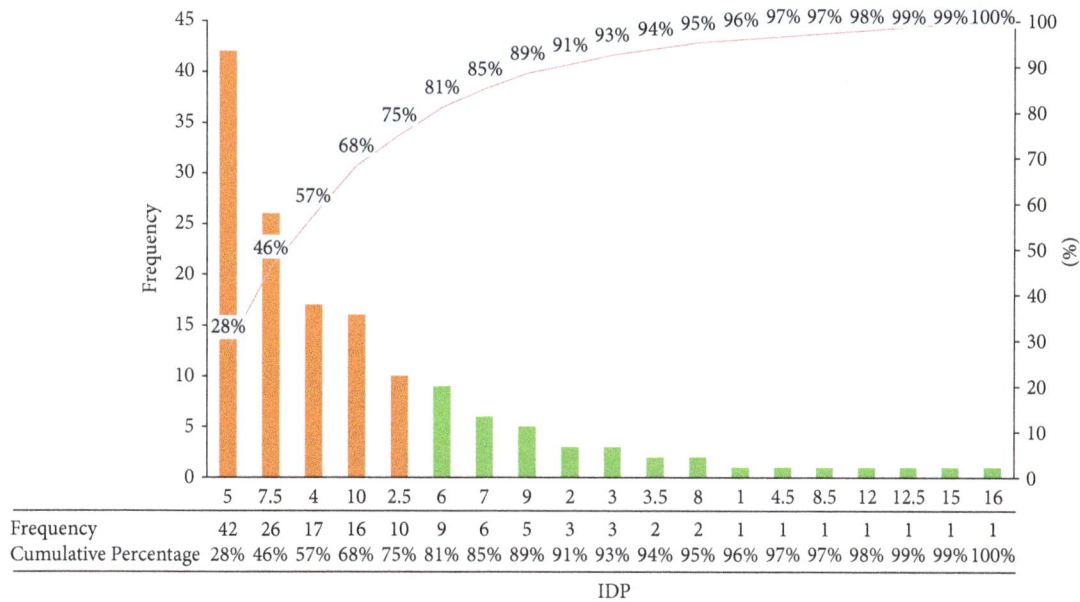

Frequency	42	26	17	16	10	9	6	5	3	3	2	2	1	1	1	1	1	1	1
IDP	5	7.5	4	10	2.5	6	7	9	2	3	3.5	8	1	4.5	8.5	12	12.5	15	16
Cumulative Percentage	28%	46%	57%	68%	75%	81%	85%	89%	91%	93%	94%	95%	96%	97%	97%	98%	99%	99%	100%

FIGURE 2: Pareto Chart for identifying the popular Initial Dose Prescribed by the Physician (IDP). 75% of the patients receive the popular doses (5, 7.5, 4, 10, 2.5 mg).

patient which is a case of achieving a complete correlation between the two variables. It provides a visual aid as to how distant the points are in the space from the complete correlation between the variables.

It is evident that most physicians tend to prescribe doses at popular discrete dose values. A Pareto chart measures this tendency as shown in in Figure 2.

As it is presented in Figure 2, 75% of patients in the dataset received dose values of 2.5, 4, 5, 7.5, and 10 mg/day (bars colored in orange). We focused on the patients who have received those common doses. This was done to minimize the effect on rare unusual doses on our model and to increase the robustness of the model for the more common doses. This

was necessary due to the relatively small size of the dataset. The distribution of the therapeutic dose at each level of the IDP is presented in Figure 3. Additionally, in Figure 4, a boxplot for each level is created.

Using the initial dose which was prescribed by the clinicians and the value of the therapeutic dose, the amount of percentage error is calculated. The frequency of patients with differing percentage error is presented in Figure 4. By a subjective definition of a clinically significant percentage difference, the patients who are at high risk/low risk of misdosing can be identified. Taking Figure 5 as an example, it is assumed that 20% difference is a significant difference and it is shown by dark vertical lines. The bars in Figure 5

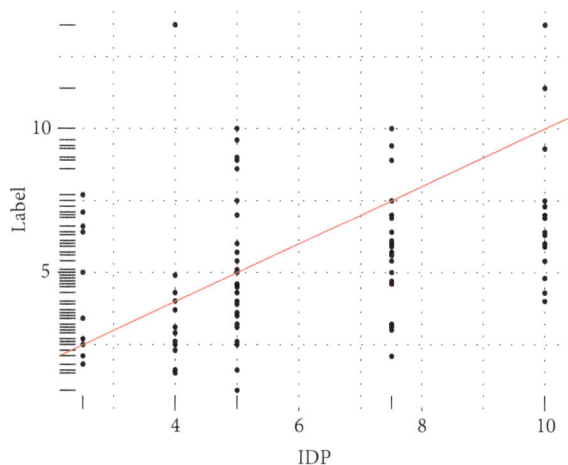

FIGURE 3: Distribution of the Initial Dose Prescribed by the Physician (IDP) versus the therapeutic dose (Label) for the popular doses against the ideal dosing setting.

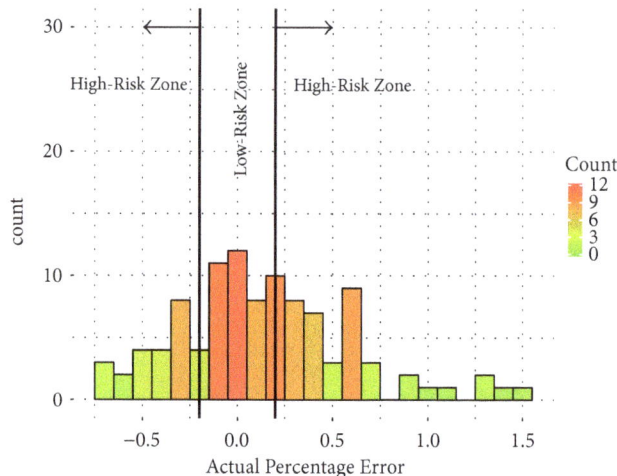

FIGURE 5: Defining the high-risk and low-risk dosing zones with the respect to the amount of generated percentage error by the Initial Dose Prescribed by the Physicians (IDP).

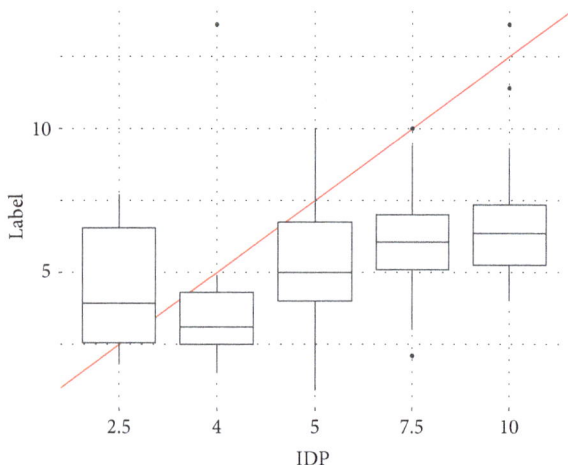

FIGURE 4: Comparing the distribution of therapeutic dose for popular Initial Dose Prescribed by the Physicians (IDP) using boxplots.

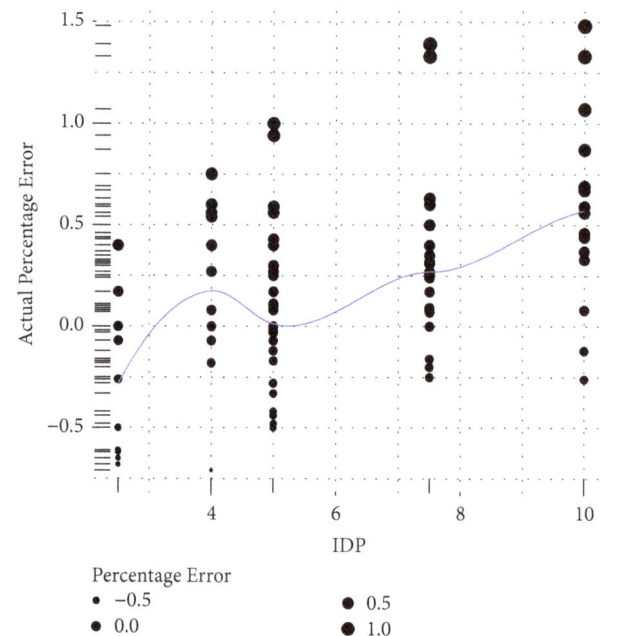

FIGURE 6: Distribution of percentage error at each level of popular Initial Doses Prescribed by the Physicians (IDP) (the sizes of the points are proportional with the amount of error generated at each dosing level).

are color-coded based on the intensity of their corresponding volume.

Another point of interest is to identify the ranges of prescribed initial dose where higher values of percentage error occur. In Figure 3, the relationship between the initial dose and the percentage error is presented. Additionally, using a polynomial local regression, the fitted curve describing their relationship along with its prediction confidence interval is presented in Figure 6. The size of each point in Figure 6 is proportional to the amount of percentage error. It is evident from Figure 6 that the frequency of higher values of percentage error tends to increase at larger values of initial dose.

Our goal is to develop a prediction model which assigns potential risk of misdosing to any prescribed initial dose. Therefore, in order to identify the linear dependency among the variables, a Pearson correlation matrix was created in

Figure 7 and the corresponding p values are presented in Figure 8. The values in Figures 7 and 8 are color-coded to facilitate the process of comparing the relative magnitude of numbers in the figure with the dark red being the highest value and the dark blue being the lowest value. In order to avoid collinearity in modeling, variables that had a correlation more than or equal to 85% were defined as highly correlated; only one of them was entered in the modeling phase. The data points which had missing values for their therapeutic dose were eliminated from the dataset.

	Label	Percentage Error	IDP	AGE	Ht	Wt	CrCl	Albumi	AST	ALT
Label	1.00									
Percentage Error	−0.57	1.00								
IDP	0.36	0.47	1.00							
AGE	−0.22	−0.08	−0.36	1.00						
Ht	0.15	−0.12	0.13	−0.12	1.00					
Wt	0.29	−0.02	0.40	−0.06	0.39	1.00				
CrCl	0.15	0.08	0.28	−0.56	0.39	0.07	1.00			
Albumi	−0.16	0.11	−0.04	0.24	−0.15	0.02	−0.19	1.00		
AST	−0.11	0.05	−0.03	0.00	0.21	0.10	0.02	−0.14	1.00	
ALT	−0.08	0.17	0.12	−0.10	0.16	0.24	0.20	−0.14	0.74	1.00

FIGURE 7: The Pearson correlation matrix. The values are color-coded to identify the highly correlated variables.

	Label	Percentage Error	IDP	AGE	Ht	Wt	CrCl	Albumi	AST	ALT
Label	$0.00E+00$									
Percentage Error	$2.77E-10$	$0.00E+00$								
IDP	$1.49E-04$	$5.63E-07$	$0.00E+00$							
AGE	$2.58E-02$	$3.94E-01$	$1.60E-04$	$0.00E+00$						
Ht	$1.16E-01$	$2.42E-01$	$1.97E-01$	$2.30E-01$	$0.00E+00$					
Wt	$2.91E-03$	$8.74E-01$	$2.38E-05$	$5.72E-01$	$3.81E-05$	$0.00E+00$				
CrCl	$1.36E-01$	$4.24E-01$	$4.34E-03$	$6.07E-10$	$4.65E-05$	$4.53E-01$	$0.00E+00$			
Albumi	$1.05E-01$	$2.79E-01$	$6.68E-01$	$1.24E-02$	$1.16E-01$	$8.63E-01$	$5.72E-02$	$0.00E+00$		
AST	$2.62E-01$	$6.35E-01$	$7.72E-01$	$9.89E-01$	$3.46E-02$	$3.22E-01$	$8.42E-01$	$1.49E-01$	$0.00E+00$	
ALT	$4.24E-01$	$8.12E-02$	$2.38E-01$	$3.33E-01$	$9.59E-02$	$1.50E-02$	$3.99E-02$	$1.57E-01$	$6.05E-19$	$0.00E+00$

FIGURE 8: Corresponding p values to the Pearson correlation matrix in Figure 7.

The missing values for other variables were imputed using KNN ($K = 5$) method since 81% of the data points in the dataset were complete. The choice of K in the KNN resulted from the cross-validation process. There existed a significant number of variables compared to the number of data points in the dataset, so we needed to select the best subset of variables. Using shrinkage methods, the process of variable selection and developing a prediction model took place simultaneously. Accordingly, the categorical variables in the dataset were transformed into multiple binary dummy variables with one level kept out as the reference (baseline). In the data preprocessing phase, entering the two-level categorical variables with highly imbalanced ratio of levels (when the volume of one level is less than 10% of the entire values of the variable) was avoided. After dividing the data randomly to derivation and validation cohorts (60%/40%) the optimal prediction model was developed using LASSO (Least Absolute Shrinkage and Selection Operator) and the entire analysis was implemented in R 3.0.2. A brief overview of the shrinkage regression models is presented below.

2.1. *Shrinkage Regression.* An alternative approach to least square method, and ridge regression, towards estimating a linear model's coefficients, is LASSO (Least Absolute Shrinkage and Selection Operator) [18]. The objective in LASSO is to minimize the residual sum of square subjects through the summation of the absolute values of coefficients which are less than a constant.

$$\text{argmin} \quad \left\{ \sum_{i=1}^{N} \left(y_i - \beta_0 - \sum_j \beta_j x_{ij} \right)^2 \right\}$$
$$\text{Subject to} \quad \sum_j \left| \beta_j \right| \le \lambda. \tag{1}$$

One of the most important characteristics associated with LASSO is that it enforces some coefficients to be exactly equal to zero and, hence, it results in a sparse model. However, by choosing a significantly small λ, this property will be nullified (and LASSO regression will be the regular least square model). Therefore, an appropriate choice of λ is quite critical. Because of this important attribute, the variable selection and modeling phases take place simultaneously. This idea can be considered as a major improvement over

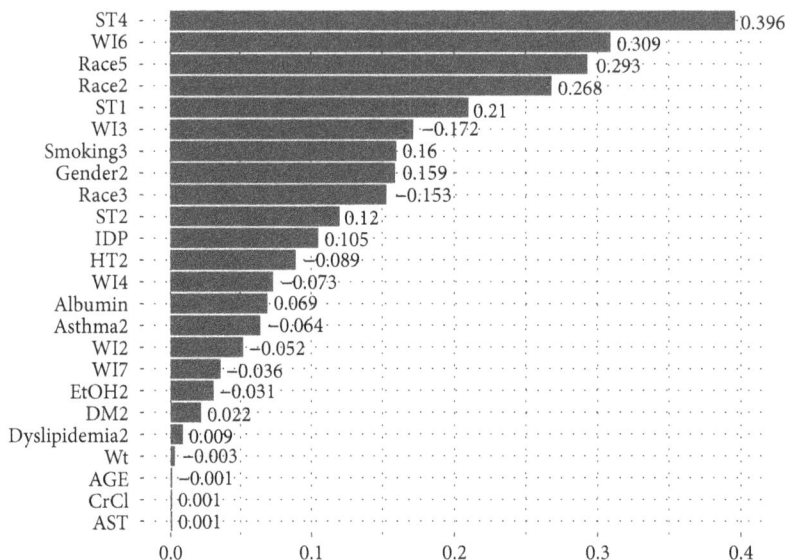

FIGURE 9: Model coefficients resulting from LASSO with involving IDP (the numbers attached to the variable names are the codes created after converting the variables into dummy variables. The codes are defined in Table 1.).

ridge regression where some coefficients will tend to zero but not exactly zero (see (2)).

$$\text{argmin} \quad \left\{ \sum_{i=1}^{N} \left(y_i - \beta_0 - \sum_j \beta_j x_{ij} \right)^2 \right\}$$

$$\text{Subject to} \quad \sum_j \beta_j^2 \le \lambda. \tag{2}$$

Another major advantage of LASSO is its interpretability. As opposed to some more complex nonlinear models such as neural networks, LASSO will result in an interpretable model which is very important especially in clinical studies. For a detailed study on LASSO see Tibshirani's [19] original paper.

3. Results

The optimal value of λ was selected by performing the k-fold cross-validation ($k = 10$). The resulting prediction model's coefficients are presented in Figure 9.

After developing the prediction model using the training set, its performance was evaluated on the testing set. Therefore, for every data point in the testing set the amount of percentage error was estimated. By defining a given threshold for determination of the significant percentage error, it can be decided whether the IDP was acceptable or would have needed modification. Therefore, the threshold represents the user's choice in defining the level of significance in percentage difference which triggers that action for dose revision.

According to the estimated percentage error, the prescribed initial dose can be revised.

$$\text{Revised Dose} = \left(1 - \frac{\text{Estimated Percentage Error}}{100} \right) \times \text{IDP}. \tag{3}$$

Therefore, the resulting revised initial dose values were compared against the original initial dose along with the Gage model in terms of RMSE.

The RMSE is used as the leading indicator of modeling performance and was selected since it is more appropriate to use (than Mean Absolute Error) when the error has a Gaussian distribution. According to the most cited dataset in the literature for warfarin dosing, IWPC dataset [20], the assumption of the errors having the Gaussian distribution in a larger setting was proven and therefore most prediction models in this context in the literature are compared based on the RMSE.

Additionally, in order to examine the impact of involving IDP in the modeling process, a new prediction model was developed with IDP being eliminated from the model. The developed model coefficients are presented in Figure 10.

Based on the results presented in Table 3, the estimated initial doses will result in more accurate estimations than the original dose values (RMSE = 2.38), the prediction values made by Gage model (RMSE = 2.05), and the linear model without using the initial dose in modeling (RMSE = 2.68).

4. Discussion

The proposed methodology has been developed and tested on the data of patients and physicians at the UIH, a tertiary urban hospital with an ethnically diverse patient population. The dataset is relatively small, but the 60% training set was able to develop a model which had better predictive power than traditional models. The methodology is novel for two reasons. First, this is the only model in the literature which uses information from clinicians, their first dose, to help estimate the best dose. Secondly, this model used a LASSO methodology to help deal with a less-than-ideal number of variables versus data points.

TABLE 3: Comparing the performance of the revised values of IDP with the original values of IDP, the Gage CL model, and the linear model without IDP. The percentage change in the table represents the percentage decrease in RMSE after revising the IDP.

Threshold	RMSE of the revised IDP	RMSE of the Original IDP (percent change)	RMSE of the Gage model (percent change)	RMSE of the linear model without involving IDP (percent change)
0.1	1.65	2.391 (31%)	2.063 (20%)	2.661 (38%)
0.15	1.76	2.378 (26%)	2.047 (14%)	2.667 (34%)
0.2	1.77	2.392 (26%)	2.051 (13.7%)	2.682 (34%)
0.25	1.9	2.375 (20%)	2.05 (7.3%)	2.68 (29.1%)
0.3	1.96	2.39 (18%)	2.05 (4.4%)	2.681 (26.9%)
0.35	1.96	2.39 (18%)	2.05 (4.4%)	2.681 (26.9%)
0.4	2.06	2.368 (13%)	2.05 (−0.5%)	2.679 (23.1%)

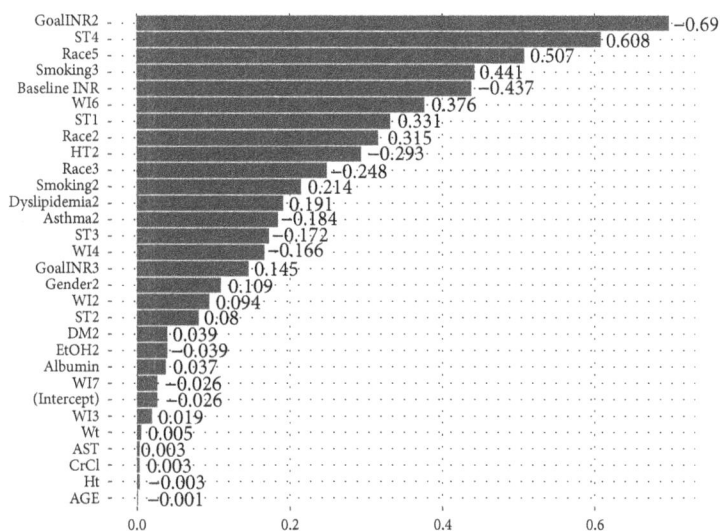

FIGURE 10: Model coefficients resulting from LASSO without involving IDP (the numbers attached to the variable names are the codes created after converting the variables into dummy variables. The codes are defined in Table 1.).

The goal of this project was to provide evidence of the feasibility of this approach. We have shown that there is some information content in the first dose ordered, as inclusion provides a better fit in our own model without the initial dose, as well as a better fit than traditional models. The reason that this occurred was not studied, but it suggests the previous models do not contain some variables or factors which ordering clinicians may be considering when dosing. Since the main focus of this study is to propose a new template for dosing by involving the suggested dose by the physician into the modeling process, for future deployment of such template, it is suggested to explore the performance of other predictive models after fully evaluating the model (power tests, diagnostic tests, etc.) as well. Additionally, on larger datasets, we suggest adjusting the K-fold cross-validation approach with lower number for K in order to avoid overfitting the model.

The final model produced by the LASSO procedure does not include some elements of the traditional clinical Gage equation, the use of the medications amiodarone, sulfamethoxazole, and azole antifungal agents. This may be due to the small population size and infrequency of use of these medications. Using this methodology on a larger dataset may or may not have the same finding. Our model includes the IDP which is not used in the Gage equation, and although it is less of a factor (see Figure 9) it does include the presence of diabetes mellitus. The Gage equation uses the presence or absence of liver disease, while our equation includes the lab values of AST and albumin, which can be considered a proxy for liver disease.

This type of analysis could be used for an active clinical decision support system once validated more thoroughly. All prior dosing data at a given institution which includes a proven maintenance dose can be used to develop the model. Once developed, a clinician's first dose, along with the noted patient variables would be used to determine a percentage error estimate. If this was less than some institutionally agreed upon threshold, no advice would be given to the clinician regarding their dose selection. If the initial dose was greater than the threshold away from the estimate, a dosing reminder or a new order could be introduced to the ordering clinician. This would only interrupt clinicians when there was a high likelihood of error.

The model is based on patient specific data from a given institution as well as the IDP for that institution. Because of this, it will need to be derived for each institution and as changes in initial dosing (IDP) occur, the model would likely change as the IDP does play a role in the predicted dose. If clinicians begin to dose purely on the model itself, it is likely that the added predictive power of adding the IDP will be lost as the variance between a predicted dose and the actual dose clearly contains useful information. It is however unlikely that this will occur at most hospitals soon as clinicians often disregard suggested dosing. As variations occur in physician compliance with initial dosing recommendations, patient mix, and changes in clinical practice, the model will need to be continuously adjusted. A reliance on prior clinical practice and prior patient mix will not likely produce the most accurate predictions.

The major limitation of this work is the relatively small dataset. The degree of fit and the novel use of the clinicians' first dose are intriguing and suggest larger studies to better validate the method. As this method is presently designed to help with the first dose, it can be used in conjunction with other models for subsequent decision support, with or without pharmacogenomics testing. It should work with any ethnic mixture of patients as the machine learning models are based on the patients seen at the particular institution, not a cohort from a published study which is likely different than the patients seen at an institution.

5. Conclusions

In this paper, an intelligent clinical decision support system for prescribing the initial dose of warfarin is presented. The maintenance dose of warfarin is estimated using shrinkage methods and including the actual initial ordered dose. This estimate was more accurate than the original dose given and the values predicted by the Gage clinical model. This approach is promising and warrants further study that may produce a functional clinical decision support system to assist with initial dosing of warfarin. The major limitation of this analysis is the small sample size used in its derivation. This limits the generalizability of our findings; however, the method is novel and should be tested in larger datasets. The proposed methodology serves as a modeling template for other healthcare institutions. Therefore, based on each institution's attributes (local patient's attributes/physicians' preferred dosing methods), customized models can be derived, which function more efficiently than generic models in the literature.

Disclosure

The content is solely the responsibility of the authors and does not necessarily represent the official views of the National Institutes of Health or the Agency for Healthcare Research and Quality.

Conflicts of Interest

The authors declare that they have no conflicts of interest in the research.

Acknowledgments

The authors acknowledge the Research Open Access Publishing (ROAAP) Fund of the University of Illinois at Chicago for financial support towards the open access publishing fee for this article. They also would like to thank Miss Elnaz Douzali and Angeline Kampert for their support and assistance in this project. Dr. Nutescu is supported by the National Heart, Lung, and Blood Institute of the National Institutes of Health under Award no. K23HL112908. Dr. Galanter is supported from the Agency for Healthcare Research and Quality by Grant no. U19HS021093.

References

[1] I. M. S. I. for H. Informatics, "The use of medicines in the United States: Review of 2011," 2011.

[2] J. Hirsh, V. Fuster, J. Ansell, and J. L. Halperin, "American Heart Association/American College of Cardiology Foundation guide to warfarin therapy," *Journal of the American College of Cardiology*, vol. 41, no. 9, pp. 1633–1652, 2003.

[3] B. F. Gage, C. Eby, J. A. Johnson et al., "Use of pharmacogenetic and clinical factors to predict the therapeutic dose of warfarin," *Clinical Pharmacology & Therapeutics*, vol. 84, no. 3, pp. 326–331, 2008.

[4] International Warfarin Pharmacogenetics Consortium, "Estimation of the warfarin dose with clinical and pharmacogenetic data," *The New England Journal of Medicine*, vol. 360, no. 8, pp. 753–764, 2009.

[5] J. A. Johnson, L. Gong, M. Whirl-Carrillo et al., "Clinical pharmacogenetics implementation consortium guidelines for CYP2C9 and VKORC1 genotypes and warfarin dosing," *Clinical Pharmacology & Therapeutics*, vol. 90, no. 4, pp. 625–629, 2011.

[6] E. Grossi, G. M. Podda, M. Pugliano et al., "Prediction of optimal warfarin maintenance dose using advanced artificial neural networks," *Pharmacogenomics*, vol. 15, no. 1, pp. 29–37, 2014.

[7] M. Buscema, E. Grossi, M. Intraligi, N. Garbagna, A. Andriulli, and M. Breda, "An optimized experimental protocol based on neuro-evolutionary algorithms: Application to the classification of dyspeptic patients and to the prediction of the effectiveness of their treatment," *Artificial Intelligence in Medicine*, vol. 34, no. 3, pp. 279–305, 2005.

[8] C.-F. Zambon, V. Pengo, R. Padrini et al., "VKORC1, CYP2C9 and CYP4F2 genetic-based algorithm for warfarin dosing: an Italian retrospective study," *Pharmacogenomics*, vol. 12, no. 1, pp. 15–25, 2011.

[9] A. Sharabiani, A. Bress, E. Douzali, and H. Darabi, "Revisiting warfarin dosing using machine learning techniques," *Computational and Mathematical Methods in Medicine*, vol. 2015, Article ID 560108, 9 pages, 2015.

[10] A. Sharabiani, *Medical Decision Making for Warfarin Dosing Using Machine Learning Methods, [Doctoral dissertation]*, 2015.

[11] M. J. Rieder, A. P. Reiner, B. F. Gage et al., "Effect of VKORC1 haplotypes on transcriptional regulation and warfarin dose,"

The New England Journal of Medicine, vol. 352, no. 22, pp. 2285–2293, 2005.

[12] M. Wadelius, L. Y. Chen, J. D. Lindh et al., "The largest prospective warfarin-treated cohort supports genetic forecasting," *Blood*, vol. 113, no. 4, pp. 784–792, 2009.

[13] N. A. Limdi, T. M. Beasley, M. R. Crowley et al., "VKORC1 polymorphisms, haplotypes and haplotype groups on warfarin dose among African-Americans and European-Americans," *Pharmacogenomics*, vol. 9, no. 10, pp. 1445–1458, 2008.

[14] E. Cosgun, N. A. Limdi, and C. W. Duarte, "High-dimensional pharmacogenetic prediction of a continuous trait using machine learning techniques with application to warfarin dose prediction in African Americans," *Bioinformatics*, vol. 27, no. 10, pp. 1384–1389, 2011.

[15] H. Schelleman, J. Chen, Z. Chen et al., "Dosing algorithms to predict warfarin maintenance dose in Caucasians and African Americans," *Clinical Pharmacology & Therapeutics*, vol. 84, no. 3, pp. 332–339, 2008.

[16] H. Schelleman, N. A. Limdi, and S. E. Kimmel, "Ethnic differences in warfarin maintenance dose requirement and its relationship with genetics," *Pharmacogenomics*, vol. 9, no. 9, pp. 1331–1346, 2008.

[17] N. A. Limdi and D. L. Veenstra, "Warfarin pharmacogenetics," *Pharmacotherapy*, vol. 28, no. 9, pp. 1084–1097, 2008.

[18] A. Sharabiani, H. Darabi, A. Bress, L. Cavallari, E. Nutescu, and K. Drozda, "Machine learning based prediction of warfarin optimal dosing for African American patients," in *Proceedings of the IEEE International Conference on Automation Science and Engineering (CASE '13)*, pp. 623–628, Madison, Wis, USA, August 2013.

[19] W. Hernandez, E. R. Gamazon, K. Aquino-Michaels et al., "Ethnicity-specific pharmacogenetics: the case of warfarin in African Americans," *The Pharmacogenomics Journal*, vol. 14, no. 3, pp. 223–228, 2014.

[20] https://www.pharmgkb.org/downloads/.

10

Medical Image Fusion based on Sparse Representation and PCNN in NSCT Domain

Jingming Xia,[1] **Yiming Chen** (iD)**,**[1] **Aiyue Chen,**[1] **and Yicai Chen**[2]

[1]*School of Electronics and Information Engineering, Nanjing University of Information Science and Technology, Nanjing 210044, China*
[2]*School of Mechanical Engineering, North China Electric Power University, Hebei 071000, China*

Correspondence should be addressed to Yiming Chen; 1770213116@qq.com

Academic Editor: Michele Migliore

The clinical assistant diagnosis has a high requirement for the visual effect of medical images. However, the low frequency subband coefficients obtained by the NSCT decomposition are not sparse, which is not conducive to maintaining the details of the source image. To solve these problems, a medical image fusion algorithm combined with sparse representation and pulse coupling neural network is proposed. First, the source image is decomposed into low and high frequency subband coefficients by NSCT transform. Secondly, the K singular value decomposition (K-SVD) method is used to train the low frequency subband coefficients to get the overcomplete dictionary D, and the orthogonal matching pursuit (OMP) algorithm is used to sparse the low frequency subband coefficients to complete the fusion of the low frequency subband sparse coefficients. Then, the pulse coupling neural network (PCNN) is excited by the spatial frequency of the high frequency subband coefficients, and the fusion coefficients of the high frequency subband coefficients are selected according to the number of ignition times. Finally, the fusion medical image is reconstructed by NSCT inverter. The experimental results and analysis show that the algorithm of gray and color image fusion is about 34% and 10% higher than the contrast algorithm in the edge information transfer factor QAB/F index, and the performance of the fusion result is better than the existing algorithm.

1. Introduction

Medical imaging attracts more and more attention due to the increasing requirements of clinic investigation and disease diagnosis [1]. Imaging of different modalities can reflect different information about the lesion. For example, CT images have a clear bone image, but soft tissue imaging is blurred; MRI images can obtain multiangle and multiplane detail information of soft tissue, but the skeleton imaging is blurred; PET images can present metabolic activity of human cells, but the anatomical structure is not clear. Therefore, the medical images of different modalities are fused to improve the accuracy and recognition of lesion location, which provides a more effective imaging reference for clinical diagnosis of modern medicine [2].

Compared with wavelet transform and Contourlet transform, NSCT transform has the advantages of multiscale and multidirection analysis, and anisotropy and translation invariance [3]. However, the low frequency subband coefficients obtained by NSCT decomposition are not sparse, and the fusion of them directly is not conducive to maintain the characteristics of the source image. Sparse Representation (SR) can extract deeper structural features between low frequency subband coefficients and express or approximate it in a linear combination of a few atoms [4]. Compared with other artificial neural networks, PCNN has an incomparable advantage over other traditional artificial neural networks [5]. The PCNN model has global coupling and pulse synchronization, which can combine the input high frequency subband coefficients with human visual characteristics to obtain richer detail information [6]. Therefore, NSCT transform, sparse representation, and PCNN model image fusion method are gaining more and more attention. Chun-hui and Yun-ting [7] propose a fast image fusion algorithm based on sparse representation and nonsubsampled Contourlet transform. This algorithm greatly improves the efficiency of image

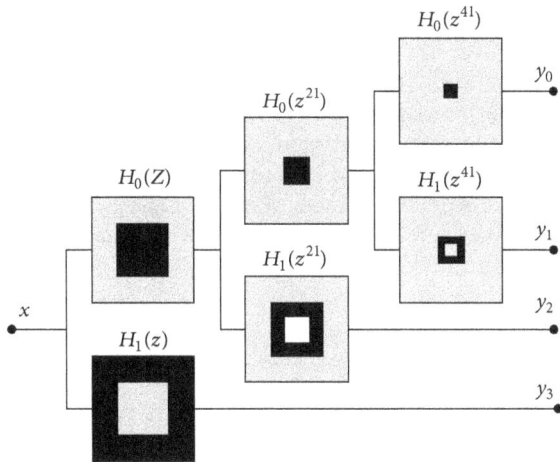

FIGURE 1: NSPFB filter decomposition.

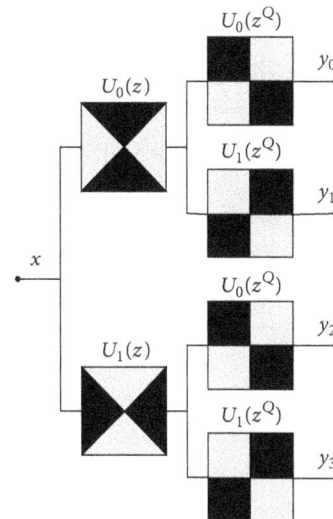

FIGURE 2: NSDFB filter decomposition.

fusion, but it gives only four-directional sparse representation in the low frequency subband, which cannot fully represent the characteristics and details of the source image. Shabanzade and Ghassemian [8] propose a multimodal image fusion algorithm based on NSCT and sparse representation. This algorithm uses sparse representation to perfectly approximate the low frequency subband coefficients. However, the rule based on the larger local energy or variance is used for high frequency subband coefficients, which cannot effectively solve the problem of image detail smoothing caused by sparse representation. Gong et al. [9] propose an image fusion method based on the improved NSCT transform and PCNN model, and this method can preserve the image structure better so that the fusion image is more in line with the human visual nervous system. However, the mutual information of the fusion image is relatively less. Mohammed et al. [10] propose a medical image fusion algorithm based on sparse representation and dual input PCNN model. This algorithm has a high fusion performance and adapts to the human visual nerve system. However, it needs to train medical image database to get an overcomplete dictionary; in addition, PCNN model applies a dual input, which presents the high complexity and low integration efficiency of the algorithm.

In order to obtain the medical fusion image with high fusion performance and high fusion efficiency, and to help it adapt to human visual nervous system, this paper, by aiming at the above research situation and existing problems and combining the sparse representation with PCNN simplified model, proposes the medical image fusion algorithm based on NSCT and SR-PCNN, hereinafter referred to as NSCT-SR-PCNN fusion algorithm.

2. Nonsubsampled Contourlet Transform

The NSCT transform consists of two steps: the nondownsampling pyramid (NSP) decomposition and the nondownsampling direction filter bank (NSDFB). NSP decomposition is the process of decomposing the source image into low and high frequency subbands through the nonsubsampling tower filter bank to ensure the characteristic of NSCT multiscale

transformation. The NSPFB filter is decomposed as shown in Figure 1.

3. Sparse Representation

Sparse representation means that the natural signal can be represented or approximated by a linear combination of a small number of atoms in the overcomplete dictionary $D \in R^{n \times k}$; then the sparse coefficient of the signal x can be obtained by

$$
\begin{aligned}
\min_{A} \quad & \|A\|_0, \\
\text{s.t.} \quad & \|X - DA\|_2^2 < \varepsilon,
\end{aligned}
\tag{1}
$$

where D is a prespecified dictionary; A is a sparse coefficient vector; $\|A\|_0$ stands for the count of nonzero entries in A; ε is the bounded representation error. NSCT-SR-PCNN algorithm uses K-SVD method to train the dictionary and uses the orthogonal matching tracking optimization (OMP) algorithm to estimate the sparse coefficient A [11].

4. Pulse Coupled Neural Network

PCNN simplified model is a feedback neural network model proposed by simulating the signal processing mechanism of cat visual cortex [12]. In the simplified model, the partial simplification of the parameters makes the generality of the model well guaranteed. However, there is a great difference in the response of the visual system to the different feature regions in the image. In the PCNN model, this difference is mainly reflected in the setting of the parameters, and the flexible changes in the parameters still affect the final fusion results. Therefore, this paper uses the most commonly used discrete mathematical iterative model. The simplified model is shown in Figure 3.

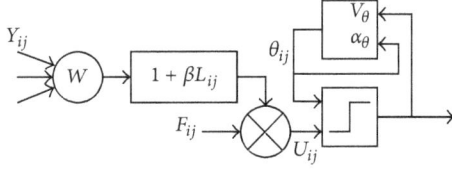

FIGURE 3: PCNN simplified model.

The mathematical expression of the PCNN simplified model can be expressed by

$$F_{ij}[n] = I_{ij}$$

$$L_{ij}[n] = \exp(-\alpha_L) L_{ij}[n-1]$$

$$+ V_L \sum_{k,l} W_{ijkl} Y_{ij}[n-1]$$

$$U_{ij}[n] = F_{ij}[n](1+\beta) L_{ij}[n] \qquad (2)$$

$$\theta_{ij}[n] = \exp(-\alpha_\theta)\theta_{ij}[n-1] + V_\theta Y_{ij}[n-1]$$

$$Y_{ij}[n-1] = \begin{cases} 1, & U_{ij}[n] > \theta_{ij}[n] \\ 0, & U_{ij}[n] \le \theta_{ij}[n], \end{cases}$$

where n is the number of iterations; I_{ij} is the external input; Y_{ij} is the output of neuron; U_{ij} is the internal behavior of neurons; F_{ij} is feedback input excitation; L_{ij} is the input of neuron's link; W_{ijkl} is the weight coefficient of the connection between neurons; β is the link strength coefficient; θ_{ij} is the output of variable threshold function; V_L and α_L are, respectively, the signal amplification factor and attenuation time constant of neuron's link; V_θ and α_θ are, respectively, the signal amplification factor and decay time constant of variable threshold function.

5. Medical Image Fusion Algorithm Based on NSCT-SR-PCNN

NSCT-SR-PCNN algorithm firstly uses NSCT transform to decompose the source image after registration to obtain the low frequency and high frequency subband of the source image; secondly the fusion method based on sparse representation is used to fuse the low frequency subband, and the fusion method based on PCNN simplified model is used to fuse the high frequency subband; finally NSCT inverse transform is used to reconstruct the fused subband coefficients to obtain the medical image of fusion. The specific implementation process of NSCT-SR-PCNN medical image fusion algorithm is shown in Figure 4.

5.1. The Rules of Low Frequency Subband Coefficient Fusion. Low frequency subband coefficient fusion is achieved by using sparse representation fusion. First of all, blocks taken from the image to be fused form a training sample set, and secondly K-SVD algorithm is used to train a complete dictionary, and then the Batch-OMP [13] optimization algorithm is used to estimate the sparse coefficient; finally, the sparse coefficients are adaptively fused according to image features. The specific steps are as follows.

Step 1. Use the NSCT transforms to decompose, respectively, the source images A and B with $M \times N$ size after registration to obtain the low frequency and high frequency subband coefficients.

Step 2. Segment the low frequency subband coefficients L_A and L_B by using the sliding window with the steps of S pixels and the size $n \times n$, and obtain the $(N + n - 1) \times (M + n - 1)$ subblocks; transform the image subblocks into column vectors to form the sample training matrix V_A and V_B.

Step 3. Average the sample training matrices V_A and V_B to obtain the mean matrices $\hat{V}_A$ and $\hat{V}_B$; average of the sample training matrices V_A and V_B is removed to obtain the sparse representation of the sample matrices V'_A and V'_B.

Step 4. Use the K-SVD algorithm to iterate the sample matrix to obtain the overcomplete dictionary matrix D of the low frequency subband coefficient.

Step 5. Use the Batch-OMP optimization algorithm to estimate the sparse coefficients of V'_A and V'_B and obtain the sparse coefficient matrices α_A and α_B. According to the value of L_1 norm, the sparse coefficient matrix of column i is fused by applying the rules of

$$\overset{i}{\alpha}_F = \begin{cases} \overset{i}{\alpha}_A + \dfrac{1}{2}\overset{i}{\alpha}_B, & \text{if } \sum_{k=1}^{n}\left\|\overset{k}{\alpha}_A\right\|_1 > \sum_{k=1}^{n}\left\|\overset{k}{\alpha}_B\right\|_1, \ \overset{i}{\alpha}_A < \overset{i}{\alpha}_B, \ \overset{i}{\alpha}_A \cdot \overset{i}{\alpha}_B < 0 \\[3mm] \overset{i}{\alpha}_B + \dfrac{1}{2}\overset{i}{\alpha}_A, & \text{if } \sum_{k=1}^{n}\left\|\overset{k}{\alpha}_A\right\|_1 < \sum_{k=1}^{n}\left\|\overset{k}{\alpha}_B\right\|_1, \ \overset{i}{\alpha}_A > \overset{i}{\alpha}_B, \ \overset{i}{\alpha}_A \cdot \overset{i}{\alpha}_B < 0 \\[3mm] \dfrac{\overset{i}{\alpha}_A + \overset{i}{\alpha}_B}{2} + \dfrac{1}{2}\overset{i}{\alpha}_A, & \text{if } \sum_{k=1}^{n}\left\|\overset{k}{\alpha}_A\right\|_1 = \sum_{k=1}^{n}\left\|\overset{k}{\alpha}_B\right\|_1, \ \overset{i}{\alpha}_A > \overset{i}{\alpha}_B, \ \overset{i}{\alpha}_A \cdot \overset{i}{\alpha}_B < 0 \\[3mm] \dfrac{\overset{i}{\alpha}_A + \overset{i}{\alpha}_B}{2} + \dfrac{1}{2}\overset{i}{\alpha}_B, & \text{if } \sum_{k=1}^{n}\left\|\overset{k}{\alpha}_A\right\|_1 = \sum_{k=1}^{n}\left\|\overset{k}{\alpha}_B\right\|_1, \ \overset{i}{\alpha}_A < \overset{i}{\alpha}_B, \ \overset{i}{\alpha}_A \cdot \overset{i}{\alpha}_B < 0 \\[3mm] \alpha^F, & \text{otherwise} \end{cases} \qquad (3)$$

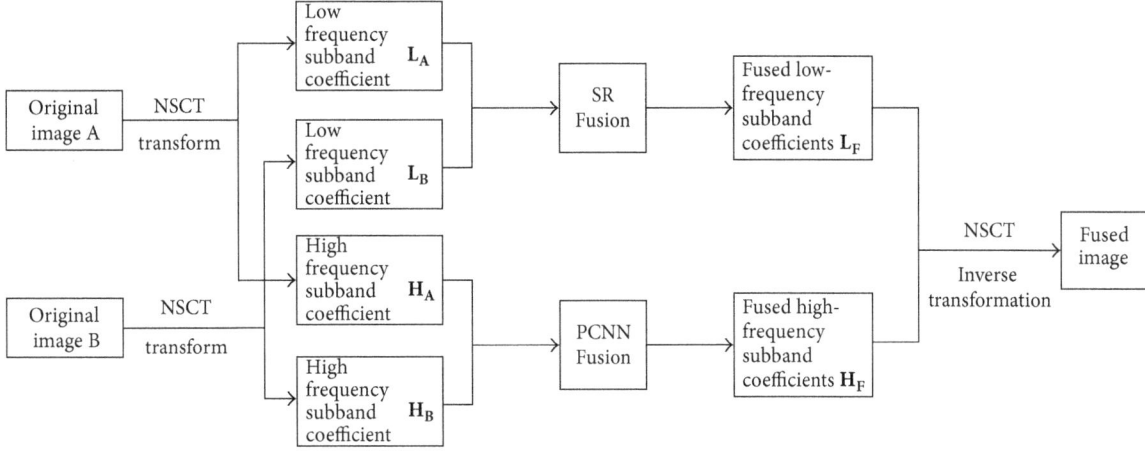

FIGURE 4: NSCT-SR-PCNN medical image fusion algorithm flow.

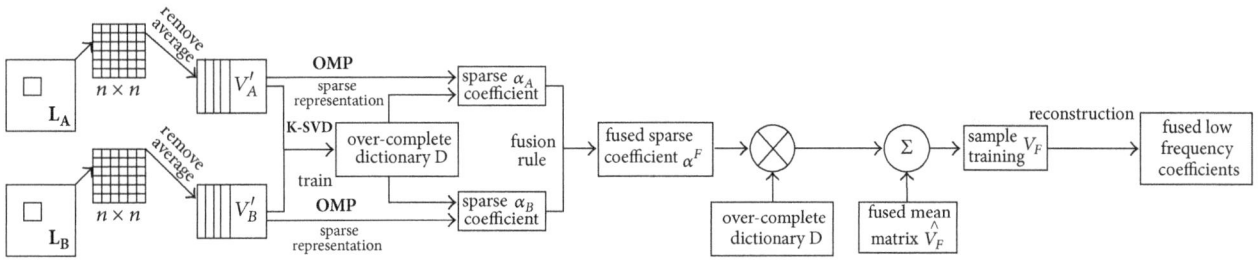

FIGURE 5: Low frequency subband coefficient SR fusion process.

Among them, α^F can be seen from

$$
\alpha^F = \begin{cases} \alpha_A^i, & \text{if } \sum_{k=1}^n \left\| \alpha_A^k \right\|_1 > \sum_{k=1}^n \left\| \alpha_B^k \right\|_1 \\[2mm] \alpha_B^i, & \text{if } \sum_{k=1}^n \left\| \alpha_A^k \right\|_1 < \sum_{k=1}^n \left\| \alpha_B^k \right\|_1 \\[2mm] \dfrac{\alpha_A^i + \alpha_B^i}{2}, & \text{if } \sum_{k=1}^n \left\| \alpha_A^k \right\|_1 = \sum_{k=1}^n \left\| \alpha_B^k \right\|_1. \end{cases} \tag{4}
$$

Step 6. The choice of the fusion mean matrix is given by

$$
\hat{V}_F = \begin{cases} \hat{V}_A, & \text{if } \sum_{k=1}^n \left\| \alpha_A^k \right\|_1 > \sum_{k=1}^n \left\| \alpha_B^k \right\|_1 \\[2mm] \hat{V}_B, & \text{if } \sum_{k=1}^n \left\| \alpha_A^k \right\|_1 < \sum_{k=1}^n \left\| \alpha_B^k \right\|_1 \\[2mm] \dfrac{\hat{V}_A + \hat{V}_B}{2}, & \text{if } \sum_{k=1}^n \left\| \alpha_A^k \right\|_1 = \sum_{k=1}^n \left\| \alpha_B^k \right\|_1. \end{cases} \tag{5}
$$

Step 7. Multiply the overcomplete dictionary matrix D with the fusion sparse coefficient matrix α^F and then add fusion mean matrix $\hat{V}_F$. The fusion sample training matrix V_F is given by

$$
V_F = D\alpha_F + \hat{V}_F. \tag{6}
$$

Step 8. Convert the columns of the fusion sample training matrix V_F into data subblocks, and reconstruct the data subblocks to obtain the fusion coefficients of the low frequency subbands.

The implementation of low frequency subband coefficients fusion based on sparse representation is shown in Figure 5.

5.2. The Rules of High Frequency Subband Coefficient Fusion. According to the characteristics of human visual system, the spatial frequency (SF) reflects the local area characteristics and details of the image. The high frequency subband coefficient fusion selects SF as the neuron feedback input to stimulate the PCNN simplified model. The neuron feedback input is expressed by

$$
F_{ij} = \text{SF}_{ij} = \sqrt{RF_{ij}^2 + CF_{ij}^2} \tag{7}
$$

Among them are the window size 3×3, RF_{ij}, and CF_{ij}; from formula (8) we can see:

$$
RF_{ij} = \sqrt{\frac{1}{M \times N} \sum_{i=1}^M \sum_{j=2}^N \left[X(i,j) - X(i,j-1) \right]^2}
$$

$$
\tag{8}
$$

$$
CF_{ij} = \sqrt{\frac{1}{M \times N} \sum_{i=2}^M \sum_{j=1}^N \left[X(i,j) - X(i-1,j) \right]^2}
$$

In the PCNN model, the value of β determines the strength of the coupling relationship of the neurons, and the high frequency subband coefficient fusion selects the Laplacian energy (EOL), the visibility (VI), and the standard deviation (SD) that can measure the neighborhood characteristic information, respectively, as the linking strength values of PCNN corresponding neurons, and EOL, VI, and SD are expressed by

$$\text{EOL} = \sum_{(u,v)\in w} \left(f_{uu} + f_{vv}\right)^2$$

$$\text{VI} = \frac{1}{N} \sum_{(u,v)\in w} \left(\frac{1}{m_k}\right)^\alpha \cdot \frac{|f(u,v) - m_k|}{m_k} \qquad (9)$$

$$\text{SD} = \sqrt{\frac{\sum_{i=1}^{l} \sum_{j=1}^{l} \left(f(u,v) - m_k\right)^2}{l \cdot l}},$$

where (u,v) is a pixel point of the image; $f(u,v)$ is the pixel value; w is the window of size $l \times l$; m_k is the pixel gray level average; N is the number of pixels in the window; α is a constant.

For fusion based on PCNN simplified model, SF is used as the neuron feedback input to excite each neuron, and EOL, VI, and SD are selected as the linking strength values of the corresponding neurons; then the corresponding ignition map is obtained by the PCNN ignition, and the new ignition map of the source image is constructed by the weighting function. Finally, the fusion coefficient is selected according to the number of ignition frequencies. Specific implementation steps are as follows.

Step 9. According to formula (7), calculate the neighborhood spatial frequency SF_A and SF_B of the high frequency subband coefficients HA and HB and then normalize SF_A and SF_B, and mark them as SF'_A and SF'_B, respectively; SF'_A and SF'_B are used as neuron feedback input to motivate the PCNN simplified model.

Step 10. According to formula (9), calculate EOL, VI, and SD of high frequency subband coefficients HA and HB (which is recorded as β_{AE}, β_{AV}, β_{AS}, β_{BE}, β_{BV}, and β_{BS}) and take them, respectively, as the linking strength value of corresponding neurons.

Step 11 (initialization setting). $L_{ij}(0) = U_{ij}(0) = 0$, $\theta_{ij}(0) = 1$; at this time the neuron is in the flameout state; that is, $Y_{ij}(0) = 0$, so the number of pulses generated is $O_{ij}(0) = 0$.

Step 12. According to formula (2), calculate $L_{ij}[n]$, $U_{ij}[n]$, $\theta_{ij}[n]$, and $Y_{ij}[n]$.

Step 13. The output of the PCNN simplified model iteration run is as follows: O_{AE}, O_{AV}, O_{AS}, O_{BE}, O_{BV}, and O_{BS}; use the weighting function to obtain the new ignition map O_A and O_B which corresponds to high frequency subband coefficients

HA and HB: $O_A = w_1 O_{AE} + w_2 O_{AV} + w_3 O_{AS}$, $O_B = w_4 O_{BE} + w_5 O_{BV} + w_6 O_{BS}$; w_i $(i = 1, 2, 3, 4, 5, 6)$ is given by

$$w_1 = \frac{O_{AE}}{\left(O_{AE} + O_{AV} + O_{AS}\right)}$$

$$w_2 = \frac{O_{AV}}{\left(O_{AE} + O_{AV} + O_{AS}\right)}$$

$$w_3 = \frac{O_{AS}}{\left(O_{AE} + O_{AV} + O_{AS}\right)}$$

$$w_4 = \frac{O_{BE}}{\left(O_{BE} + O_{BV} + O_{BS}\right)} \qquad (10)$$

$$w_5 = \frac{O_{BV}}{\left(O_{BE} + O_{BV} + O_{BS}\right)}$$

$$w_6 = \frac{O_{BS}}{\left(O_{BE} + O_{BV} + O_{BS}\right)}.$$

Step 14. Compare the ignition time output threshold values (ignition frequencies) at the new ignition map pixel; the high frequency subband fusion coefficient $H_F(i,j)$ is given by

$$H_F(i,j)$$

$$= \begin{cases} H_A(i,j), & \text{if } O_A(i,j) > O_B(i,j) \\ H_B(i,j), & \text{if } O_A(i,j) < O_B(i,j) \\ \dfrac{H_A(i,j) + H_B(i,j)}{2}, & \text{if } O_A(i,j) = O_B(i,j). \end{cases} \qquad (11)$$

The adaptive fusion implementation process based on PCNN simplified model is shown in Figure 6.

6. The Results and Analysis of Experiments

In order to verify the effectiveness of the proposed algorithm, five kinds of contrast algorithms are selected to conduct gray and color medical image fusion experiments. The medical images of each group are obtained from http://www.med .harvard.edu/AANLIB/home.html page. Objective evaluation of quality is made in terms of 7 indexes, such as the information entropy (IE), spatial frequency (SF), mean gradient (AG) [14], clarity (MC), mutual information (MI), standard deviation (SD) [15], and edge information delivery factor ($Q^{AB/F}$ high weight evaluation index) [16–19]. The visual information fidelity (VIFF) and structural similarity model (SSIM) were used to evaluate the visual effect of human eyes. The contrast algorithm 1 is a medical image fusion study based on NSCT transform (referred to as NSCT fusion algorithm) proposed in the paper [20]. The contrast algorithm 2 is the multifocus image fusion (referred to as the SR fusion algorithm) based on the fragmented complete sparse representation proposed in the paper [21]. The contrast

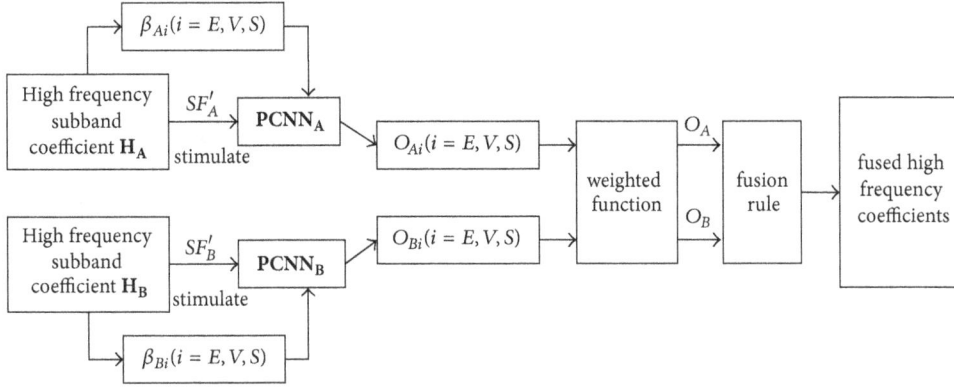

FIGURE 6: High frequency subband coefficient PCNN fusion process.

algorithm 3 is the image fusion by using pulse coupled neural network (referred to as PCNN fusion algorithm), proposed by the paper [22]. The contrast algorithm 4 is a multifocus image fusion based on NSCT and sparse representation (referred to as NSCT-SR fusion algorithm) proposed in the paper [11]. The contrast algorithm 5 is an improved algorithm based on NSCT and adaptive PCNN medical image fusion (referred to as NSCT-PCNN fusion algorithm) proposed in the paper [23]. NSCT transformation parameters setting: the class of decomposition is 4, the scale decomposition filter selects "pyrexc" filter, and the direction filter selects "vk" filter [24]; SR parameters setting: sliding window size is 8×8, step size is 1, the number of dictionary training iteration is 30 times, and sparse error is 0.01; PCNN parameters setting: $V_L = 1$, $V_\theta = 20$, $\alpha_L = 1$, $\alpha_\theta = 0.2$, $N_{\max} = 100$, and

$$w = \begin{bmatrix} 0.707 & 1 & 0.707 \\ 1 & 0 & 1 \\ 0.707 & 1 & 0.707 \end{bmatrix} \quad (12)$$

(see [25]).

6.1. Gray Image Fusion Experiment. Gray image fusion experiment is conducted by selecting the images of four groups of brain under different states as the images to be fused. The results of the fusion of the various algorithms are shown in Figures 7–10, and the objective evaluation indexes for quality of the various algorithms are shown in Tables 1–4.

NSDFB is a two-channel nondownsampling filter bank, and it decomposes the high frequency subband image decomposed by NSP in level-one NSDFB direction, so it can produce 2^l different directional subband image. NSDFB filter is decomposed as shown in Figure 2.

The NSCT-SR-PCNN algorithm has better fusion and better fusion performance than the five contrast algorithms, from the human visual effects in Figures 7–10 or the evaluation index from Tables 1–4. The reason is that, for NSCT algorithm, NSCT decomposition of the low frequency subband coefficient is not sparse, and direct low frequency coefficient fusion is not conducive to the retention of the source image features; for SR algorithm and the PCNN algorithm, the

image fusion is based on the spatial domain implementation, and the spatial domain fusion method fails to express details, so the fusion image has low contrast, fuzzy details, and block artifact, and other problems. For NSCT-SR algorithm, it solves the problem that low frequency subband coefficient is not sparse, but the fusion of high frequency subband is only conducted based on the direction featured principle, which cannot completely present the details of the image information. For NSCT-PCNN algorithm, it can adapt to the human visual system, but the low frequency subband coefficients have no sparseness. For NSCT-SR-PCNN algorithm, it not only solves the problem of the detail loss of the wavelet transform and the sparseness loss of low frequency subband coefficient of the NSCT, but also improves the comprehensive performance of the fusion results by using the spatial frequency of the high frequency subband coefficients to impel input and by using EOL, VI, and SD to strengthen their links with the corresponding neurons. NSCT-SR-PCNN algorithm can obtain better performance for CT/MRI, MR-PD/MR-T1 and MR-T1/MR-T2 medical image fusion in the comprehensive analysis of evaluation indexes. The NSCT-SR-PCNN algorithm can achieve better performance for CT/MRI, MR-PD/MR-T1 and MR-PD/MR-T2 medical image fusion according to edge information delivery factor of $Q^{AB/F}$ index.

6.2. Color Image Fusion Experiment. Color image fusion experiment selects three groups of brain under different images as the images to be fused. The fusion results of various algorithms are shown in Figures 11–13, and the objective evaluation index for quality of various algorithms is shown in Tables 5–7.

Compared with the five contrast algorithms in terms of the human visual effect of Figures 11–13 or the comprehensive analysis of the evaluation index and the $Q^{AB/F}$ index of the edge information delivery factor, the NSCT-SR-PCNN algorithm can provide better performance for MR-PD/PET, MR-T1/PET, and MR-T2/PET medical image fusion. Based on the experimental data, the NSCT-SR-PCNN algorithm proposed in this paper can make the fusion image obtain high fusion performance in the aspect of texture clarity, gray scale variation, and contrast ratio and can realize no color loss or distortion in transmission.

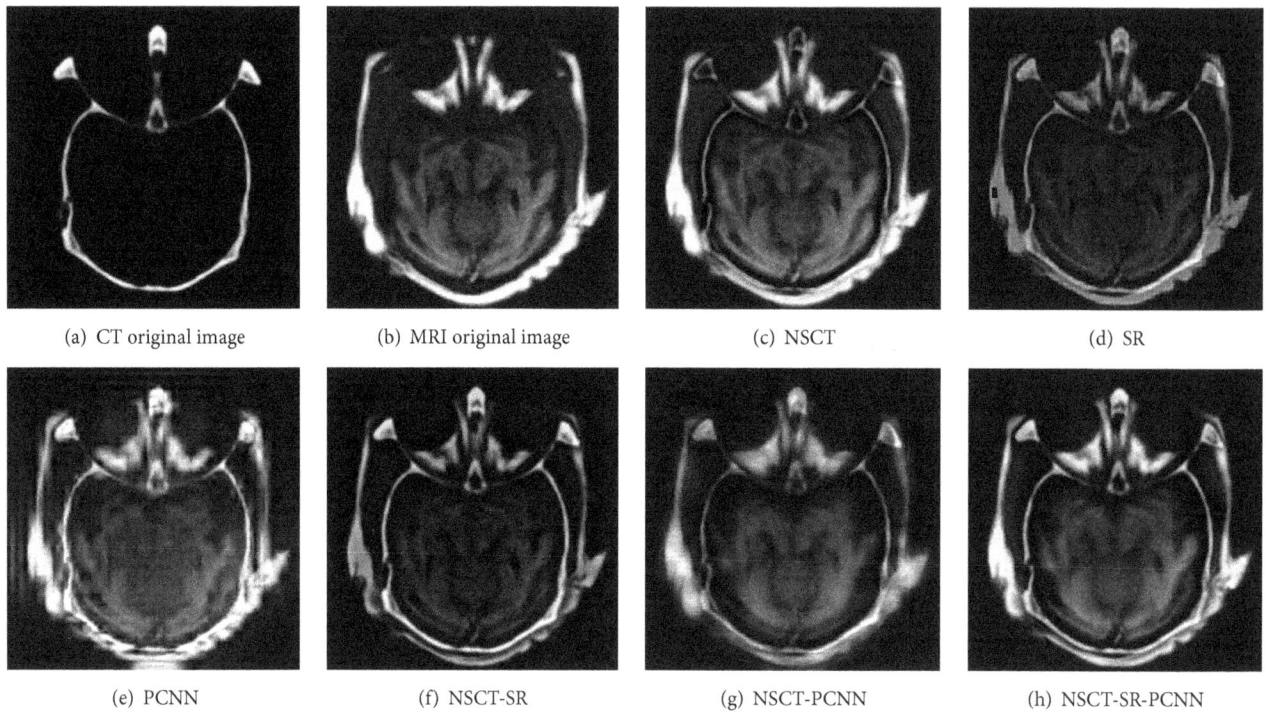

(a) CT original image   (b) MRI original image   (c) NSCT   (d) SR

(e) PCNN   (f) NSCT-SR   (g) NSCT-PCNN   (h) NSCT-SR-PCNN

FIGURE 7: CT/MRI medical image fusion results.

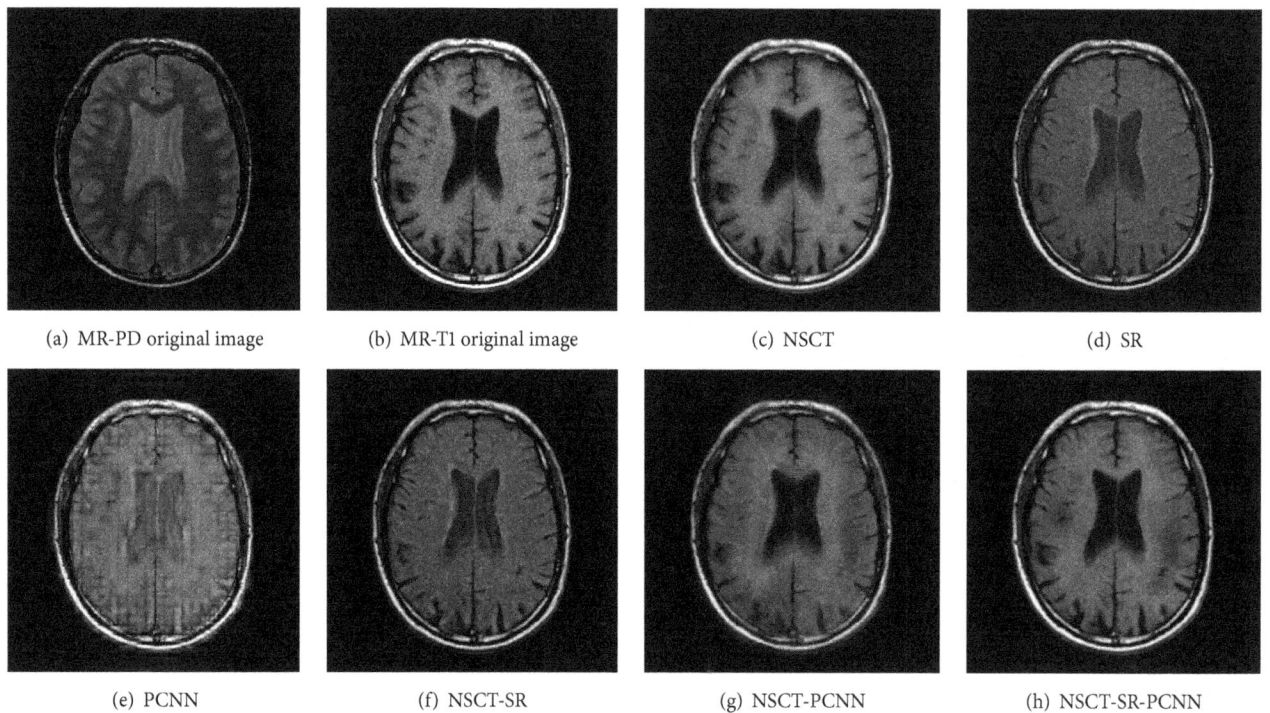

(a) MR-PD original image   (b) MR-T1 original image   (c) NSCT   (d) SR

(e) PCNN   (f) NSCT-SR   (g) NSCT-PCNN   (h) NSCT-SR-PCNN

FIGURE 8: MR-PD/MR-T1 medical image fusion results.

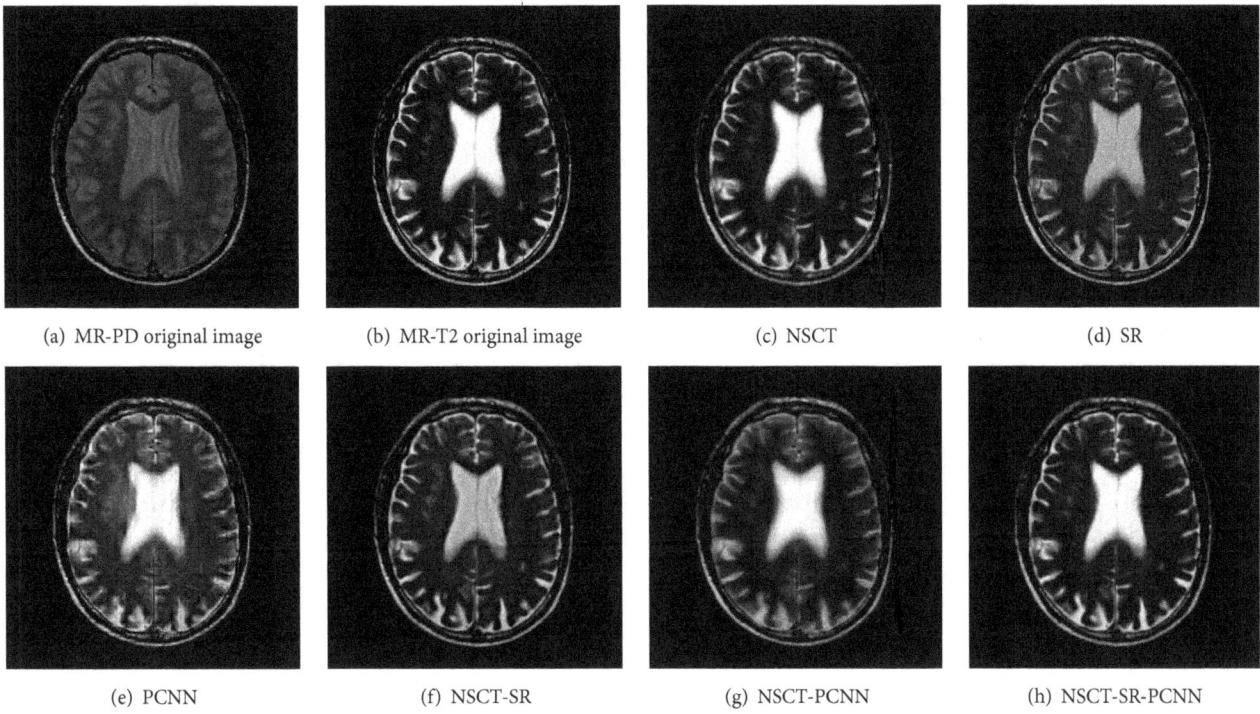

(a) MR-PD original image   (b) MR-T2 original image   (c) NSCT   (d) SR

(e) PCNN   (f) NSCT-SR   (g) NSCT-PCNN   (h) NSCT-SR-PCNN

FIGURE 9: MR-PD/MR-T2 medical image fusion results.

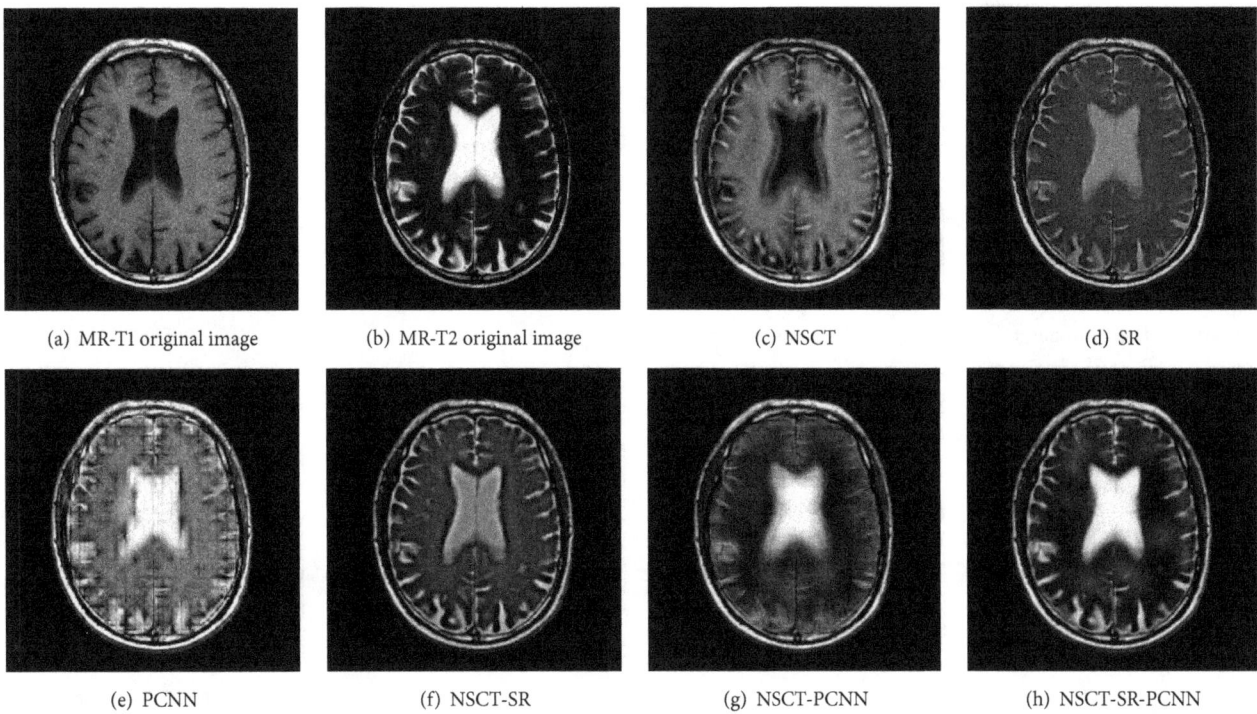

(a) MR-T1 original image   (b) MR-T2 original image   (c) NSCT   (d) SR

(e) PCNN   (f) NSCT-SR   (g) NSCT-PCNN   (h) NSCT-SR-PCNN

FIGURE 10: MR-T1/MR-T2 medical image fusion results.

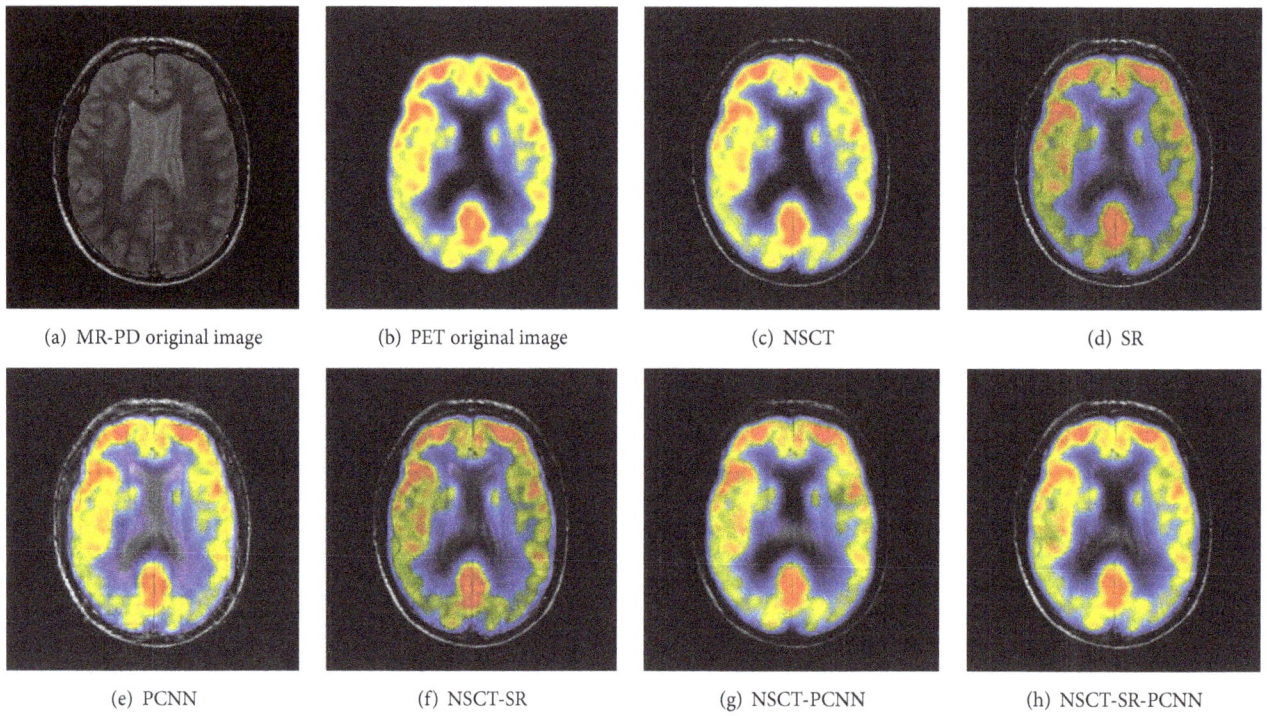

(a) MR-PD original image   (b) PET original image   (c) NSCT   (d) SR

(e) PCNN   (f) NSCT-SR   (g) NSCT-PCNN   (h) NSCT-SR-PCNN

FIGURE 11: MR-PD/PET medical image fusion results.

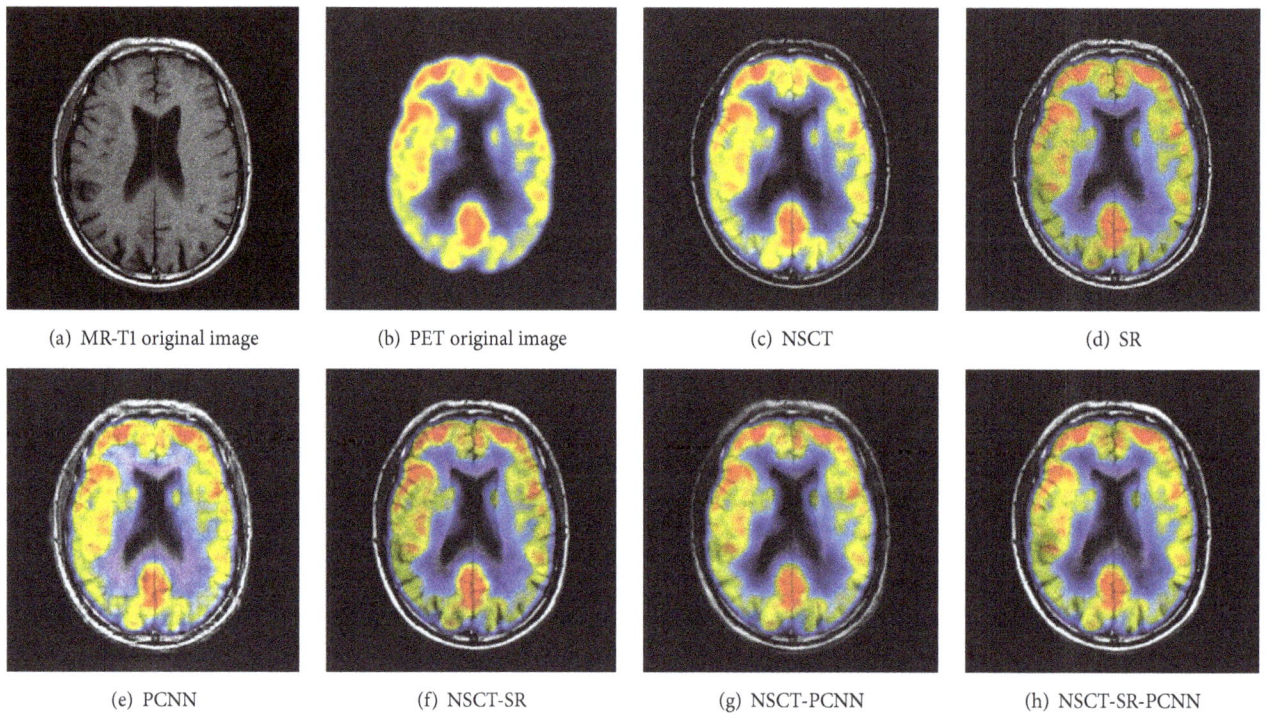

(a) MR-T1 original image   (b) PET original image   (c) NSCT   (d) SR

(e) PCNN   (f) NSCT-SR   (g) NSCT-PCNN   (h) NSCT-SR-PCNN

FIGURE 12: MR-T1/PET medical image fusion results.

TABLE 1: Quality evaluation of CT/MRI medical image fusion.

Evaluation index	NSCT	SR	PCNN	NSCT-SR	NSCT-PCNN	NSCT-SR-PCNN
IE	0.1312	**0.1498**	0.1000	**0.3965**	0.0620	**0.1634**
MC	**2.6621**	2.3780	**2.9962**	2.3718	2.4343	**2.4396**
MI	**3.4885**	**2.8146**	1.8082	2.1005	1.7618	**2.2426**
SD	**56.6060**	37.9078	**59.5349**	44.0044	46.2033	**55.4061**
$Q^{AB/F}$	**0.6572**	0.5441	0.4020	**0.6794**	0.3502	**0.6899**
VIFF	0.6598	0.5688	0.3922	**0.7074**	0.4201	**0.6677**
SSIM	**0.9385**	0.8775	0.6674	0.8520	0.7896	**0.9567**

TABLE 2: Quality evaluation of MR-PD/MR-T1 medical image fusion.

Evaluation index	NSCT	SR	PCNN	NSCT-SR	NSCT-PCNN	NSCT-SR-PCNN
IE	**0.9999**	0.9904	0.9579	0.9922	**0.9999**	0.9963
MC	2.2233	2.4200	**4.3005**	2.4234	**2.7476**	2.6054
MI	**3.0047**	**2.4785**	2.1328	2.3858	2.2826	**2.5474**
SD	**54.6893**	45.1990	**56.0878**	45.4664	46.5353	**51.4444**
$Q^{AB/F}$	**0.5648**	**0.5669**	0.4345	0.5399	0.4205	**0.5887**
VIFF	0.5722	0.5675	0.3408	0.4964	0.4228	**0.5991**
SSIM	1.4165	**1.5332**	0.9745	1.4869	1.3444	**1.4279**

TABLE 3: Quality evaluation of MR-PD/MR-T2 medical image fusion.

Evaluation index	NSCT	SR	PCNN	NSCT-SR	NSCT-PCNN	NSCT-SR-PCNN
IE	0.9730	**0.9768**	**0.9928**	**0.9777**	**0.9859**	0.9768
MC	**2.5614**	**2.5205**	**3.0647**	2.4164	2.4802	**2.5033**
MI	2.3808	**2.7229**	2.3961	**2.5019**	**2.4154**	2.5378
SD	**56.4522**	46.3235	**59.0546**	47.5818	**52.1596**	**56.6857**
$Q^{AB/F}$	**0.6120**	**0.6491**	0.4912	**0.6385**	0.4612	**0.6530**
VIFF	0.7091	0.7528	0.5534	0.6966	0.6267	**0.8150**
SSIM	1.6297	1.6524	1.5168	1.6552	1.6306	**1.7148**

TABLE 4: Quality evaluation of MR-T1/MR-T2 medical image fusion.

Evaluation index	NSCT	SR	PCNN	NSCT-SR	NSCT-PCNN	NSCT-SR-PCNN
IE	0.9936	0.9907	**0.9979**	0.9920	**0.9974**	0.9956
MC	2.7955	2.6224	**3.2850**	2.6689	**2.8966**	2.8338
MI	1.8604	**2.4779**	2.1623	**2.2494**	2.0621	**2.2047**
SD	53.9478	47.4264	**72.9638**	49.5285	**54.9129**	58.7637
$Q^{AB/F}$	0.4321	**0.5076**	0.4357	**0.5754**	0.4007	**0.5732**
VIFF	0.3003	0.4529	0.3316	0.3400	0.3400	**0.4769**
SSIM	1.2341	**1.3590**	1.2475	1.2379	1.2379	**1.2812**

TABLE 5: Quality evaluation of MR-PD/PET medical image fusion.

Evaluation index	NSCT	SR	PCNN	NSCT-SR	NSCT-PCNN	NSCT-SR-PCNN
IE	**0.9977**	0.9761	0.9677	0.9791	**0.9954**	0.9801
SF	**6.0266**	5.7013	**6.9747**	5.8537	5.7295	**5.9952**
AG	4.8934	**4.9109**	**6.9312**	4.8133	4.2310	**4.9744**
MC	**1.9402**	1.7960	**2.5601**	1.8627	1.8753	**1.9409**
MI	**2.7632**	**2.7705**	2.6597	2.6677	2.6979	**2.7879**
SD	**70.2719**	50.0841	**70.9987**	50.8343	63.5030	**67.2682**
$Q^{AB/F}$	**0.5414**	**0.5411**	0.4311	0.5295	0.3908	**0.5718**

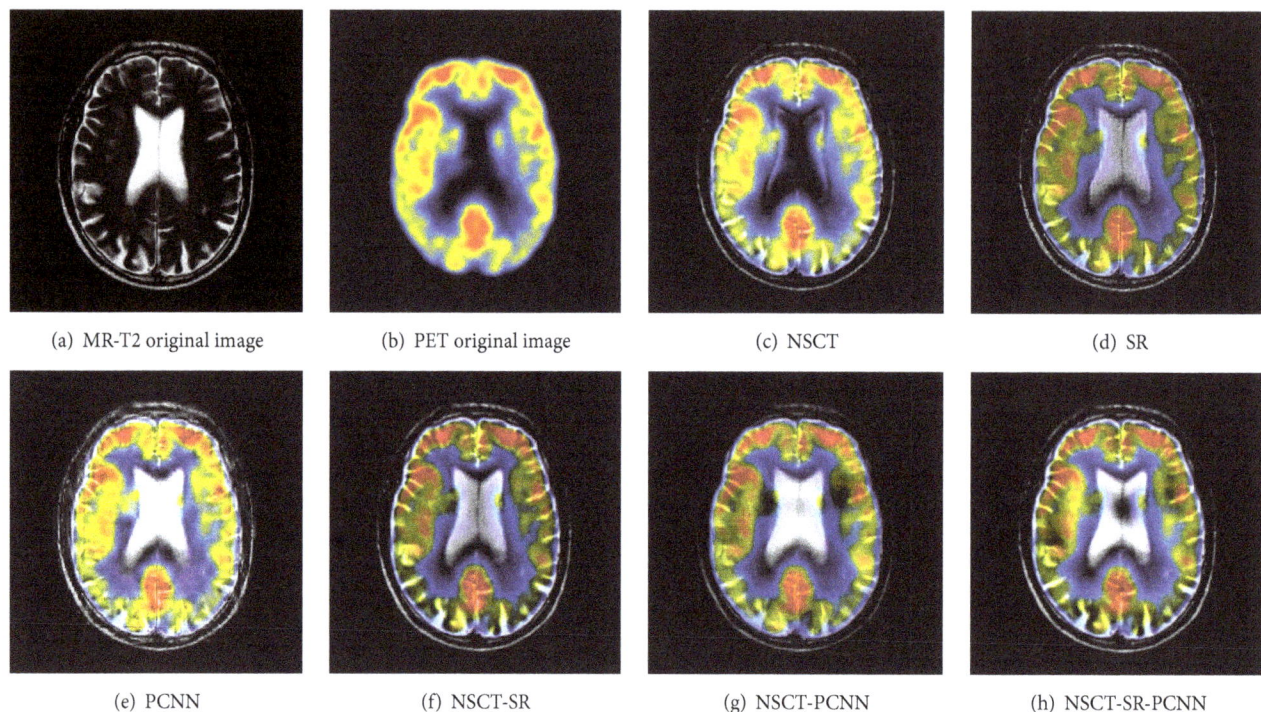

(a) MR-T2 original image   (b) PET original image   (c) NSCT   (d) SR

(e) PCNN   (f) NSCT-SR   (g) NSCT-PCNN   (h) NSCT-SR-PCNN

Figure 13: MR-T2/PET medical image fusion results.

Table 6: Quality evaluation of MR-T1/PET medical image fusion.

Evaluation index	NSCT	SR	PCNN	NSCT-SR	NSCT-PCNN	NSCT-SR-PCNN
IE	**0.9992**	0.9879	0.9755	0.9897	**0.9975**	**0.9923**
SF	6.6819	**6.9951**	**7.9528**	6.9423	6.7408	**6.9475**
AG	6.5924	**8.0276**	**9.9589**	7.5923	6.2566	**7.5961**
MC	2.2740	2.3869	**3.0047**	2.3844	**2.4070**	**2.4067**
MI	2.5493	**2.7738**	2.5631	**2.7455**	2.5485	**2.7559**
SD	**70.8814**	60.3674	**77.6841**	62.4699	63.5939	**67.0245**
$Q^{AB/F}$	0.4333	**0.5505**	0.4521	**0.5611**	0.3908	**0.5681**

Table 7: Quality evaluation of MR-T2/PET medical image fusion.

Evaluation index	NSCT	SR	PCNN	NSCT-SR	NSCT-PCNN	NSCT-SR-PCNN
IE	**0.9953**	0.9697	0.9622	0.9734	**0.9935**	0.9769
SF	6.7434	**6.9677**	**8.0595**	6.6804	6.7986	**6.9365**
AG	6.7453	**8.0305**	**10.3970**	7.1794	6.0200	**7.4678**
MC	2.2195	**2.2513**	**3.0121**	2.1432	2.2898	**2.3136**
MI	2.5588	**2.7566**	2.5835	**2.6558**	**2.6199**	2.6076
SD	**70.6653**	54.3247	**82.1519**	56.6147	63.2384	**65.1174**
$Q^{AB/F}$	0.3985	**0.5125**	0.3832	**0.5449**	0.3166	**0.5451**

7. Conclusion

The NSCT-SR-PCNN algorithm effectively combines NSCT transform, sparse representation, and pulse coupled neural network to overcome the shortcomings of wavelet transform, which cannot reflect the holistic characteristics, and solves the problem that the low frequency subband coefficient is not sparse. In addition, this algorithm collects the image texture, the degree of change in edge and details, and other information, which improves the comprehensive performance of the fusion results. The experimental data show that although not all the evaluation indexes of NSCT-SF-PCNN algorithm rank the first, the evaluation indexes of the NSCT-SF-PCNN algorithm are all in the top three and the top four; besides this, the comprehensive indexes are the number one, and the edge information delivery factor $Q_{AB/F}$ of the high weight evaluation index is higher than that of the five contrast algorithms, and the edge and detail information of the source image is better preserved, and the human visual effect is better. Certainly, the NSCT-SR-PCNN algorithm also needs to be improved. For example, through the online dictionary learning method, to obtain a complete dictionary D still requires further study.

Conflicts of Interest

The authors declare that they have no conflicts of interest.

Acknowledgments

This work was funded by the National Natural Science Foundation (41505017).

References

[1] Y. Fei, G. Wei, and S. Zongxi, "Medical image fusion based on feature extraction and sparse representation," *International Journal of Biomedical Imaging*, vol. 2017, Article ID 3020461, 11 pages, 2017.

[2] J. Zhen-yi and W. Yuan-jun, "Multi-modality medical image fusion method based on non-subsampled contourlet transform," *Chinese Journal of Medical Physics*, vol. 33, no. 5, pp. 445–450, 2016.

[3] M. N. Do and M. Vetterli, "Contourlets: A directional multiresolution image representation," in *Proceedings of the ICIP 2002 International Conference on Image Processing*, vol. 1, pp. 357–360, Rochester, NY, USA, 2001.

[4] S. Zhao-yu, H. Rong, and O. Ning, "Image fusion based on multi-scale sparse representation," *Computer Engineering and Design*, vol. 36, no. 1, pp. 232–235, 2015.

[5] R. Eckhorn, H. J. Reitboeck, and M. Arndt, "A neural network for feature linking via synchronous activity," *Canadian Journal of Microbiology*, vol. 46, no. 8, pp. 759–763, 1989.

[6] H. J. Reitboeck, R. Eckhorn, M. Arndt, and P. Dicke, "A Model for Feature Linking via Correlated Neural Activity," in *Synergetics of Cognition*, pp. 112–125, Springer, Berlin, Germany, 1990.

[7] Z. Chun-hui and G. Yun-ting, "Fast image fusion algorithm based on sparse representation and non-subsampled contourlet transform," *Journal of Electronics and Information Technology*, vol. 7, no. 38, pp. 1773–1780, 2016.

[8] F. Shabanzade and H. Ghassemian, "Multimodal image fusion via sparse representation and clustering-based dictionary learning algorithm in NonSubsampled Contourlet domain," in *Proceedings of the 8th International Symposium on Telecommunications, IST 2016*, pp. 472–477, Tehran, Iran, September 2016.

[9] J. Gong, B. Wang, L. Qiao, J. Xu, and Z. Zhang, "Image Fusion Method Based on Improved NSCT Transform and PCNN Model," in *Proceedings of the 9th International Symposium on Computational Intelligence and Design, ISCID 2016*, pp. 28–31, Hangzhou, China, December 2016.

[10] A. Mohammed, K. L. Nisha, and P. S. Sathidevi, "A novel medical image fusion scheme employing sparse representation and dual PCNN in the NSCT domain," in *Proceedings of the 2016 IEEE Region 10 Conference, TENCON 2016*, pp. 2147–2151, Singapore, November 2016.

[11] O. Ning, Z. Xue-ying, and Y. Hua, "Multi-focus image fusion based on NSCT and sparse representation," *Computer Engineering and Design*, vol. 38, pp. 177–182, 2017.

[12] C. M. Gray and W. Singer, "Stimulus specific neuronal oscillations in the cat visual cortex: A cortical functional unit," *Soc.neurosci.abst*, 1987.

[13] Z. Hai-feng, L. Yu-miao, L. Ming, and C. Si-bao, "Medical Image Compression Based on Fast Sparse Representation," *Computer Engineering*, vol. 40, no. 4, pp. 233–236, 2014.

[14] W. Yuan-jun, J. Bo-yu, and J. Zhen-yi, "Review of multimodal medical image fusion technology based on wavelet transformation," *Chinese Journal of Medical Physics*, vol. 30, no. 6, pp. 4530–4536, 2013.

[15] X. Wei-liang, D. Wen-zhan, and L. Jun-feng, "Medical image fusion algorithm based on lifting wavelet transform and PCNN," *Journal of Zhejiang Sci-Tech University*, vol. 35, no. 6, pp. 891–898, 2016.

[16] C. S. Xydeas and V. Petrović, "Objective image fusion performance measure," *IET Journals and Magazines on Electronics Letters*, vol. 36, no. 4, pp. 308-309, 2000.

[17] G. Qu, D. Zhang, and P. Yan, "Information measure for performance of image fusion," *IET Journals and Magazines on Electronics Letters*, vol. 38, no. 7, pp. 313–315, 2002.

[18] G. Piella and H. Heijmans, "A new quality metric for image fusion," in *Proceedings of the 10th International Conference on Image Processing*, vol. 3, pp. 173–176, IEEE, Barcelona, Spain, September 2003.

[19] Z. Liu, E. Blasch, Z. Xue, J. Zhao, R. Laganiére, and W. Wu, "Objective assessment of multiresolution image fusion algorithms for context enhancement in Night vision: A comparative study," *IEEE Transactions on Pattern Analysis and Machine Intelligence*, vol. 34, no. 1, pp. 94–109, 2012.

[20] T. Xiu-hua and X. Wang, "Research on NSCT-based Medical Image Fusion," *Computer Applications and Software*, vol. 30, no. 4, pp. 287–290, 2013.

[21] C. Yao-jia, Z. Yong-ping, and T. Jian-yan, "Multi-focus Image Fusion Based on Blocked Sparse Representation," *Video Engineering*, vol. 36, no. 13, pp. 48–52, 2012.

[22] C. Hao, Z. Juan, and L. Yan-ying, "Image fusion based on pulse coupled neural network," *Optics and Precision Enginee Ring*, vol. 18, no. 4, pp. 995–1001, 2010.

[23] C. Jun-qiang and H. Dan-fei, "A Medical Image Fusion Improved Algorithm Based on NSCT and Adaptive PCNN," *Journal of Changchun University of Science and Technology*, vol. 38, no. 3, pp. 152–155, 2015.

[24] S. Li, B. Yang, and J. Hu, "Performance comparison of different multi-resolution transforms for image fusion," *Information Fusion*, vol. 12, no. 2, pp. 74–84, 2011.

[25] Y. Tian, Y. Li, and F. Ye, "Multimodal medical image fusion based on nonsubsampled contourlet transform using improved PCNN," in *Proceedings of the 13th IEEE International Conference on Signal Processing, ICSP 2016*, vol. 13, pp. 799–804, Chengdu, China, November 2016.

11

Arrhythmia Classification of ECG Signals using Hybrid Features

Syed Muhammad Anwar [ID],[1] Maheen Gul [ID],[2] Muhammad Majid [ID],[2] and Majdi Alnowami [ID][3]

[1]Department of Software Engineering, University of Engineering and Technology, Taxila, Pakistan
[2]Department of Computer Engineering, University of Engineering and Technology, Taxila, Pakistan
[3]Department of Nuclear Engineering, King Abdulaziz University, Jeddah, Saudi Arabia

Correspondence should be addressed to Syed Muhammad Anwar; s.anwar@uettaxila.edu.pk

Guest Editor: Dominique J. Monlezun

Automatic detection and classification of life-threatening arrhythmia plays an important part in dealing with various cardiac conditions. In this paper, a novel method for classification of various types of arrhythmia using morphological and dynamic features is presented. Discrete wavelet transform (DWT) is applied on each heart beat to obtain the morphological features. It provides better time and frequency resolution of the electrocardiogram (ECG) signal, which helps in decoding important information of a quasiperiodic ECG using variable window sizes. RR interval information is used as a dynamic feature. The nonlinear dynamics of RR interval are captured using Teager energy operator, which improves the arrhythmia classification. Moreover, to remove redundancy, DWT subbands are subjected to dimensionality reduction using independent component analysis, and a total of twelve coefficients are selected as morphological features. These hybrid features are combined and fed to a neural network to classify arrhythmia. The proposed algorithm has been tested over MIT-BIH arrhythmia database using 13724 beats and MIT-BIH supraventricular arrhythmia database using 22151 beats. The proposed methodology resulted in an improved average accuracy of 99.75% and 99.84% for class- and subject-oriented scheme, respectively, using three-fold cross validation.

1. Introduction

Cardiac arrhythmias are a type of irregular heartbeats in which the heart rhythm is either too fast (tachycardia) or too slow (bradycardia). A small change in electrocardiogram (ECG) morphology or dynamics may lead to severe arrhythmia attacks, which can reduce the ability of the heart to pump blood and causes shorting of breath, pain in chest, tiredness, and loss of consciousness. There are several types of arrhythmia, and some of these are dangerous which may lead to cardiac arrest and sudden death if not detected and monitored in time [1]. There are other types of arrhythmias which are not essentially life-threatening, but still require proper analysis to avoid future clinical problems. A few categories of arrhythmia appear infrequently in the ECG signal and hence require long electrocardiogram recordings in order to be detected. A manual analysis of longer ECG recordings requires time and great effort. The automatic

detection and classification of these arrhythmias offer great assistance to physicians [2, 3]. Moreover, early diagnosis of arrhythmias would help in proper treatment and support sustained life. Therefore, several techniques have been proposed for automatic detection and classification of various types of arrhythmia [4–10].

A method for classification of sixteen types of arrhythmia based on ECG morphology and dynamics was proposed in [11]. Morphological features were extracted using discrete wavelet transform (DWT) and independent component analysis (ICA), while ECG dynamic features were extracted by calculating RR interval. These features were then classified using support vector machine with an average accuracy of 99.6%. Five types of heartbeats, namely, normal, premature ventricular contractions (PVC), atrial premature contractions (APC), left bundle branch block (LBBB), and right bundle branch block (RBBB) were recognized in [4]. Stationary wavelet transform (SWT) was applied on each ECG signal to make it noise free. The high-order statistics of ECG signals and three timing intervals were considered as features, which were then fed to a hybrid bees algorithm for training the radial basis function and resulted in an average accuracy of 95.18%.

Some techniques rely on fiducial features, which are temporal and dynamic features that directly depend upon the ECG characteristics, e.g., wave onset point, peaks (maxima/minima), and offset [5]. Nonfiducial features that are directly derived from the fiducial features or obtained by segmenting the ECG signal into several parts have also been used [6]. These features are not found good enough when used independently for accurate classification of ECG arrhythmia. A combination of both fiducial and nonfiducial features was used for defining a biological marker for person identification [7, 12].

The extracted features have usually been analyzed either in time domain or frequency domain. Some of the most important time domain features, including RR interval, ST segment, and T height, require identification of key time points within the signal [13]. An approach for heartbeat classification with dynamic rejection thresholds was proposed using QRS morphology, frequency information, AC power of QRS detail coefficients, and RR intervals as features to represent ECG beats [8]. A support vector machine (SVM) was used to classify with an improved accuracy of 97.2% and minimum rejection cost. A combination of time and frequency information has also been used in [9, 11, 14–16], giving better extraction of information from a quasiperiodic ECG signal using wavelet transform, which provides a good time and frequency resolution. Five important types of arrhythmia, namely, nonectopic, ventricular ectopic, supraventricular ectopic, unclassifiable beats, and fusion betas, were analyzed and detected in [9]. Features were extracted using DWT, and only significant coefficients were selected by applying independent component analysis which in combination with neural network yielded an accuracy of 99.28%.

All methods discussed above have the following shortcomings:

(1) Performances of most of the methods have been tested only on smaller data sets, and there is a need to verify their performance on larger databases

(2) Selected classes of arrhythmia have been evaluated, and there is a need to test all arrhythmia classes

(3) The classification accuracy on sparsely occurring arrhythmia classes is not good

In this paper, a novel technique for ECG beat classification of arrhythmia is proposed that considers a hybrid of enhanced morphological and dynamic features to overcome these shortcomings. Morphological features are obtained using DWT on each heartbeat. The resulting features consist of DWT approximation coefficient and detail coefficients at level 4. Independent component analysis is applied on both approximation and detail coefficients independently to extract only important coefficients. In addition, four types of RR interval features are calculated to represent the dynamic

features of ECG heartbeats. Moreover, to enhance the dynamic features of ECG heartbeats corrupted with Gaussian noise, Teager energy operator (TEO) [17] is used. All these features are combined and fed to a neural network (NN) for automatic classification of heartbeats into different arrhythmia types according to both class-oriented scheme (18 classes) and subject-oriented scheme (5 classes).

The rest of the paper is organized as follows. Firstly, the proposed methodology is explained in detail in Section 2. Class- and subject-oriented evaluation of the proposed system is presented in Section 3, followed by conclusion in Section 4.

2. Methodology

The proposed methodology is presented in Figure 1, which consists of four major phases, namely, preprocessing, heartbeat segmentation, feature extraction, and feature classification. The details of these phases are presented in the following subsections.

2.1. ECG Signal Preprocessing. Mostly ECG signals are affected by baseline wander or power line interface (PLI). Different methods were introduced to remove these types of noises from the ECG signal [18]. Experiments showed that baseline wander significantly affects the detection of arrhythmia and makes the ECG signal analysis difficult for an expert [19]. PLI is a type of noise that occurs due to broken electrodes, offset voltages in the electrodes, movement of patient, respiration errors, or electrode resistance while recording the ECG signal. It is a low frequency noise and typically exists in the frequency range of 0–0.3 Hz. For baseline wander removal, the expected value of the signal was subtracted from the raw ECG signal to obtain the noise-free ECG signal using

$$x[n] = x_r[n] - \mu, \qquad (1)$$

where $x[n]$ is the denoised signal, $x_r[n]$ represents the raw ECG signal, and μ is the expected value of the raw EEG signal.

2.2. Heartbeat Segmentation. Three basic constituents of a heart cycle are QRS complex, T wave, and P wave, termed as fiducial points. The correct splitting of the ECG signal into heartbeat segments involves recognition of borders and peak locations of these fiducial points. The information about the R-peak locations given in the dataset was used to obtain these heartbeat segments. A single heartbeat consisted of 200 samples including the R-peak and the samples around the peak. This segment size contained maximum information of a single heartbeat and is shown in Figure 2.

2.3. Feature Extraction. In feature extraction, improved features based on DWT, RR interval, and Teager energy operator were selected, which were able to represent the morphological and dynamic changes in the ECG signal with more significance.

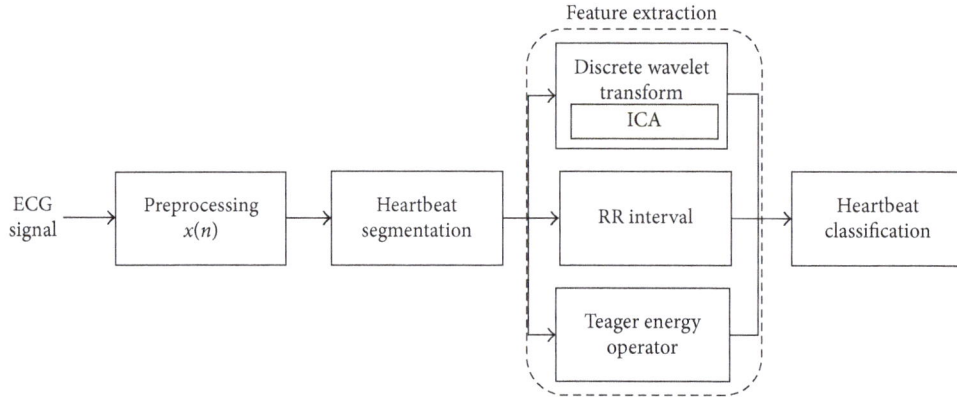

FIGURE 1: Block diagram of the proposed arrhythmia classification scheme using hybrid features.

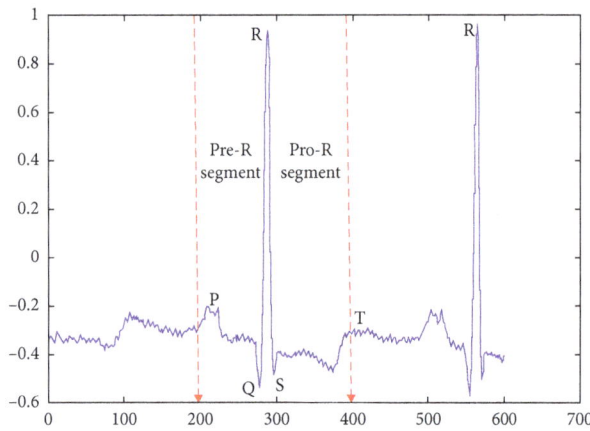

FIGURE 2: Heartbeat segmentation of ECG signal from MITDB database.

2.3.1. Discrete Wavelet Transform (DWT).

Statistical features of biomedical signals usually change over position or time. Wavelet transform offers signal representation in both time and frequency domains, which makes it capable for analyzing quasiperiodic signals like ECG. Wavelet transform was employed in processing of the ECG signals for feature extraction [1], denoising [11], and heartbeat recognition [20]. In the proposed method, DWT was used as a feature extraction technique. After applying DWT, the ECG signal decomposed into low-frequency approximation components and high-frequency detail components.

The most commonly used wavelets which provide orthogonality properties are Daubechies, Coiflets, Symlets, and Discrete Meyer [21]. Each heartbeat was disintegrated using the finite impulse response (FIR) approximation of the Discrete Mayers wavelet transform. The frequency range of fourth-level approximation subband was 011.25 Hz, and the frequency range for fourth level detail subband was 11.2522.5 Hz. A total of 200 coefficients were extracted as wavelet features, which were processed using ICA for dimensionality reduction. Six major ICA components were selected from each of the two DWT subbands, resulting in a total of twelve morphological features from the two subbands.

2.3.2. RR Interval Features.

R is a point corresponding to the highest peak of the ECG waveform, and RR interval is the time between the successive QRS complexes. The ECG signal has a nonlinear dynamic behavior, and during arrhythmia, nonlinear dynamic components change more significantly than the linear counterparts. RR interval is simple, easy to calculate, and less prone to noise. Four types of RR interval features, namely, previous-RR, post-RR, average-RR, and local-RR interval, were derived from the RR sequence, to characterize the dynamic features of the heartbeat. The calculation of these features uses the following equations:

$$
\begin{aligned}
RR_{pre}(i) &= R(i) - R(i-1), \\
RR_{post}(i) &= R(i+1) - R(i), \\
RR_{local} &= \frac{1}{10} \sum_{i=-5}^{5} RR(i), \\
RR_{ave} &= \frac{1}{N_{RR}} \sum_{i=1}^{N_{RR}} RR(i),
\end{aligned}
\tag{2}
$$

where i shows the location of the current R-peak and RR_{pre}, RR_{post}, RR_{local}, and RR_{ave} represent the previous, post, local, and average RR interval, respectively. $R(i)$ is the current R-peak, $R(i-1)$ and $R(i+1)$ represent the previous and post R-peaks, respectively, and N_{RR} shows the total number of RR intervals in an ECG segment.

2.3.3. Teager Energy Operator (TEO).

An independent analysis of RR interval does not capture the nonlinear nature of RR interval inconsistency. TEO was utilized to represent the nonlinear behavior of the RR interval, which is a nonlinear operator for energy tracking [17]. It measures the instantaneous frequency, amplitude envelope, and the energy of the system that generated the signal. The energy required by a source to generate signals with different frequencies and same energy and amplitude would be different. More energy is needed to generate a high-frequency signal as compared with a low-frequency signal. TEO reflects the source energy; hence, any instability in the conduction path and impulse generation gets revealed in the Teager energy function. For a discrete time signal $x[n]$, the Teager–Kaiser nonlinear energy (NE) and the average nonlinear energy (ANE) in the time domain are given as

$$\mathrm{NE}\{x[n]\} = x^2[n] - x[n-1]x[n+1], \qquad (3)$$

$$\mathrm{ANE} = \frac{1}{N}\sum \mathrm{NE}\{x[n]\}, \qquad (4)$$

where N represents the total number of samples in ECG heartbeat.

2.4. Neural Network (NN) Classifier. An artificial neural network consists of interconnected neurons which send and receive messages between each other. These interconnections are assigned weights, which represent a network state and are updated during the learning process. A feedforward neural network with 10 hidden layers was used for the classification of arrhythmia in this study. The network was implemented on MATLAB R2013a. The number of neurons in each hidden layer was limited to 50, which allowed training this network on a core-i5 CPU-based system with a RAM of 8 GB. An activation function based on rectified linear unit (ReLU) was used for the hidden layers, and a sigmoid function was used at the output layer. Back propagation with stochastic gradient decay was used for updating the network weights. The learning rate was optimized to a value of 0.63, using grid search for accuracy and to avoid over fitting.

3. Experimental Results

The details of the dataset used and the experimental results are presented in the following subsections.

3.1. Dataset. The MIT-BIH arrhythmia database (MITDB) [22] and MIT-BIH supraventricular arrhythmia database (SVDB) [23] from physionet were used for evaluation of the performance of the proposed algorithm. The MITDB includes 48 ECG recordings of 47 subjects, whereas the SVDB contains 78 half-hour ECG recordings. The data in SVDB were recorded to increase the supraventricular arrhythmias examples in MITDB. The databases contain an annotation file with locations of the "QRS" complex and the type of the heartbeat for each record. These class annotations for heartbeats were exploited as reference annotations for evaluation purpose of the proposed model.

3.2. Evaluation Strategy. Two different types of evaluation strategies were considered, namely, class-oriented [24] and subject-oriented [9]. In class-oriented strategy, all signals from both databases were segmented down using already annotated QRS locations. The resulting segments were divided into 18 different types of beats, namely, normal beat (NOR "N"), atrial premature contraction (APC "A"), fusion of ventricular and normal beat (FVN "F"), left bundle branch block (LBBB "L"), unclassifiable beat (UN "Q"), premature ventricular contraction (PVC "V"), right bundle branch

block beat (RBBB "R"), ventricular flutter wave (VF "!"), atrial escape beat (AE "e"), fusion of paced and normal beat (FPN "f"), nodal (junctional) premature beat (NP "J"), isolated QRS-like artifact (—), aberrated atrial premature beat (AP "a"), ventricular escape beat (VE "E"), nodal (junctional) escape beat (NE "j"), nonconducted P-wave (blocked APB "x"), paced beat (PACE "/"), and supraventricular premature beat (SP "S").

In addition, subject-oriented strategy was also evaluated. All 126 records from both the datasets were divided into a similar training and testing ratio as for the class-oriented scheme, but performance was reported according to ANSI/AAMI EC57:1998 standard [25]. The original 18 classes of heartbeats were grouped into five bigger classes, namely, nonectopic beats (N), ventricular ectopic beat (V), supraventricular ectopic beat (S), unknown beat (Q), and fusion beat (F). The mapping from the MITDB and SVDB classes to the ANSI/AAMI heartbeat classes is presented in Table 1.

The ECG signal from MITDB and SVDB datasets are first denoised to remove baseline wander. The denoised signal was segmented into different heartbeats of same length (200 samples each) by using R-peak location information in the given annotations. In total, 35875 beats form both databases (13724 from MIT-BIH arrhythmia dataset and 22151 beats from MIT-BIH supraventricular arrhythmia dataset) were considered. FIR approximation of Mayers wavelet was applied on each heartbeat segment. ICA was applied on the resulting 4th level approximation and 4th level detail coefficients independently to remove the redundancy between feature coefficients. In addition, dynamic features of the ECG signal were represented by four types of RR interval features, and Teager energy operator was used to represent the nonlinear dynamics of the ECG signal.

A 3-fold cross-validation method was used for training and testing of the classifier. The complete dataset ($35,875$ beats) was subsampled into two sets, one having 70% of the total samples and the other with the remaining heartbeats from each of the classes (50% data was selected for training from atrial escape beat (e), due to very low number of beats). 70% of total heartbeats were utilized for training purpose, and the rest of the heartbeats were used in testing and evaluation of the performance of the classifier. The process was repeated three times with different heartbeats used for training and testing. The average results of the three folds were calculated to assess the general performance of the proposed method. Sensitivity (Se), specificity (Sp), positive predictive value (PPV), and accuracy (Acc) were calculated to analyze the performance.

3.2.1. Class-Oriented Evaluation. In class-oriented evaluation scheme, a neural network was trained to predict the class of test heartbeats among 18 different classes of arrhythmia. The specificity, sensitivity, and PPV of each individual class are summarized in Table 2, which shows that the proposed approach demonstrates a reasonable individual-class performance, showing greater specificity, good sensitivity, and PPV. Moreover, it has given better results on classes whose

TABLE 1: Mapping from MIT-BIH arrhythmia database (MITDB)/supraventricular arrhythmia database (SVDB) heartbeat classes to ANSI/AAMI heartbeat classes.

AAMI classes	MITDB/SVDB classes	Total
Nonectopic beat (N)	NOR, LBBB, RBBB, AE, NE	30929
Supraventricular ectopic beat (S)	APC, AP, APB, NP, SP	1538
Ventricular ectopic beat (V)	PVC, VE, VF	2035
Fusion beat (F)	F	14
Unknown beat (Q)	UN, FPN, PACE, |	1329

TABLE 2: A summary of performance analysis of the proposed method on each arrhythmia class in the "class-oriented" scheme.

Heartbeat type	Fold I				Fold II				Fold III				Average			
	Sp	Se	PPV	Acc	Sp	Se	PPV	Acc	Sp	Se	PPV	Acc	Sp	Se	PPV	Acc
Normal beat (NOR)	100	100	99.8	99.4	100	100	99.9	99.7	99.8	100	99.7	99.7	99.9	100	99.8	99.6
Atrial premature contraction	100	97	100	100	100	96.5	100	100	100	97.5	100	100	100	97	100	100
Fusion of ventricular and normal beat	100	100	100	100	100	100	100	92.7	100	100	100	100	100	100	100	97.5
Left bundle branch block (LBBB)	100	97.5	100	100	100	97	100	99.3	100	96.5	100	100	100	97	100	99.7
Unclassifiable beat (UN)	100	100	100	100	100	100	100	100	100	100	100	100	100	100	100	100
Right bundle branch block beat (RBBB)	99.8	99.4	99.4	99.7	99.9	99.2	99.4	99.4	99.9	99.3	99.4	99.4	99.8	99.3	99.4	99.5
Premature ventricular contraction (PVC)	100	99.1	99.6	99.7	100	99.2	99.6	99.5	100	99.3	99.6	99.6	100	99.2	99.6	99.6
Ventricular flutter wave (VF)	100	100	100	100	100	100	100	100	100	100	100	100	100	100	100	100
Aberrated atrial premature beat (AP)	100	100	100	100	100	100	100	100	100	100	100	100	100	100	100	100
Nodal (junctional) premature beat (NP)	100	92.6	100	100	100	92.8	100	100	100	92.7	100	100	100	92.8	100	100
Atrial escape beat (AE)	100	100	100	100	100	100	100	100	100	100	100	100	100	100	100	100
Fusion of paced and normal beat (FPN)	100	100	100	100	99.9	100	100	100	100	100	100	100	100	100	100	100
Isolated QRS-like artifact (Iso)	99.9	100	97.2	100	99.9	100	98.1	100	99.9	99.1	99.1	99.1	99.9	98.1	98.1	99.5
Ventricular escape beat (VE)	100	100	100	100	99.9	100	95.2	100	99.9	100	98.5	100	100	95.2	100	100
Nodal (junctional) escape beat	99.9	100	95	100	99.9	100	97.5	100	100	100	100	100	100	100	100	100
Paced beat (PACE)	99.9	100	99.2	100	100	100	100	100	99.9	100	99.6	100	100	99.2	100	100
Nonconducted P-wave (blocked APB)	100	100	100	100	100	100	100	100	100	100	100	100	100	100	100	100
Supraventricular premature beat (SP)	100	100	100	100	100	100	100	100	100	100	100	100	100	99.4	100	100
Average	99.9	99.9	99.4	99.9	99.9	99.3	99.4	99.3	99.9	99.9	99.8	99.9	99.9	98.7	99.8	99.75

presence was low like "Q," "e," and "x." The performance evaluation measures are shown for all three folds in Table 2, where the best accuracy achieved was 99.9%. In addition, 98.7% average sensitivity, 99.9% average specificity, 99.8% average PPV, and 99.75% overall accuracy were achieved. The confusion matrix is presented in Table 3, which shows the correctly classified and misclassified arrhythmia classes.

A comparison of the classification accuracy of the proposed approach and state-of-the-art methods based on class-oriented strategy is presented in Table 4. An improvement in accuracy with increased number of classes and reduced feature dimension is observed. In addition, other performance parameters such as sensitivity, specificity, and PPV have also shown improvement. These results depict that the proposed method is more generalized and computationally efficient for arrhythmia classification. An assessment based solely on "class-oriented" scheme is not a faithful measure for the performance analysis of a real-time heartbeat classification system. The performance of the subject-oriented scheme is also analyzed for practical evaluation.

3.2.2. Subject-Oriented Evaluation. In subject-oriented scheme, results have reported according to the ANSI/ AAMI standard. The specificity, sensitivity, PPV and

accuracy of each individual class in ANSI/AAMI standard is shown in Table 5. The hybrid feature approach demonstrated reasonable individual-class performances, showing greater specificity, good sensitivity, positive PPV, and accuracy for all classes. The fusion beats showed lower PPV in Fold II, which can be attributed to smaller number of beats in this class. The peak accuracy achieved was 99.9% with 99.7% average sensitivity, 99.9% average specificity, 99.1% of average PPV, and 99.8% average accuracy. Table 6 shows the confusion matrix depicting an improved performance on all classes with an average accuracy of 99.8%. A comparative analysis is presented in Table 7 with state-of-the-art techniques for subject-oriented classification. A significant improvement is observed, when taking this fact into account that 18 arrhythmia classes were classified. The comparison is reported for methods using the MIT-BIH data for adding credence to the results.

4. Conclusion

In this paper, a new technique for automatic heartbeat classification of all types of arrhythmia was presented. An improved hybrid feature representation of heartbeat segments was used based on a mixture of a set of derived morphological and dynamic features. The classification was done using twelve ICA projection coefficients computed

TABLE 3: Confusion matrix for the proposed method using a neural network based classifier (class-oriented scheme).

Predicted labels	N	A	F	L	Q	R	V	!	a	J	E	f	—	E	J	/	X	S
Actual labels																		
N	8656	0	0	0	0	0	0	0	0	0	0	0	0	0	0	0	0	0
A	2	65	0	0	0	0	0	0	0	0	0	0	0	0	0	0	0	0
F	0	0	14	0	0	0	0	0	0	0	0	0	0	0	0	0	0	0
L	8	0	0	260	0	0	0	0	0	0	0	0	0	0	0	0	0	0
Q	0	0	0	0	5	0	0	0	0	0	0	0	0	0	0	0	0	0
R	2	0	0	0	0	314	0	0	0	0	0	0	0	0	0	0	0	0
V	4	0	0	0	0	0	564	0	0	0	0	0	0	0	0	0	0	0
!	0	0	0	0	0	0	0	21	0	0	0	0	0	0	0	0	0	0
a	0	0	0	0	0	0	0	0	1	0	0	0	0	0	0	0	0	0
J	1	0	0	0	0	0	0	0	0	13	0	0	0	0	0	0	0	0
e	0	0	0	0	0	0	0	0	0	0	1	0	0	0	0	0	0	0
f	0	0	0	0	0	0	0	0	0	0	0	33	0	0	0	0	0	0
—	0	0	0	0	0	2	0	0	0	0	0	0	105	0	0	0	0	0
E	1	0	0	0	0	0	0	0	0	0	0	0	0	20	0	0	0	0
j	0	0	0	0	0	0	0	0	0	0	0	0	0	0	40	0	0	0
/	0	0	0	0	0	0	0	0	0	0	0	2	0	0	0	254	0	0
x	0	0	0	0	0	0	0	0	0	0	0	0	0	0	0	0	2	0
S	0	0	0	0	0	0	2	0	0	0	0	0	0	0	0	0	0	376

TABLE 4: Comparison of the proposed scheme with state-of-the-art methods using class-oriented scheme.

	Features	Dimension	Classes	Accuracy	Sensitivity	Specificity	PPV
Proposed	*DWT + RR + TEO*	17	18	99.75	98.7	99.9	99.8
Zidelmal et al. [8]	Frequency content + RR + QRS	13	2	97.2	99	—	—
Ye et al. [11]	WT + ICA + RR	18	16	99.3	91.3	—	—
Ebrahimzadeh et al. [4]	HOS + timing interval	24	5	95.18	95.61	98.8	90.6
Pathoumvanh et al. [24]	DCT	5	5	99.11	97.01	99.44	—
Rabee and Barhumi [26]	Multi resolution WT	251	14	99.2	96.2	100	—
Alajlan et al. [27]	HOS of 2nd-order-cumulant	604	2	94.96	92.19	95.19	—
de Oliveira et al. [14]	Waveform + RR	—	2	95	95	99.87	98
Li et al. [19]	Timing interval + waveform amplitude	—	2	98.2	93.1	—	81.4

TABLE 5: Performance of the proposed method on each arrhythmia class in the "subject-oriented" scheme.

	Fold I				Fold II				Fold III				Average			
Heartbeat type	Sp	Se	PPV	Acc	Sp	Se	PPV	Acc	Sp	Se	PPV	Acc	Sp	Se	PPV	Acc
Nonectopic beats (N)	99.9	100	94.2	100	99.7	99.9	99.8	99.9	100	100	99.8	100	99.9	99.9	97.9	99.9
Supraventricular ectopic beats (S)	100	99.8	100	100	99.9	100	99.8	100	100	99.9	100	100	99.9	99.6	99.9	100
Ventricular ectopic beats (V)	100	99.6	100	100	100	99.5	100	99.9	100	99.7	100	100	100	99.6	100	99.9
Fusion beats (F)	99.9	100	99.9	100	99.9	100	92.8	98.9	99.9	100	100	100	99.9	100	97.6	99.6
Unclassifiable beats (Q)	100	99.6	100	99.8	100	99.4	100	100	100	99.5	100	99.7	100	99.5	100	99.8
Average	99.9	99.8	98.8	99.9	99.9	99.7	99.6	97.7	99.9	99.8	99.9	99.9	99.9	99.7	99.1	99.8

TABLE 6: Confusion matrix for Fold II using NN (subject-oriented scheme).

Predicted labels	N	S	V	F	Q
Actual labels					
N	9280	1	0	0	0
S	1	458	0	1	0
V	2	0	604	0	0
F	0	0	0	14	0
Q	2	0	0	0	398

from the DWT features, plus four RR interval features, and Teager energy value. Two types of evaluation schemes, class- and subject-oriented, were implemented for analyzing the system. On the standard benchmark of MIT-BIH arrhythmia database and MIT-BIH supraventricular arrhythmia database, an average accuracy of 99.75% with a peak accuracy in a single fold of 99.9% in the class-oriented evaluation was achieved. An accuracy of 99.8% in the subject-oriented evaluation was achieved. In future, an automatic patient customization scheme will be considered, allowing

TABLE 7: Comparison of the proposed scheme with state-of-the-art methods using subject-oriented scheme.

	Features	Dimensions	Classes	Accuracy	Sensitivity	Specificity
Proposed	*DWT + RR interval + TEO*	17	5 (18)	99.8	99.7	99.9
Ye et al. [11]	WT + ICA + RR	18	5 (16)	86.4	91.3	—
Martis et al. [9]	DWT + ICA	12	5 (15)	99.28	97.97	99.83
Mar et al. [15]	RR interval series and WT	—	3	93	80	82
de Lannoy et al. [5]	Waveform + HOS + RR	249	5 (16)	94	—	—

the heartbeat classification method to be able to adjust to individual physiological features using wearable sensors.

Conflicts of Interest

The authors declare that there are no conflicts of interest regarding the publication of this paper.

Authors' Contributions

Syed Muhammad Anwar and Maheen Gul contributed equally to the study.

References

[1] H. V. Huikuri, A. Castellanos, and R. J. Myerburg, "Sudden death due to cardiac arrhythmias," *New England Journal of Medicine*, vol. 345, no. 20, pp. 1473–1482, 2001.

[2] P. de Chazal and R. B. Reilly, "A patient-adapting heartbeat classifier using ECG morphology and heartbeat interval features," *IEEE Transactions on Biomedical Engineering*, vol. 53, no. 12, pp. 2535–2543, 2006.

[3] A. Mustaqeem, S. M. Anwar, M. Majid, and A. R. Khan, "Wrapper method for feature selection to classify cardiac arrhythmia," in *Proceedings of 39th Annual International Conference of the IEEE Engineering in Medicine and Biology Society (EMBC)*, pp. 3656–3659, IEEE, Jeju Island, South Korea, July 2017.

[4] A. Ebrahimzadeh, B. Shakiba, and A. Khazaee, "Detection of electrocardiogram signals using an efficient method," *Applied Soft Computing*, vol. 22, pp. 108–117, 2014.

[5] G. de Lannoy, D. François, J. Delbeke, and M. Verleysen, "Weighted conditional random fields for supervised inter-patient heartbeat classification," *IEEE Transactions on Biomedical Engineering*, vol. 59, no. 1, pp. 241–247, 2012.

[6] S. Poungponsri and X.-H. Yu, "An adaptive filtering approach for electrocardiogram (ECG) signal noise reduction using neural networks," *Neurocomputing*, vol. 117, pp. 206–213, 2013.

[7] E. J. d. S. Luz, D. Menotti, and W. R. Schwartz, "Evaluating the use of ECG signal in low frequencies as a biometry," *Expert Systems with Applications*, vol. 41, no. 5, pp. 2309–2315, 2014.

[8] Z. Zidelmal, A. Amirou, D. Ould-Abdeslam, and J. Merckle, "ECG beat classification using a cost sensitive classifier," *Computer Methods and Programs in Biomedicine*, vol. 111, no. 3, pp. 570–577, 2013.

[9] R. J. Martis, U. R. Acharya, and L. C. Min, "ECG beat classification using PCA, LDA, ICA and discrete wavelet transform," *Biomedical Signal Processing and Control*, vol. 8, no. 5, pp. 437–448, 2013.

[10] A. Mustaqeem, S. M. Anwar, and M. Majid, "Multiclass classification of cardiac arrhythmia using improved feature selection and SVM invariants," *Computational and Mathematical Methods in Medicine*, vol. 2018, Article ID 7310496, 10 pages, 2018.

[11] C. Ye, B. V. Kumar, and M. T. Coimbra, "Heartbeat classification using morphological and dynamic features of ECG signals," *IEEE Transactions on Biomedical Engineering*, vol. 59, no. 10, pp. 2930–2941, 2012.

[12] M. Abo-Zahhad, S. M. Ahmed, and S. N. Abbas, "Biometric authentication based on PCG and ECG signals: present status and future directions," *Signal, Image and Video Processing*, vol. 8, no. 4, pp. 739–751, 2014.

[13] E. Ullah, A. D. Bakhshi, M. Majid, and S. Bashir, "Empirical mode decomposition for improved least square t-wave alternans estimation," in *Proceedings of 15th International Bhurban Conference on Applied Sciences and Technology (IBCAST)*, pp. 334–338, IEEE, Islamabad, Pakistan, January 2018.

[14] L. S. de Oliveira, R. V. Andreão, and M. Sarcinelli-Filho, "Premature ventricular beat classification using a dynamic bayesian network," in *Proceedings of Annual International Conference of the IEEE Engineering in Medicine and Biology Society, EMBC*, pp. 4984–4987, IEEE, Boston, MA, USA, August-September 2011.

[15] T. Mar, S. Zaunseder, J. P. Martínez, M. Llamedo, and R. Poll, "Optimization of ECG classification by means of feature selection," *IEEE Transactions on Biomedical Engineering*, vol. 58, no. 8, pp. 2168–2177, 2011.

[16] M. M. Tantawi, K. Revett, A.-B. Salem, and M. F. Tolba, "A wavelet feature extraction method for electrocardiogram (ECG)-based biometric recognition," *Signal, Image and Video Processing*, vol. 9, no. 6, pp. 1271–1280, 2015.

[17] F. Jabloun, A. E. Cetin, and E. Erzin, "Teager energy based feature parameters for speech recognition in car noise," *IEEE Signal Processing Letters*, vol. 6, no. 10, pp. 259–261, 1999.

[18] S. Khan, S. M. Anwar, W. Abbas, and R. Qureshi, "A novel adaptive algorithm for removal of power line interference from ECG signal," *Science International*, vol. 28, no. 1, pp. 139–143, 2016.

[19] P. Li, C. Liu, X. Wang, D. Zheng, Y. Li, and C. Liu, "A low-complexity data-adaptive approach for premature ventricular contraction recognition, signal," *Image and Video Processing*, vol. 8, no. 1, pp. 111–120, 2014.

[20] S. Kadambe, R. Murray, and G. F. Boudreaux-Bartels, "Wavelet transform-based QRS complex detector," *IEEE Transactions on Biomedical Engineering*, vol. 46, no. 7, pp. 838–848, 1999.

[21] P. S. Addison, "Wavelet transforms and the ECG: a review," *Physiological Measurement*, vol. 26, no. 5, p. R155, 2005.

[22] G. B. Moody and R. G. Mark, "The MIT-BIH arrhythmia database on cd-rom and software for use with it," in

Proceedings of Computers in Cardiology 1990, pp. 185–188, IEEE, Chicago, IL, USA, 1990.

[23] A. L. Goldberger, L. A. Amaral, L. Glass et al., "Physiobank, physiotoolkit, and physionet," *Circulation*, vol. 101, no. 23, pp. e215–e220, 2000.

[24] S. Pathoumvanh, K. Hamamoto, and P. Indahak, "Arrhythmias detection and classification base on single beat ECG analysis," in *Proceedings of 4th Joint International Conference on Information and Communication Technology, Electronic and Electrical Engineering (JICTEE)*, pp. 1–4, IEEE, Chiang Rai, Thailand, March 2014.

[25] Association for the Advancement of Medical Instrumentation and others, Testing and reporting performance results of cardiac rhythm and st segment measurement algorithms, *ANSI/AAMI EC38*, vol. 1998, 1998.

[26] A. Rabee and I. Barhumi, "ECG signal classification using support vector machine based on wavelet multiresolution analysis," in *Proceedings of 11th International Conference on Information Science, Signal Processing and their Applications (ISSPA)*, pp. 1319–1323, IEEE, Montreal, Canada, July 2012.

[27] N. Alajlan, Y. Bazi, F. Melgani, S. Malek, and M. A. Bencherif, "Detection of premature ventricular contraction arrhythmias in electrocardiogram signals with kernel methods," *Signal, Image and Video Processing*, vol. 8, no. 5, pp. 931–942, 2014.

12

Explicit Theoretical Analysis of How the Rate of Exocytosis Depends on Local Control by Ca^{2+} Channels

Francesco Montefusco [iD][1] **and Morten Gram Pedersen** [iD][1,2,3]

[1]*Department of Information Engineering, University of Padova, Padova, Italy*
[2]*Department of Mathematics "Tullio Levi-Civita", University of Padova, Padova, Italy*
[3]*Padova Neuroscience Center, University of Padova, Padova, Italy*

Correspondence should be addressed to Francesco Montefusco; montefusco@dei.unipd.it and Morten Gram Pedersen; pedersen@dei.unipd.it

Academic Editor: Jan Rychtar

Hormones and neurotransmitters are released from cells by calcium-regulated exocytosis, and local coupling between Ca^{2+} channels (CaVs) and secretory granules is a key factor determining the exocytosis rate. Here, we devise a methodology based on Markov chain models that allows us to obtain analytic results for the expected rate. First, we analyze the property of the secretory complex obtained by coupling a single granule with one CaV. Then, we extend our results to a more general case where the granule is coupled with n CaVs. We investigate how the exocytosis rate is affected by varying the location of granules and CaVs. Moreover, we assume that the single granule can form complexes with inactivating or non-inactivating CaVs. We find that increasing the number of CaVs coupled with the granule determines a much higher rise of the exocytosis rate that, in case of inactivating CaVs, is more pronounced when the granule is close to CaVs, while, surprisingly, in case of non-inactivating CaVs, the highest relative increase in rate is obtained when the granule is far from the CaVs. Finally, we exploit the devised model to investigate the relation between exocytosis and calcium influx. We find that the quantities are typically linearly related, as observed experimentally. For the case of inactivating CaVs, our simulations show a change of the linear relation due to near-complete inactivation of CaVs.

1. Introduction

Molecules, e.g., neurotransmitters and proteins, are released from the cell by exocytosis [1]. In this paper, we focus on regulated exocytosis in the endocrine cells that release different kinds of hormones regulating various physiological processes [2]. When hormone secretion is defectively regulated, several diseases may develop. For example, in diabetes, the two main pancreatic hormones, insulin and glucagon, are not released appropriately for fine-tuning glucose homeostasis [3, 4]. Therefore, it is crucial to achieve a better understanding of the main mechanisms underlying hormone exocytosis that determines the control of different physiological processes.

In most endocrine cells, the hormones are contained in secretory granules that, in response to a series of cellular mechanisms culminating with an increase in the intracellular Ca^{2+} levels, fuse with the cell membrane and release the hormone molecules. The main mechanisms regulating hormone exocytosis are shared with exocytosis of synaptic vesicles underlying neurotransmitter release in neurons [1, 5]. The granules contain v-SNARE proteins that can form the so-called SNARE complexes with t-SNAREs inserted in the cell membrane [1]. SNARE complexes interact with other proteins, notably, Ca^{2+}-sensing proteins such as synaptotagmins, which trigger exocytosis upon Ca^{2+} binding. Therefore, the local Ca^{2+} concentration at the Ca^{2+} sensor of the exocytotic machinery is a key factor determining the probability rate of exocytosis of the secretory granule [6].

Recently, we have devised a detailed model of Ca^{2+} dynamics and exocytosis for the glucagon-secreting pancreatic alpha-cells and showed how exocytosis is dependent on calcium dynamics, in particular, on calcium levels surrounding the Ca^{2+} channels (CaVs) [7], the so-called nanodomains [8]. Here, in order to characterize the local interactions between the single granule and the surrounding CaVs, we will exploit a strategy that is similar to the methodology devised in our recent paper to describe the large conductance BK potassium current that is controlled locally by CaVs [9]. We showed that the number and the type of CaVs coupled with the BK channel affect the electrical activity of neurons and other excitable cells, such as pancreatic beta-cells and pituitary cells. Therefore, we will implement mathematical modelling for characterizing the local interactions between granules and CaVs and, specifically, Markov chain models that could provide important insight into the exocytosis rate. In particular, by using the Markov chain theory [10], we will achieve analytic results for the expected rate and show how coupling different numbers and types of CaVs with the granule determines different responses.

2. Methods

2.1. CaV Channel Model. We model the Ca^{2+} channel by using the 3-state Markov chain of Figure 1(a), where C corresponds to the closed state, O to the open state, and B to the inactivated (blocked) state of the calcium channel [11]. Then, the CaV model takes values in the state space $S = \{C, O, B\}$ and its transition rate or generator matrix M_{CaV} is given by

$$M_{CaV} = \begin{bmatrix} -\alpha & \alpha & 0 \\ \beta & -\beta-\delta & \delta \\ 0 & \gamma & -\gamma \end{bmatrix}, \quad (1)$$

where α and β represent the voltage-dependent Ca^{2+} channel opening rate and closing rate, respectively, and have the following forms:

$$\alpha(V) = \alpha_0 e^{-\alpha_1 V},$$
$$\beta(V) = \beta_0 e^{-\beta_1 V}. \quad (2)$$

The rate for channel inactivation, δ, is Ca^{2+}-dependent and has the following form:

$$\delta = \delta_0 \times [Ca_{CaV}], \quad (3)$$

where Ca_{CaV} is the Ca^{2+} concentration at the Ca^{2+} sensor for inactivation and is given using reaction-diffusion theory [8, 12, 13] by

$$Ca_{CaV} = \frac{i_{Ca_{max}}}{8\pi r_{Ca} D_{Ca} F} \exp\left[\frac{-r_{Ca}}{\sqrt{D_{Ca}/(k_B^+[B_{total}])}}\right], \quad (4)$$

where $i_{Ca_{max}} = \bar{g}_{Ca}(V - V_{Ca})$ is the single-channel Ca^{2+} current with $\bar{g}_{Ca}$ the single-channel conductance and V_{Ca} the reverse potential, and r_{Ca} represents the distance of the sensor for Ca^{2+}-dependent inactivation from the channel pore. Finally, γ is the constant reverse reactivation rate. Table 1 reports the parameter values for the CaV model defined by above equations.

The deterministic description of the 3-state Markov chain model for the CaV channel is given by the following ODE system:

$$\frac{dc}{dt} = \beta o - \alpha c,$$

$$\frac{do}{dt} = \alpha c + \gamma b - (\beta + \delta)o, \quad (5)$$

$$b = 1 - c - o = 1 - h,$$

where the italic lowercase letters represent the corresponding state variables of the ODE model (h represents the fraction of Ca^{2+} channels not inactivated).

Finally, in order to investigate the relationship between exocytosis and Ca^{2+} loading, we compute the total charge entering via the Ca^{2+} channel at a given step voltage with time window, t_s, as

$$Q_{Ca} = \int_0^{t_s} o(\tau) \cdot i_{Ca_{max}} d\tau. \quad (6)$$

2.2. Exocytosis Model. We assume a single granule, adjacent to the plasma membrane and primed for exocytosis, that can be in one of four different states depending on the number of Ca^{2+} ions bound to the Ca^{2+} sensor on the granule, likely synaptotagmin [14]: in G_0 with no bound Ca^{2+} ions, or in G_1 with one, or in G_2 with two, or in G_3 with three bound ions. Once it is in G_3, the granule can fuse with the membrane and release its hormone content, assuming the final state Y [6, 15]. Therefore, we use a five-state Markov chain model for describing exocytosis as shown in Figure 1(b), where the model takes values in the state space $S = \{G_0, G_1, G_2, G_3, Y\}$, and its transition rate or generator matrix M_G is given by

$$M_G = \begin{bmatrix} -3k_{Ca} & 3k_{Ca} & 0 & 0 & 0 \\ k_- & -2k_{Ca}-k_- & 2k_{Ca} & 0 & 0 \\ 0 & 2k_- & -k_{Ca}-2k_- & k_{Ca} & 0 \\ 0 & 0 & 3k_- & -u-3k_- & u \\ 0 & 0 & 0 & 0 & 0 \end{bmatrix}, \quad (7)$$

where

$$k_{Ca} = k_+ \times [Ca_G] \quad (8)$$

represents the Ca^{2+} binding rate, with Ca_G the Ca^{2+} concentration at the granule sensor given by Equation (4) with $r = r_G$ being the distance from the CaV to the Ca^{2+} sensor on the granule. In the following, the distance from the CaV to the granule means the distance from the CaV to the Ca^{2+} sensor on the granule, which will be of the order of tens of nm. For comparison, secretory granules have diameters on the order 100–500 nm [16–19]. We assume a constant number of Ca^{2+} sensor molecules, which is therefore included in the binding parameter k_{Ca}. The parameter k_- is the unbinding rate, and u is the fusion rate. Table 1 reports the parameter values.

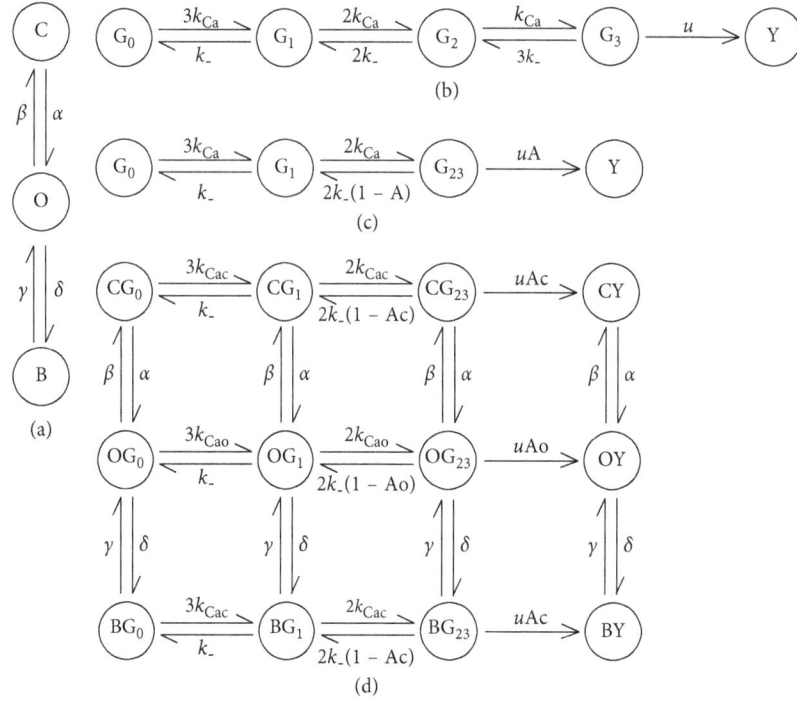

FIGURE 1: Markov chain models for Ca^{2+} channel (CaV), exocytosis of single granule and granule-CaV complex. (a) Markov chain model for CaV, where C is the closed state, O the open state, and B the inactivated or blocked state. (b) Markov chain model for exocytosis of a single granule adjacent to the plasma membrane, where G_0 correspond to the state with no bound Ca^{2+} ions, G_1 with one, G_2 with two, and G_3 with three. (c) Markov chain model for the approximated exocytosis model where the dynamics of states G_2 and G_3 are described by the auxiliary variable G_{23} using quasi-steady state approximation for the corresponding ODE model. (d) Markov chain model for the granule-CaV complex where the granule dynamics are described by the model shown in panel (c) and the CaV dynamics by the model shown in panel (a).

TABLE 1: Model parameters.

Parameter	Value	Unit
CaV model parameters		
α_0	0.6	ms^{-1}
α_1	−0.1	mV^{-1}
β_0	0.2	ms^{-1}
β_1	0.0375	mV^{-1}
γ	0.002	ms^{-1}
δ_0	0.0025	$\mu M^{-1} \cdot ms^{-1}$
Parameters for calculating Ca^{2+} concentration at different distances		
r_{Ca}	7	nm
r_G	10, 20, 30, 50	nm
D_{Ca}	250	$\mu m^2 \cdot s^{-1}$
F	9.6485	$C\ mol^{-1}$
k_B	500	$\mu M^{-1} \cdot s^{-1}$
B_{total}	30	μM
V_{Ca}	60	mV
$\bar{g}_{Ca}$	2.8	pS
Ca_c	0.1	μM
Ca_b	0.1	μM
Exocytosis model parameters		
k_+	1.85	$\mu M^{-1} \cdot s^{-1}$
k_-	50	s^{-1}
u	1000	s^{-1}

The deterministic description of the 5-state Markov chain model for exocytosis is given by the following ODE system:

$$\frac{dg_0}{dt} = -3k_{Ca}g_0 + k_-g_1, \tag{9}$$

$$\frac{dg_1}{dt} = -(2k_{Ca} + k_-)g_1 + 3k_{Ca}g_0 + 2k_-g_2, \tag{10}$$

$$\frac{dg_2}{dt} = -(k_{Ca} + 2k_-)g_2 + 2k_{Ca}g_1 + 3k_-g_3, \tag{11}$$

$$\frac{dg_3}{dt} = -(u + 3k_-)g_3 + k_{Ca}g_2, \tag{12}$$

$$y = 1 - g_0 - g_1 - g_2 - g_3. \tag{13}$$

For the above ODE model of Equations (9)–(13), we exploit quasi steady-state approximation for state g_3, since its dynamics are fastest (the value of u is much higher than those of the other parameters). Then, by renaming the state variables as

$$g_{23} = g_2 + g_3, \tag{14}$$

by setting Equation (12) equal to zero yielding

$$g_3 = Ag_{23}, \quad \text{with} \quad A = \frac{k_{Ca}}{k_{Ca} + 3k_- + u}, \tag{15}$$

and by summing Equations (11) and (12), we achieve a single ODE model for describing the dynamics of state variable g_2 and g_3 as follows:

$$\frac{dg_{23}}{dt} = -(2k_-(1-A) + uA)g_{23} + 2k_{Ca}g_1. \qquad (16)$$

The corresponding Markov chain model takes values in the state space $S = \{G_0, G_1, G_{23}, Y\}$ (Figure 1(c)) and is described by the following generating matrix, $M_{G_{ap}}$:

$$M_{G_{ap}} = \begin{bmatrix} -3k_{Ca} & 3k_{Ca} & 0 & 0 \\ k_- & -2k_{Ca}-k_- & 2k_{Ca} & 0 \\ 0 & 2k_-(1-A) & -2k_-(1-A)-uA & uA \\ 0 & 0 & 0 & 0 \end{bmatrix}.$$
$$(17)$$

Note that state Y of the Markov chain described by $M_{G_{ap}}$ is an absorbing state: the process can never leave Y after entering it, reflecting that fusion is an irreversible process. Then $M_{G_{ap}}$ can be rewritten as

$$M_{G_{ap}} = \begin{bmatrix} D_{3\times3} & \mathbf{d}_{3\times1} \\ \mathbf{0}_{1\times3} & 0 \end{bmatrix}, \qquad (18)$$

where

$$D_{3\times3} = \begin{bmatrix} -3k_{Ca} & 3k_{Ca} & 0 \\ k_- & -2k_{Ca}-k_- & 2k_{Ca} \\ 0 & 2k_-(1-A) & -2k_-(1-A)-uA \end{bmatrix}, \qquad (19)$$

describes only the transitions between the transient states G_0, G_1, and G_{23} and $\mathbf{d} = [0, 0, uA]^T$ is a vector containing the transition intensities from the transient states to the absorbing state Y. The row vector $\mathbf{0} \in \mathbb{R}^{1\times3}$ consists entirely of 0's since no transitions from Y to the transient states can occur. The remaining element of the matrix $M_{G_{ap}}$ is 0 and gives the transition rate out of the absorbing state.

Using phase-type distribution results for Markov chains [10], we obtain an explicit formula for calculating the expected event rate λ_Y to reach the absorbing state Y, given the initial probability row vector π for the transient states $(\pi = (\pi_{G_0}, \pi_{G_1}, \pi_{G_{23}}))$, as

$$\lambda_Y = \frac{1}{\pi(-D^{-1})\mathbf{1}}, \qquad (20)$$

where $\mathbf{1} \in \mathbb{R}^{3\times1}$.

2.3. Granule-CaV Complex Model with 1:1 and 1:n Stoichiometries

2.3.1. 1:1 Stoichiometry.
By coupling the CaV and exocytosis models, we obtain the 12-state Markov chain model of Figure 1(d). The model takes values in the state space

$$S = \{CG_0, OG_0, BG_0, CG_1, OG_1, BG_1, CG_{23}, OG_{23}, BG_{23}, CY, OY, BY\},$$
$$(21)$$

and its transition matrix, $D_{G:CaV}$, is as follows:

$$D_{G:CaV_{9\times9}} = \begin{bmatrix} M_{CaV} - 3\text{diag}(k_{Ca_c}, k_{Ca_o}, k_{Ca_c}) & 3\text{diag}(k_{Ca_c}, k_{Ca_o}, k_{Ca_c}) & \mathbf{0}_{3\times3} \\ \text{diag}(k_-, k_-, k_-) & M_{CaV} - \text{diag}(2k_{Ca_c}+k_-, 2k_{Ca_o}+k_-, 2k_{Ca_c}+k_-) & 2\text{diag}(k_{Ca_c}, k_{Ca_o}, k_{Ca_c}) \\ \mathbf{0}_{3\times3} & 2k_-\text{diag}((1-A_c), (1-A_o), (1-A_c)) & M_{CaV} - \text{diag}(2k_-(1-A_c)+uA_c, 2k_-(1-A_o)+uA_o, 2k_-(1-A_c)+uA_c) \end{bmatrix}, \quad (22)$$

where M_{CaV} is defined by Equation (1), $k_{Ca_c}(A_c)$ by Equation (8) (Equation (15)) with $Ca_G = Ca_c$, i.e., the concentration at the granule when the associated CaV is closed (or inactivated, i.e., $Ca_c = Ca_b$), and $k_{Ca_o}(A_o)$ by Equation (8) (Equation (15)) with $Ca_G = Ca_o$, i.e., the concentration at the granule when the associated CaV is open, computed by Equation (4). Then, the expected exocytosis rate for the single granule, λ_{Y_1}, can be estimated by using Equation (20), assuming initially the granule in state G_0 and the CaV closed, i.e., the complex in the state CG_0 ($\pi = (1, \mathbf{0}_{1\times8})$), as

$$\lambda_{Y_1} = \frac{1}{\pi(-D_{G:CaV}^{-1})\mathbf{1}}, \qquad (23)$$

where $\mathbf{1} \in \mathbb{R}^{9\times1}$.

We also consider the particular case with non-inactivating CaV (i.e., the Ca^{2+} channel can be only in C or in O). In this case, $M_{CaV} \in \mathbb{R}^{2\times2}$ and is defined by Equation (1) with $\delta = \gamma = 0$, and then $D_{G:CaV}$, given by Equation (22), belongs to $\mathbb{R}^{6\times6}$.

2.3.2. 1:n Stoichiometry.
In the following, we assume the case where the granule is coupled with more than one CaV. In particular, by considering k Ca^{2+} channels, we have a Markov chain model with $n_S = \sum_{i=0}^{k}(k+1-i) = (k^2/2) + (3k/2) + 1$ possible states describing the k CaVs. In particular, the CaVs model takes values in the state space $S = \{C_{k-i-j}O_iB_j\}$ with $j \in \{0, \ldots, k\}$ and $i \in \{0, \ldots, k-j\}$, and its generating matrix, M_{kCaV}, is given by

$$
M_{k\mathrm{CaV}_{n_S \times n_S}} = \begin{bmatrix} M_{0_{(k+1)\times(k+1)}} & \begin{matrix} 0_{1\times k} \\ \delta \operatorname{diag}(1,\ldots,k) \end{matrix} & 0 & \cdots & \cdots & \cdots & \cdots\,\cdots & 0 \\ \begin{matrix} 0_{k\times 1} & \gamma I_k \\ 0 \end{matrix} & \ddots & \ddots & 0 & \cdots & \cdots & \cdots\,\cdots & \vdots \\ & \ddots & \ddots & \ddots & 0 & \cdots & \cdots\,\cdots & \vdots \\ \vdots & \cdots & 0 & 0_{(k+1-j)\times 1}\;\; j\gamma I_{(k+1-j)} \;\; M_{j_{(k+1-j)\times(k+1-j)}} & \begin{matrix} 0_{1\times(k-j)} \\ \delta \operatorname{diag}(1,\ldots,k-j) \end{matrix} & 0 & \cdots & \vdots \\ \vdots & \cdots & \cdots & \cdots & 0 & \ddots & \ddots & 0 \\ \vdots & \cdots & \cdots & \cdots & \cdots & 0 & \ddots\;\;\ddots & \delta \\ \vdots & \cdots & \cdots & \cdots & \cdots & \cdots & 0 \;\; k\gamma & M_{k_{1\times 1}} \end{bmatrix},
$$

$$(24)$$

where

$$
M_{0_{(k+1)\times(k+1)}} = \begin{bmatrix} -k\alpha & k\alpha & 0 & \cdots & & \cdots & & \cdots & \cdots\,\cdots & 0 \\ \beta & \ddots & \ddots & 0 & & \cdots & & \cdots & \cdots\,\cdots & \vdots \\ 0 & \ddots & \ddots & \ddots & & 0 & & \cdots & \cdots\,\cdots & \vdots \\ \vdots & \cdots & 0 & (i-1)\beta & -(k-(i-1))\alpha-(i-1)(\beta+\delta) & (k-(i-1))\alpha & 0 & \cdots & & \vdots \\ \vdots & \cdots\,\cdots & \cdots & & 0 & & \ddots & \ddots & \ddots & 0 \\ \vdots & \cdots\,\cdots & \cdots & & \cdots & & & 0 & \ddots\;\;\ddots & \alpha \\ 0 & \cdots\,\cdots & \cdots & & \cdots & & & 0 & k\beta & -k(\beta+\delta) \end{bmatrix},
$$

$$(25)$$

$$
M_{j_{(k+1-j)\times(k+1-j)}} = \begin{bmatrix} -(k-j)\alpha-j\gamma & (k-j)\alpha & 0 & \cdots & & \cdots & & \cdots & \cdots\;\;\cdots & 0 \\ \beta & \ddots & \ddots & 0 & & \cdots & & \cdots & \cdots\;\;\cdots & \vdots \\ 0 & \ddots & \ddots & \ddots & & 0 & & \cdots & \cdots\;\;\cdots & 0 \\ \vdots & \cdots & 0 & (i-1)\beta & -(k-(i-1)-j)\alpha-(i-1)(\beta+\delta)-j\gamma & (k-(i-1)-j)\alpha & 0 & \cdots & & \vdots \\ \vdots & \cdots\;\;\cdots & \cdots & & 0 & & \ddots & \ddots & \ddots & 0 \\ \vdots & \cdots\;\;\cdots & \cdots & & \cdots & & & 0 & \ddots\;\;\ddots & \alpha \\ 0 & \cdots\;\;\cdots & \cdots & & \cdots & & & 0 & (k-j)\beta & -(k-j)(\beta+\delta)-j\gamma \end{bmatrix},
$$

$$(26)$$

and $M_{k_{1\times 1}} = -k\gamma$.

Then, by coupling the CaVs and exocytosis models, we obtain a $4n_S$-state Markov chain model. The model takes values in the state space $S = \{C_{k-i-j}O_iB_jG_l, \ldots, C_{k-i-j}O_iB_j G_{23}, C_{k-i-j}O_iB_jY\}$, with $j \in \{0,\ldots,k\}$, $i \in \{0,\ldots,k-j\}$ and $l \in \{0,1\}$, and its transition matrix, $D_{\mathrm{G:}k\mathrm{CaV}}$, can be written as

$$
D_{\mathrm{G:}k\mathrm{CaV}_{3n_S \times 3n_S}} = \begin{bmatrix} M_{k\mathrm{CaV}} - K_{\mathrm{Ca}_1} & K_{\mathrm{Ca}_1} & 0_{n_S \times n_S} \\ k_- I_{n_S} & M_{k\mathrm{CaV}} - K_{\mathrm{Ca}_2} - k_- I_{n_S} & K_{\mathrm{Ca}_2} \\ 0_{n_S \times n_S} & 2k_-\left(I_{n_S} - D_A\right) & M_{k\mathrm{CaV}} - 2k_-\left(I_{n_S} - D_A\right) - uD_A \end{bmatrix},
$$

$$(27)$$

where

$$
K_{\mathrm{Ca}_{1n_S \times n_S}} = \begin{bmatrix} 3k_{\mathrm{Ca}_c} & 0 & & & & & \\ 0 & 3k_{\mathrm{Ca}_o}\operatorname{diag}(1,\ldots,k) & & & & & \\ & & \ddots & & & & \\ & & & 3k_{\mathrm{Ca}_c} & 0 & & \\ & & & 0 & 3k_{\mathrm{Ca}_o}\operatorname{diag}(1,\ldots,k-j) & & \\ & & & & & \ddots & \\ & & & & & & 3k_{\mathrm{Ca}_c} \end{bmatrix},
$$

$$(28)$$

$$K_{Ca_{2n_S \times n_S}} = \begin{bmatrix} 2k_{Ca_c} & 0 & & & & & \\ 0 & 2k_{Ca_o} \operatorname{diag}(1,\ldots,k) & & & & & \\ & & \ddots & & & & \\ & & & 2k_{Ca_c} & 0 & & \\ & & & 0 & 2k_{Ca_o} \operatorname{diag}(1,\ldots,k-j) & & \\ & & & & & \ddots & \\ & & & & & & 2k_{Ca_c} \end{bmatrix}, \tag{29}$$

$$D_{A_{n_S \times n_S}} = \begin{bmatrix} A_c & 0 & & & & & \\ 0 & A_o \operatorname{diag}(1,\ldots,k) & & & & & \\ & & \ddots & & & & \\ & & & A_c & 0 & & \\ & & & 0 & A_o \operatorname{diag}(1,\ldots,k-j) & & \\ & & & & & \ddots & \\ & & & & & & A_c \end{bmatrix}. \tag{30}$$

Then, the expected exocytosis rate for the single granule coupled with k CaVs, λ_{Y_k}, can be estimated by using Equation (20), assuming initially the granule in state G_0 and the k CaVs closed, i.e., the complex is initially in state C_kG_0 $\pi = (1, 0_{1 \times (3n_S - 1)})$, which yields

$$\lambda_{Y_k} = \frac{1}{\pi(-D_{G:kCaV}^{-1})\mathbf{1}}, \tag{31}$$

where $\mathbf{1} \in \mathbb{R}^{3n_S \times 1}$.

For the particular case with non-inactivating CaVs channels, $M_{kCaV} = M_0$ by Equations (24) and (25) with $\delta = \gamma = 0$, and then, $D_{G:kCaV}$, given by Equation (27), belongs to $\mathbb{R}^{3(k+1) \times 3(k+1)}$.

In order to compare the rate for a granule coupled with different number k of CaVs, we define the relative rate, ρ_{λ_k}, as

$$\rho_{\lambda_k} = \frac{\lambda_{Y_k}}{\lambda_{Y_n}}, \tag{32}$$

with $k = 1, \ldots, n$. Moreover, in order to compare the rate at different distances from the granule to CaVs, we define the relative distance rate, ρ_{λ_d}, as

$$\rho_{\lambda_d} = \frac{\lambda_{Y_d}}{\lambda_{Y_{d_{\min}}}}, \tag{33}$$

where λ_{Y_d} is the rate computed at a given distance r_G and $\lambda_{Y_{d_{\min}}}$, the rate computed at $r_G = 10\,\text{nm}$.

3. Results and Discussion

We analyze the behavior of the devised exocytosis model where the single granule is coupled with k Ca^{2+} channels by using phase-type distribution results for Markov chains [10] (see Methods). First, we assume that a granule is coupled with one CaV and, then, we extend the results to a more general case with k CaVs. Moreover, we consider for both the cases (1 or k CaVs) that the granule forms complexes with inactivating or non-inactivating CaVs. This scenario reflects, e.g., what is observed in pancreatic beta-cells where the two main high voltage-activated Ca^{2+} channels, the L- and P/Q-type Ca^{2+} channels, are examples of inactivating and non-inactivating CaVs, respectively [20].

3.1. Granule Coupled with One Inactivating (or Non-Inactivating) CaV. Figure 2(a) shows the expected exocytosis rate, λ_{Y_1}, computed by Equation (23), for a granule at different distances from an inactivating CaV channel. Independently of the distance to the CaV, the exocytosis rate has a bell-shaped relation to voltage, as seen experimentally [20–22]. The same holds true in the case of non-inactivating CaV (Figure 2(b)). As the distance between the granule and the Ca^{2+} channel increases, the expected rate decreases substantially and nonlinearly (for instance, in Figure 2(a), compare the red and blue lines for $r_G = 20\,\text{nm}$ and $r_G = 10\,\text{nm}$, respectively). This is clearer from Figure 2(c), showing the relative distance rate ρ_{λ_d} defined by Equation (33) for different values of r_G. Note that increasing the distance by a factor of two corresponds to a more than five-fold reduction of the exocytosis rate (the relative ratio is less than 0.2, see the red plot in Figure 2(c)). This steep dependence of the distance to the channel is because the calcium levels drop rapidly, moving away from the channel [8, 23].

We perform a similar analysis for the case where a granule is coupled with a non-inactivating CaV (Figure 2(b)). We note an increase about of two orders of magnitudes for the exocytosis rate compared to the case with a granule coupled with an inactivating CaV (Figures 2(a) and 2(b)): the exocytosis proceeds more rapidly since the triggering Ca^{2+} signal is increased due to non-inactivation of Ca^{2+} currents. Also in this case, the degree of decrease for the rate is much higher than the relative increase for the distance (Figure 2(d)). However, the benefit in terms of ρ_{λ_d} by reducing the distance is slightly less than that obtained with

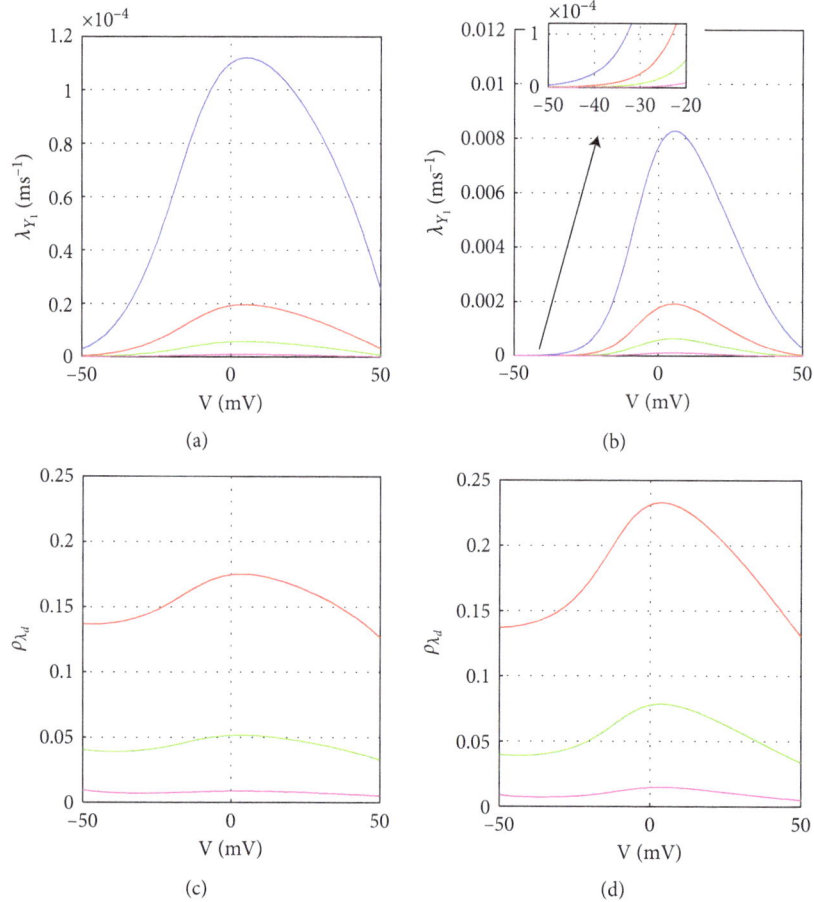

FIGURE 2: Expected exocytosis rate for single granule coupled with one (inactivating or non-inactivating) CaV. (a, b) Expected exocytosis rate λ_{Y_1} for the granule at different distances r_G from one inactivating (a) or non-inactivating (b) CaV: $r_G = 10$ nm (blue curves), $r_G = 20$ nm (red), $r_G = 30$ nm (green), and $r_G = 50$ nm (magenta). Note the different scales on the y-axes. The insert in (b) is a zoom on the lower, left part of the figure for comparison with (a). (c, d) Relative rate ρ_{λ_d} computed at different distances ($r_G = 20$ nm (red), $r_G = 30$ nm (green), and $r_G = 50$ nm (magenta)) of the granule from the inactivating (c) or not-inactivating (d) CaV and compared to the case with $r_G = 10$ nm.

inactivating CaV (compare Figures 2(c) and 2(d)): for the case with inactivating CaV, it seems that moving away from the channel, ρ_{λ_d} decreases more due to the inactivation of CaV that determines a further drop of calcium levels.

3.2. Granule Coupled with k Inactivating (or Non-Inactivating) CaVs.

Figures 3(a)–3(d) show the expected exocytosis rate λ_{Y_k} computed by Equation (31), for a granule coupled with different numbers of inactivating CaVs and at fixed distances between the granule and the CaVs. It is clear that increasing the number of CaVs coupled with the granule determines a rise of the exocytosis rate. Moreover, as the number of CaVs coupled with the granule increases, the rise in the rate is more pronounced when the distance of the granule from the CaVs is small. This is evident by considering the relative rate ρ_{λ_k} defined by Equation (32) (Figure 3(e)). For instance, consider the cyan curves computed for $k = 4$ with different types of lines denoting the different distances of the granule from the CaVs. In this case, the number of CaVs decreases by a factor of 2 (from 8 to 4) while the exocytosis rate drops more than threefold for

$r_G = 20$ nm (dashed cyan line, $\rho_{\lambda_k} < 0.3$, for $V > -10$ mV) and more than fivefold for $r_G = 10$ nm (solid cyan line, $\rho_{\lambda_k} < 0.2$, for $V > -10$ mV).

As done for the case with one CaV, we performed the same analysis with k non-inactivating CaVs coupled with the granule (Figures 3(f)–3(i)). Also in this case, it is clear that increasing the number of CaVs determines a rise of the exocytosis rate for the granule. Surprisingly and in contrast with the case with inactivating CaVs, as the number of non-inactivating CaVs increases, the relative rise in exocytosis rate is much higher at larger distances from the CaVs, as shown in Figure 3(j) reporting the relative rate ρ_{λ_k}. In case the number of CaVs is reduced from 8 to 4, the exocytosis rate decreases by 2–2.5-fold when the granule is near the CaVs (see the solid cyan curve for $r_G = 10$ nm, $0.4 < \rho_{\lambda_k} < 0.5$ with -20 mV $< V < 40$ mV), while it goes down fivefold when the granule is far from CaVs (see the dotted cyan curve for $r_G = 50$ nm, $0.2 < \rho_{\lambda_k} < 0.3$ with -20 mV $< V < 40$ mV). It seems that when the granule is surrounded by more non-inactivating CaVs, it is not necessary that the granule is very close to the CaVs for triggering exocytosis.

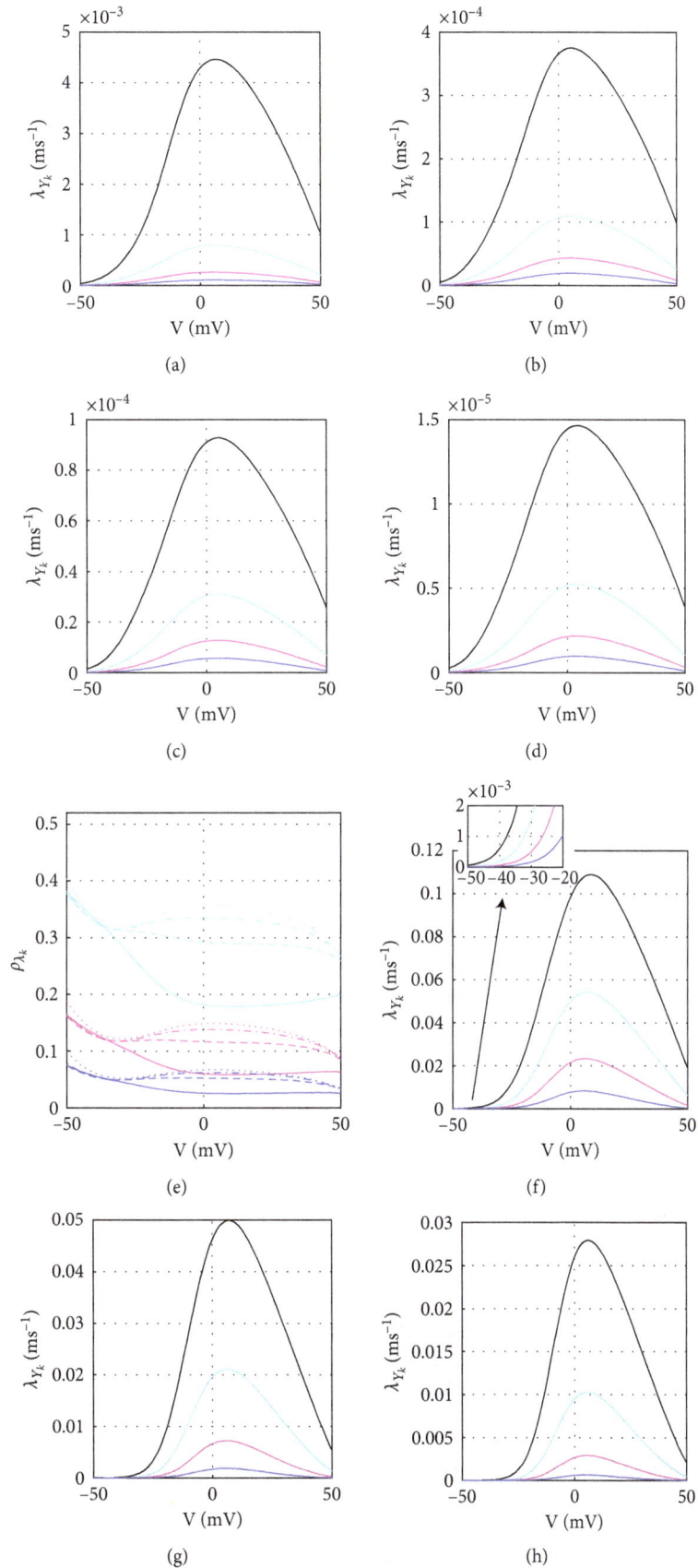

FIGURE 3: Continued.

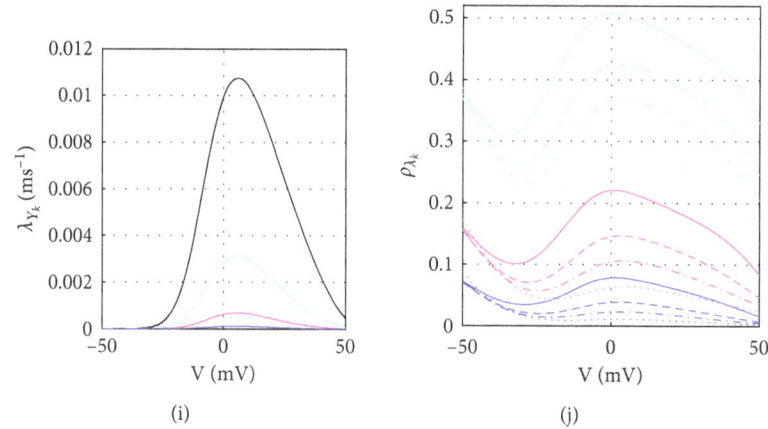

(i)

(j)

FIGURE 3: Expected exocytosis rate for single granule coupled with k (inactivating or non-inactivating) CaVs. (a–d) and (f–i) Expected exocytosis rate λ_{Y_k} for the granule at fixed distance r_G from k ($k = 1$ (blue curves), $k = 2$ (magenta), $k = 4$ (cyan), and $k = 8$ (black)) inactivating/not-inactivating CaVs: $r_G = 10$ nm (a/f), 20 nm (b/g), 30 nm (c/h), and 50 nm (d/i). The insert in (f) is a zoom on the lower, left part of the figure for comparison with (a). (e) and (j) Relative rate ρ_{λ_k} obtained from the granule coupled with k inactivating/not-inactivating CaVs (e/j), for $k = 1$ (blue), $k = 2$ (magenta), and $k = 4$ (cyan) and compared to the case with $n = 8$ CaVs. The different type of line corresponds to ρ_{λ_k} computed at fixed distance: $r_G = 10$ nm (solid line), $r_G = 20$ nm (dashed), $r_G = 30$ nm (dash-dotted), and $r_G = 50$ nm (dotted).

3.3. Relationship between Ca^{2+} Influx and Exocytosis. To investigate the relationship between exocytosis and Ca^{2+} loading, we consider a set of scenarios where the granule is coupled with different number of non-inactivating or inactivating CaVs, placed very close (10 nm) or far (100 nm) from the granule. Figure 4(a) shows the calcium current at $V = 0$ mV, for different numbers of non-inactivating CaVs, while Figure 4(b) shows the corresponding cases with inactivating CaVs. In the latter, it is evident how the calcium influx drops after few tens of ms due to the inactivation of the CaVs. Figures 4(c) and 4(d) show the probability of exocytosis p_Y ($p_Y = P(S(t) = Y)$) vs. the integral of the Ca^{2+} current, Q_{Ca}, defined by Equation (6), for the granule placed close to the CaV cluster, for different numbers of CaVs ($r_G = 10$ nm). For the case of non-inactivating CaVs (Figure 4(c)), p_Y raises linearly with Q_{Ca}, with slope that increases with the number of CaVs and then saturates due to the depletion of the granule pool as p_Y approaches 1 (see also [24]). For inactivating CaVs, we note a change of the slope of the linearity between p_Y and Q_{Ca} that is not only due to depletion (when $y \geq 0.5$) but also to near-complete inactivation of CaVs, in particular after 50 ms (Figure 4(d)). Figures 4(e) and 4(f) show p_Y vs. Q_{Ca} when the granule is placed far from CaVs ($r_G = 100$ nm). Due to the distance to CaVs, the calcium concentration at the granule increases only modestly; hence, a greater calcium influx Q_{Ca} is needed to allow the granule to move through the Markov chain from N_0 to Y and undergoes exocytosis. This causes an evident initial delay for the granule to be released, resulting in an initial convex relation between p_Y and Q_{Ca}. After this initial phase, for the case of non-inactivating CaVs (Figure 4(e)), p_Y raises linearly with Q_{Ca} with slope depending on the number of CaVs. For higher Q_{Ca}, the slope of p_Y slightly decreases in the case with $k = 8$ CaVs reflecting slight depletion of the granule pool ($p_Y \approx 0.5$ at $Q_{Ca} = 500$ fC). For inactivating CaVs

(Figure 4(f)), as for the case with $r_G = 10$ nm, we note a change of the linearity between p_Y and Q_{Ca} that is due to CaV inactivation.

4. Conclusions

In this paper, we devise a strategy that allows us to characterize the local interactions between granules and CaVs. The methodology is similar to our approach for modelling the local effect of CaVs on whole-cell BK currents [9]. We develop Markov chain models describing the dynamics of a single granule coupled with one or more inactivating (or non-inactivating) Ca^{2+} channels and use phase-type distribution results [10] for estimating the expected exocytosis rate.

We investigate how the release probability of a granule can be affected by varying the number of CaVs and the distance of the (Ca^{2+} sensor of the) granule from CaVs. In particular, from our analysis, we find that the distance between the granule and CaVs is a major factor in determining the exocytosis rate, as we recently demonstrated and quantified explicitly [23]. Further and in agreement with experiments [23], the simulations presented here show that the increase of the number of CaVs coupled with the granule determines a much higher rise of the exocytosis rate, which in the case of inactivating CaVs is more pronounced when the granule is close to CaVs (≈ 10 nm), whereas for non-inactivating CaVs the highest relative increase in rate is obtained when the CaVs are far from CaVs (≈ 50 nm).

We also study the relationship between Ca^{2+} influx and exocytosis. The results of the devised exocytosis model confirm that the granule secretion is generally linearly related to the integral of Ca^{2+} current, as experimentally observed [25–29] and theoretically justified [24]. Surprisingly, for the case of inactivating CaVs, our analysis shows a change of the linear relation between p_Y and Q_{Ca} due to

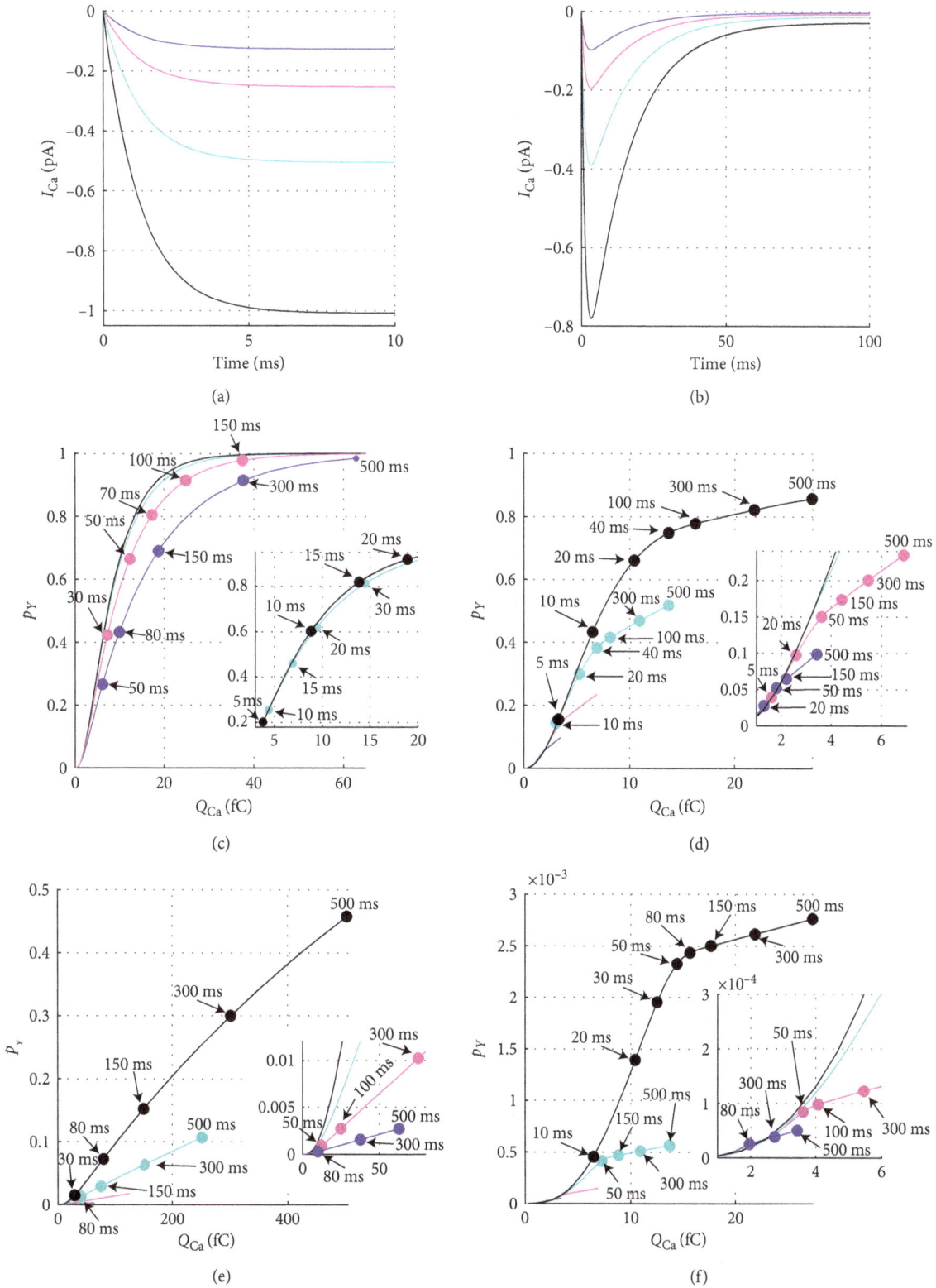

FIGURE 4: Relationship between Ca^{2+} influx and exocytosis rate. (a, b) Ca^{2+} current for the different number of non-inactivating (a) and inactivating (b) CaVs. (c, d) Probability of exocytosis, p_Y, vs. integral of Ca^{2+} currents, Q_{Ca}, computed at $V = 0$ mV by increasing the integration time, t_s, from 1 to 500 ms, for the granule at distance $r_G = 10$ nm from k not-inactivating (c) or inactivating (d) CaVs. (e, f) Legends as in (c, d) with $r_G = 100$ nm. In each panel, the different colors represent different number of CaVs: blue curve for $k = 1$; magenta for $k = 2$; cyan for $k = 4$; and black for $k = 8$. The inserts in (c–f) show a zoom-in of p_Y vs. Q_{Ca} on lower Q_{Ca} values for the granule coupled with different number k of CaVs: $k = 4$ and 8 in (c) and $k = 1, 2, 4,$ and 8 in (d–f).

near-complete inactivation of CaVs. This fact is due to the rather complex exocytosis model where the efficacy of Ca^{2+} influx in triggering exocytosis depends on the number of active CaVs, as clearly seen in the case of non-inactivating CaVs (Figures 4(c) and 4(e)), because of multiple steps of Ca^{2+} bindings before exocytosis. During inactivation, the effective number of CaVs declines, which has a similar effect as reducing the number of CaVs, and hence the slope of the relation between exocytosis and Q_{Ca} decreases. This finding reinforces the notion that a concave relation between exocytosis and Ca^{2+} influx does not necessarily reflect pool depletion [24] and provides a new example of such a scenario.

Conflicts of Interest

The authors declare that there are no conflicts of interest regarding the publication of this paper.

Acknowledgments

F.M. was supported by the University of Padova (Research Grant BIRD 2017). M.G.P. was supported by the University of Padova (Research Project SID and Research Project PROACTIVE).

References

[1] R. D. Burgoyne and A. Morgan, "Secretory granule exocytosis," *Physiological Reviews*, vol. 83, no. 2, pp. 581–632, 2003.

[2] S. Misler, "Unifying concepts in stimulus-secretion coupling in endocrine cells and some implications for therapeutics," *Advances in Physiology Education*, vol. 33, no. 3, pp. 175–186, 2009.

[3] S. E. Kahn, S. Zraika, K. M. Utzschneider, and R. L. Hull, "The beta cell lesion in type 2 diabetes: there has to be a primary functional abnormality," *Diabetologia*, vol. 52, no. 6, pp. 1003–1012, 2009.

[4] M. Frances, M. Ashcroft, and P. Rorsman, "Diabetes mellitus and the beta-cell: the last ten years," *Cell*, vol. 148, no. 6, pp. 1160–1171, 2012.

[5] S. Barg, "Mechanisms of exocytosis in insulin-secreting beta-cells and glucagon-secreting alpha-cells," *Pharmacology and Toxicology*, vol. 92, no. 1, pp. 3–13, 2003.

[6] M. G. Pedersen, A. Tagliavini, G. Cortese, M. Riz, and F. Montefusco, "Recent advances in mathematical modeling and statistical analysis of exocytosis in endocrine cells," *Mathematical Biosciences*, vol. 283, pp. 60–70, 2017.

[7] F. Montefusco and M. G. Pedersen, "Mathematical modelling of local calcium and regulated exocytosis during inhibition and stimulation of glucagon secretion from pancreatic alpha-cells," *Journal of Physiology*, vol. 593, no. 20, pp. 4519–4530, 2015.

[8] E. Neher, "Vesicle pools and Ca^{2+} microdomains: new tools for understanding their roles in neurotransmitter release," *Neuron*, vol. 20, no. 3, pp. 389–399, 1998.

[9] F. Montefusco, A. Tagliavini, M. Ferrante, and M. G. Pedersen, "Concise whole-cell modeling of BK-CaV activity controlled by local coupling and stoichiometry," *Biophysical Journal*, vol. 112, no. 11, pp. 2387–2396, 2017.

[10] P. Buchholz, K. Jan, and I. Felko, "Phase-type distributions," in *Input Modeling with Phase-Type Distributions and Markov Models*, pp. 5–28, Springer International Publishing, New York, NY, USA, 2014.

[11] A. Sherman, J. Keizer, and J. Rinzel, "Domain model for Ca^{2+}-inactivation of Ca^{2+} channels at low channel density," *Biophysical Journal*, vol. 58, no. 4, pp. 985–995, 1990.

[12] E. Neher, "Concentration profiles of intracellular Ca^{2+} in the presence of diffusible chelator," in *Calcium Electrogenesis and Neuronal Functioning*, vol. 14, pp. 80–96, Springer-Verlag, Berlin, Germany, 1986.

[13] D. H. Cox, "Modeling a Ca^{2+} channel/BK channel complex at the single-complex level," *Biophysical Journal*, vol. 107, no. 12, pp. 2797–2814, 2014.

[14] P. S. Pinheiro, S. Houy, and J. B. Sørensen, "C2-domain containing calcium sensors in neuroendocrine secretion," *Journal of Neurochemistry*, vol. 139, no. 6, pp. 943–958, 2016.

[15] T. Voets, "Dissection of three Ca^{2+}-dependent steps leading to secretion in chromaffin cells from mouse adrenal slices," *Neuron*, vol. 28, no. 2, pp. 537–545, 2000.

[16] C. P. Grabner, S. D. Price, A. Lysakowski, and A. P. Fox, "Mouse chromaffin cells have two populations of dense core vesicles," *Journal of Neurophysiology*, vol. 94, no. 3, pp. 2093–2104, 2005.

[17] S. A. Andersson, M. G. Pedersen, J. Vikman, and L. Eliasson, "Glucose-dependent docking and SNARE protein-mediated exocytosis in mouse pancreatic alpha-cell," *Pflügers Archiv—European Journal of Physiology*, vol. 462, no. 3, pp. 443–454, 2011.

[18] C. S. Olofsson, S. O. Göpel, S. Barg et al., "Fast insulin secretion reflects exocytosis of docked granules in mouse pancreatic beta-cells," *Pflügers Archiv*, vol. 444, no. 1-2, pp. 43–51, 2002.

[19] P. M. Dean, "Ultrastructural morphometry of the pancreatic beta-cell," *Diabetologia*, vol. 9, no. 2, pp. 115–119, 1973.

[20] M. Braun, R. Ramracheya, M. Bengtsson et al., "Voltage-gated ion channels in human pancreatic beta-cells: electrophysiological characterization and role in insulin secretion," *Diabetes*, vol. 57, no. 6, pp. 1618–1628, 2008.

[21] K. D. Gillis, R. Y. K. Pun, and S. Misler, "Single cell assay of exocytosis from adrenal chromaffin cells using "perforated patch recording"," *Pflugers Archiv European Journal of Physiology*, vol. 418, no. 6, pp. 611–613, 1991.

[22] K. L. Engisch and M. C. Nowycky, "Calcium dependence of large dense-cored vesicle exocytosis evoked by calcium influx in bovine adrenal chromaffin cells," *Journal of Neuroscience*, vol. 16, no. 4, pp. 1359–1369, 1996.

[23] N. R. Gandasi, P. Yin, M. Riz et al., "Ca^{2+} channel clustering with insulin-containing granules is disturbed in type 2 diabetes," *Journal of Clinical Investigation*, vol. 127, no. 6, pp. 2353–2364, 2017.

[24] M. G. Pedersen, "On depolarization-evoked exocytosis as a function of calcium entry: possibilities and pitfalls," *Biophysical Journal*, vol. 101, no. 4, pp. 793–802, 2011.

[25] T. Moser and E. Neher, "Rapid exocytosis in single chromaffin cells recorded from mouse adrenal slices," *Journal of Neuroscience*, vol. 17, no. 7, pp. 2314–2323, 1997.

[26] S. Barg, X. Ma, L. Eliasson et al., "Fast exocytosis with few Ca^{2+} channels in insulin-secreting mouse pancreatic beta-cells," *Biophysical Journal*, vol. 81, no. 6, pp. 3308–3323, 2001.

[27] Y. Z. De Marinis, S. Albert, C. E. Ward et al., "GLP-1 inhibits and adrenaline stimulates glucagon release by differential

modulation of N- and L-type Ca^{2+} channel-dependent exocytosis," *Cell Metabolism*, vol. 11, no. 6, pp. 543–553, 2010.

[28] R. Thiagarajan, J. Wilhelm, T. Tewolde, Y. Li, M. M. Rich, and K. L. Engisch, "Enhancement of asynchronous and train-evoked exocytosis in bovine adrenal chromaffin cells infected with a replication deficient adenovirus," *Journal of Neurophysiology*, vol. 94, no. 5, pp. 3278–3291, 2005.

[29] M. G. Pedersen, V. A. Salunkhe, E. Svedin, A. Edlund, and L. Eliasson, "Calcium current inactivation rather than pool depletion explains reduced exocytotic rate with prolonged stimulation in insulin-secreting INS-1 832/13 cells," *PLoS One*, vol. 9, no. 8, Article ID e103874, 2014.

13

Does the Temporal Asymmetry of Short-Term Heart Rate Variability Change during Regular Walking?

Xinpei Wang,[1] **Chang Yan,**[1] **Bo Shi,**[2] **Changchun Liu,**[1] **Chandan Karmakar,**[3] **and Peng Li**[1]

[1]*School of Control Science and Engineering, Shandong University, Jinan, Shandong 250061, China*
[2]*Department of Medical Imaging, Bengbu Medical College, Bengbu, Anhui 233030, China*
[3]*School of Information Technology, Deakin University, Burwood, VIC 3125, Australia*

Correspondence should be addressed to Peng Li; pli@sdu.edu.cn

Academic Editor: Andrzej Kloczkowski

The acceleration and deceleration patterns in heartbeat fluctuations distribute asymmetrically, which is known as heart rate asymmetry (HRA). It is hypothesized that HRA reflects the balancing regulation of the sympathetic and parasympathetic nervous systems. This study was designed to examine whether altered autonomic balance during exercise can lead to HRA changes. Sixteen healthy college students were enrolled, and each student undertook two 5-min ECG measurements: one in a resting seated position and another while walking on a treadmill at a regular speed of 5 km/h. The two measurements were conducted in a randomized order, and a 30-min rest was required between them. RR interval time series were extracted from the 5-min ECG data, and HRA (short-term) was estimated using four established metrics, that is, Porta's index (PI), Guzik's index (GI), slope index (SI), and area index (AI), from both raw RR interval time series and the time series after wavelet detrending that removes the low-frequency component of $<\sim0.03$ Hz. Our pilot data showed a reduced PI but unchanged GI, SI, and AI during walking compared to resting seated position based on the raw data. Based on the wavelet-detrended data, reduced PI, SI, and AI were observed while GI still showed no significant changes. The reduced PI during walking based on both raw and detrended data which suggests less short-term HRA may underline the belief that vagal tone is withdrawn during low-intensity exercise. GI may not be sensitive to short-term HRA. The reduced SI and AI based on detrended data suggest that they may capture both short- and long-term HRA features and that the expected change in short-term HRA is amplified after removing the trend that is supposed to link to long-term component. Further studies with more subjects and longer measurements are warranted to validate our observations and to examine these additional hypotheses.

1. Introduction

Under healthy physiological conditions, the human heart does not beat at a constant frequency; instead, heart rate changes all the time. This phenomenon has been recognized as heart rate variability (HRV) [1, 2]. For a given observation scale, the acceleration and deceleration patterns in beat-to-beat heart rate fluctuations distribute asymmetrically rather than contribute equally to HRV [3–7]. This suggests that the underlying heart rate control mechanisms—the regulation of sympathetic and parasympathetic nervous systems—are physiologically disproportionate over fixed temporal scales [8–12]. This asymmetry of acceleration

and deceleration runs is defined as heart rate asymmetry (HRA).

In clinical settings, the electrocardiograms (ECGs) are commonly collected under well-controlled conditions such as resting supine or seated position and within a short time range (e.g., 5 min or shorter). Increasing attention nowadays has been drawn to the ambulatory ECG monitoring [13], which facilitates the tracking of heart rate and HRV with activities of free living, such as walking and exercise [14]. Long-term ambulatory measurement also assists to examine whether and how HRV properties respond to these daily activities [15]. Besides, daily activities may also evoke changes that may mask the effects of interest, for example, the changes that are related to alterations of health status or different times of the day. Thus, the examination of the changes of different HRV measures with daily activities may help better understand the variation profile of these measures, providing opportunities to comprehend the knowledge of how these novel properties respond to the changing physiological conditions that eventually should be of great help to develop sensitive and specific makers for cardiovascular diseases. With such a motivation, this study focused on elucidating whether and how the daily activities alter HRA.

The high-frequency power of HRV is accepted to be related to the parasympathetic tone while HRA has shown to be positively correlated with the high-frequency power [16], offering the link between HRA and parasympathetic activity. This link has further been strengthened by the observations that parasympathetic block leads to less prevalence of HRA [16] and that the deceleration patterns have a larger contribution to short-term HRA than acceleration patterns [9, 12]. Based on these existing results, we expect to see a significantly reduced short-term HRA level during low-intensity daily exercises that are assumed to be accompanied with the withdrawal of parasympathetic modulation [17]. In the current study, we applied treadmill-based regular walking protocol to imitate daily exercises in laboratory. To examine the within-subject changes, each participant undertook a walking protocol and a rest protocol. During each protocol, ECG data were collected continuously for 5 minutes. The next section explains in detail the subjects, experimental protocols, and analysis methods. Experimental results are summarized in the Results, followed by discussions in the Discussions.

2. Methods

2.1. Subjects. Subjects include 16 college students (4 females, 12 males; age: 20.1 ± 0.6 years [mean ± standard deviation]) with their physical and mental health status confirmed by questionnaire on the history of cardiovascular diseases, diabetes, depression, and neurological disorders. No subject has been taking any medications that have known effects on ANS within two weeks before participation. Adequate sleep during the night before coming to the laboratory, as well as avoidance of vigorous exercises during the test day and the day before, was requested. Written informed consent was obtained from all subjects. The study was approved by the Ethics Committee in Clinical Study of Bengbu Medical College.

2.2. Protocols. For each subject, ECG was recorded twice in random order with the subject seating on a chair or walking on a treadmill (ZR11, Reebok, Canton, MA, USA) at a speed of 5 km/h. Both ECGs last for 5 min and a 30-min rest was scheduled between the two measurements. Holter monitors (DiCare-mlCP, Dimetek Digital Medical Tech., Ltd., Shenzhen, China) were used to collect ECG data. The sampling frequency was 200 Hz, and standard unipolar chest lead V5 was applied. All the measurements were undertaken in a quiet, temperature-controlled (23 ± 1 degree Celsius) room.

2.3. Construction of HRV Time Series. ECGs were first subjected to a visual quality inspection assisted by a self-designed MATLAB program with user interface, which confirmed that all recordings were with high signal qualities. A template-matching process was then applied to extract the R peaks [18] followed by a second-round visual inspection for the correction of misidentified peaks and ectopic beats using the same MATLAB program. During this visual inspection, false positive detection was removed while false negatives were filled with the actual location of R peaks read manually from the program. We confirmed that no ectopic beats occurred in those data. HRV time series were finally constructed by the consecutive R-R intervals.

2.4. HRA Metrics. The following four well-established metrics derived from the Poincaré plot were calculated.

2.4.1. Porta's Index (PI). Conceptually, PI renders symmetry when the numbers of points in the two regions in Poincaré plot separated by the line of identity (LI) are the same and renders asymmetry if they differ [19]. Different levels of asymmetry can be estimated by how much the numbers differ. Thus, PI can be calculated by

$$PI = \frac{a}{m} \times 100, \tag{1}$$

wherein a is the number of points above LI and m the total number of points (points on LI excluded).

2.4.2. Guzik's Index (GI). GI uses the distances between points and LI as a measure to assess whether the contributions of points in the two different regions in Poincaré plot are equal or not [20]. Specifically,

$$GI = \frac{\sum_{i=1}^{a} D_i}{\sum_{i=1}^{m} D_i} \times 100, \tag{2}$$

wherein D_i is the Euclidian distance of point i to LI. For the RR interval time series, the Poincaré plot is actually to plot the current RR interval versus its subsequent interval. Thus, $D_i = |RR_{i+1} - RR_i| / \sqrt{2}$.

2.4.3. Slope Index (SI). The average phase angles of points in the two different regions in Poincaré plot are calculated and used to assess the asymmetry [21]. Specifically,

$$SI = \frac{\sum_{i=1}^{a} |R\theta_i|}{\sum_{i=1}^{m} |R\theta_i|} \times 100, \tag{3}$$

wherein $R\theta_i = \pi/4 - \theta_i$. $\theta_i = atan(RR_{i+1}/RR_i)$ is the phase angle of point i and $\pi/4$ is the point angle of LI, that is, atan(1).

2.4.4. Area Index (AI). The average areas of sectors formed by the points and LI are calculated and used to assess the asymmetry [22]. Specifically,

$$AI = \frac{\sum_{i=1}^{a} S_i}{\sum_{i=1}^{m} S_i} \times 100, \tag{4}$$

wherein $S_i = 1/2 \times R\theta_i \times r^2$ is the area of the sector formed by point i and LI. r is the radius of the sector.

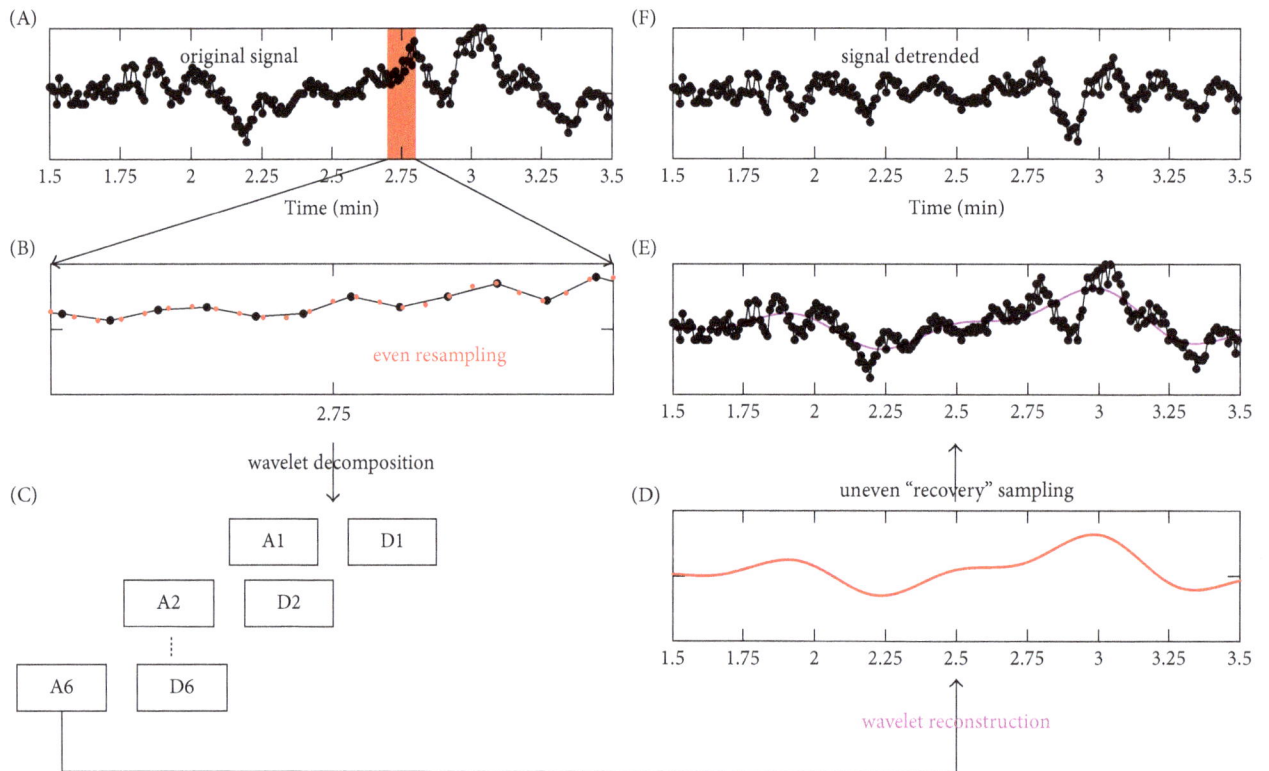

FIGURE 1: Wavelet-based nonstationary trend removal procedure. (A) The original RR interval time series. (B) The RR interval time series after the even resampling. In order to clearly demonstrate the even resampling time points (red dots) and the original time points (black dots), a segment of data from (A) is zoomed in and shown in this panel. (C) The 6-level wavelet decomposition. (D) Trend with even sampling points is obtained from wavelet reconstruction of the approximate coefficients on the 6th level. (E) The actual nonstationary trend (purple) is obtained from the uneven recovering sampling from the trend component in panel (D). (F) The detrended RR interval time series is obtained by subtracting the actual nonstationary trend from the original RR interval time series.

2.5. HRA Analysis of Short-Term HRV. The four HRA metrics were performed on HRV data collected under both conditions. The asymmetry level was further defined as the deviation of a specific HRA metric from its level for completely symmetrical data, that is, $|x - 50|$ (x denotes an HRA metric), and was denoted as ΔPI, ΔGI, ΔSI, and ΔAI, respectively. Besides, to explore the potential effect of nonstationary trend, wavelet detrending was performed and the above four asymmetrical indices were recalculated using the detrended data. To perform the wavelet detrending, raw HRV data were first evenly resampled to 4 Hz by spline interpolation. A 6-level wavelet decomposition using the coif5 wavelet was then conducted. The approximation coefficients on the 6th level were reconstructed to the original scale and were nonevenly "recovered" by spline interpolation which resulted in the trend that would be subtracted. The 6-level decomposition was used so that the frequency band of the trend would be less than ~0.03 Hz. Figure 1 intuitively demonstrates this wavelet detrending procedure.

2.6. Statistical Analysis. The Shapiro–Wilk W test suggested nonnormal distribution of all the HRA results. Therefore, the Wilcoxon signed-rank test of each pair was used to examine the within-subject differences under the two measurement conditions. In addition, Cohen's d static was calculated for

statistically significant observations to examine the effect size of the corresponding metric. A medium effect size was considered if $d \geq 0.5$ and large if $d \geq 0.8$ [23]. As secondary analysis, we also performed the Wilcoxon signed-rank tests by restricting to male subjects ($N = 12$) only. We did not perform these tests separately on females as we only had 4 females. All the statistical analyses were performed using the JMP software (Pro 13, SAS Institute, Cary, NC, USA).

3. Results

A typical RR interval time series for resting seated position and the corresponding RR interval time series from the same subject during walking are shown in Figure 2. Overall, the RR intervals become shorter (i.e., heart beats faster) during walking, such that the points distribute more compactly on the Poincaré plot than those during rest if the same scale is used. The Poincaré plots also become more compact after nonstationary trend removal, which is expected because of the effect of detrending on long-term HRA.

3.1. Asymmetry Based on Raw HRV Time Series. HRV data collected under both conditions displayed asymmetry as assessed by the four HRA metrics (all four p's < 0.001 under

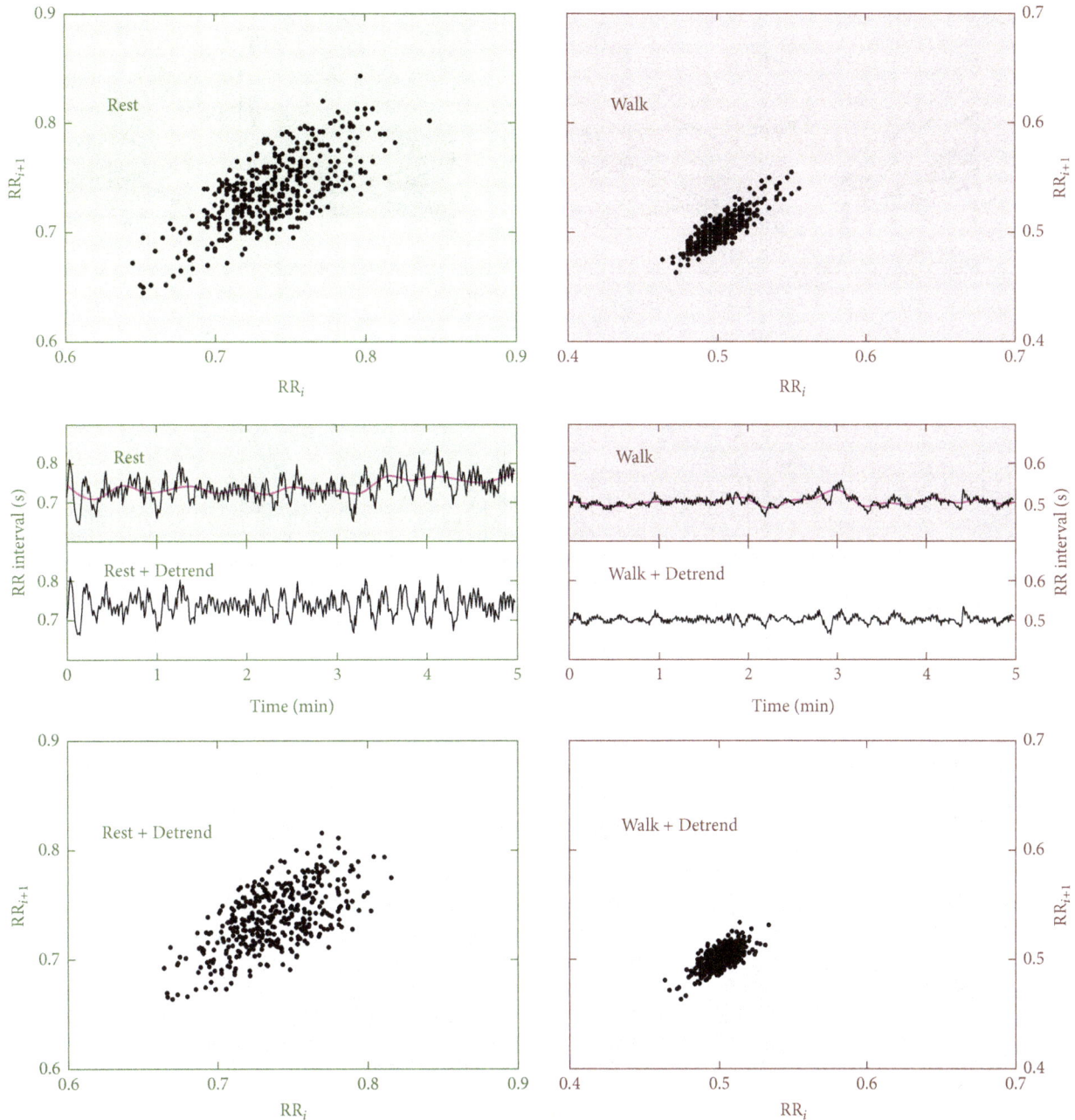

FIGURE 2: Exemplary RR interval time series (middle four panels) and the corresponding Poincaré plots (upper two and lower two panels). Left: data during seated position, right: data during walking. Data after nonstationary trend removal are shown with light-shaded background colors on lower four panels with "+Detrend" legend.

both conditions as revealed by Wilcoxon signed-rank test of each measure versus symmetrical level; i.e., index = 0). Compared to the resting seated position, a significant reduction of HRA during walking was observed by PI (Wilcoxon signed-rank test of each pair: $p = 0.001$; Cohen's $d = 1.0$; out of the 16 subjects, 14 including all the four females showed reduction; Figure 3(A1)). No significant HRA changes during walking were suggested by the remaining three metrics (all p's > 0.1; Figures 3(B1)–3(D1)). The results persisted when restricting the Wilcoxon signed-rank tests to male subjects only (Figures 3(A2)–3(D2)).

3.2. Asymmetry Based on Detrended HRV Time Series. Wavelet detrending did not change the HRA levels significantly under resting seated position (all p's > 0.05 versus results from raw HRV data as revealed by the Wilcoxon signed-rank test). Similarly, the HRA levels during walking did not show significant changes after wavelet detrending (all p's > 0.1 for PI, GI, and SI) except that assessed by AI which indicated a significant reduction ($p = 0.04$; 11 out of 16 subjects showed reduced AI after wavelet detrending). As a consequence, AI indicated significantly lower HRA during walking than that under resting seated position ($p = 0.025$; $d = 0.7$; 12 out of 16

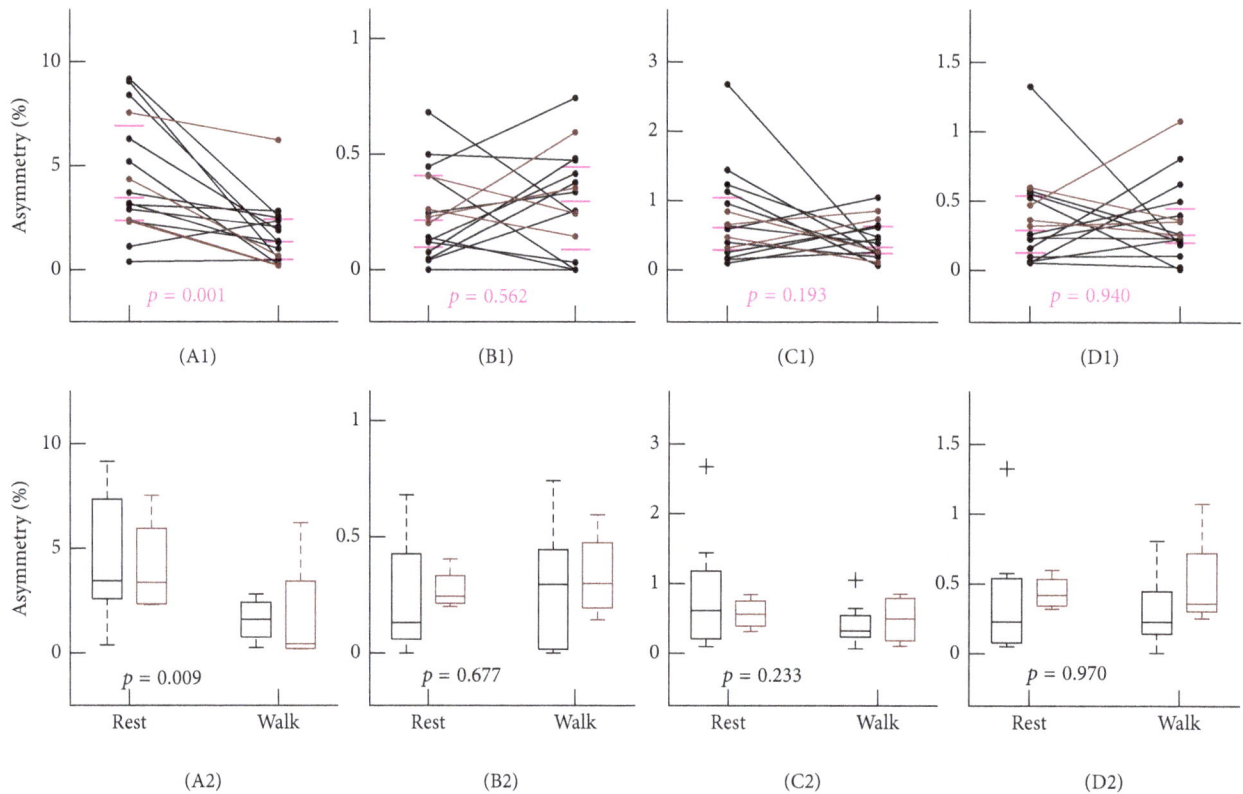

FIGURE 3: The asymmetries of short-term heart rate variability without detrending. In order to show the changes, results from the same individual were connected by lines. Horizontal bars indicate the median and [1st, 3rd] quartiles. p values were from Wilcoxon signed-rank test of each pair. ((A1) and (A2)) ΔPI; ((B1) and (B2)) ΔGI; ((C1) and (C2)) ΔSI; ((D1) and (D2)) ΔAI. *Rest*: results under resting seated position; *Walk*: results during regular walking. 14 individuals show reduction from *Rest* to *Walk* in (A1). Results from males and from females are marked in different colors (male: green; female: brown). Lower panels summarize the box plots (that show from top to bottom the max, 3rd quartile, median, 1st quartile, and min) for males and females, separately. Outliers, if there are any, are marked by "+."

subjects showed reduction; Figure 4(D1)). SI also indicated significantly lower HRA during walking ($p = 0.044$; $d = 0.4$; 12 out of 16 subjects showed reduction; Figure 4(C1)). The remaining two metrics showed consistent results as compared with those based on raw HRV data; that is, PI reduced significantly ($p = 0.050$; $d = 0.6$; 13 out of 16 subjects showed reduction) while GI showed no significant changes ($p = 0.562$; Figures 4(A1) and 4(B1)). Within the three metrics that showed statistical significance (i.e., PI, SI, and AI), the four female subjects did not display consistent changing patterns (i.e., for each metric there are both decrease and increase during walking across the four female subjects). The between-condition changes remain when restricting data to male subjects only (Figures 4(A2)–4(D2)), except that the reduction during walking in PI becomes borderline significant ($p = 0.077$; Figure 4(A2)).

4. Discussions

Asymmetry is an accepted intrinsic property of HRV. It imparts the time irreversibility of HRV—an important marker of the nonlinearity in HRV dynamics that can be perturbed by many pathologies [19]. For example, perturbed HRA has been observed in diseases including arrhythmia [21], heart failure [24], obstructive sleep apnea [25],

myocardial infarction [26, 27], postoperative myocardial ischemia [28], and type 1 diabetes [29]. Most interestingly, HRA has suggested potential for postinfarction risk prediction [30]. The current pilot study explores whether and how HRA changes during regular walking. To answer the question, we used 5 min ECG data that applied a within-subject, randomized "crossover" design to examine changes of short-term HRV during exercise [15]. ECG data of each participant were monitored two times that correspond to a resting seated position and a regular walking protocol on the treadmill, respectively. We assessed the HRA using four established HRA metrics, that is, PI, GI, SI, and AI. With the 5 min ECG data, mainly the short-term HRA is expected to be captured [12, 19, 30] while the components related to long-term HRA may only have slight contributions to results, which limits the availability of long-term HRA to be examined fairly. Therefore, in this study we focused only on short-term HRA, and in order to further get rid of the potential weak contributions of long-term HRA, we repeated the calculations of the four HRA metrics on HRV recordings after a wavelet detrending process that removes the low-frequency components of $<\sim0.03$ Hz which contribute primarily to long-term HRA.

Our pilot data on 16 healthy college students showed a reduced PI while unchanged GI, SI, and AI during walking

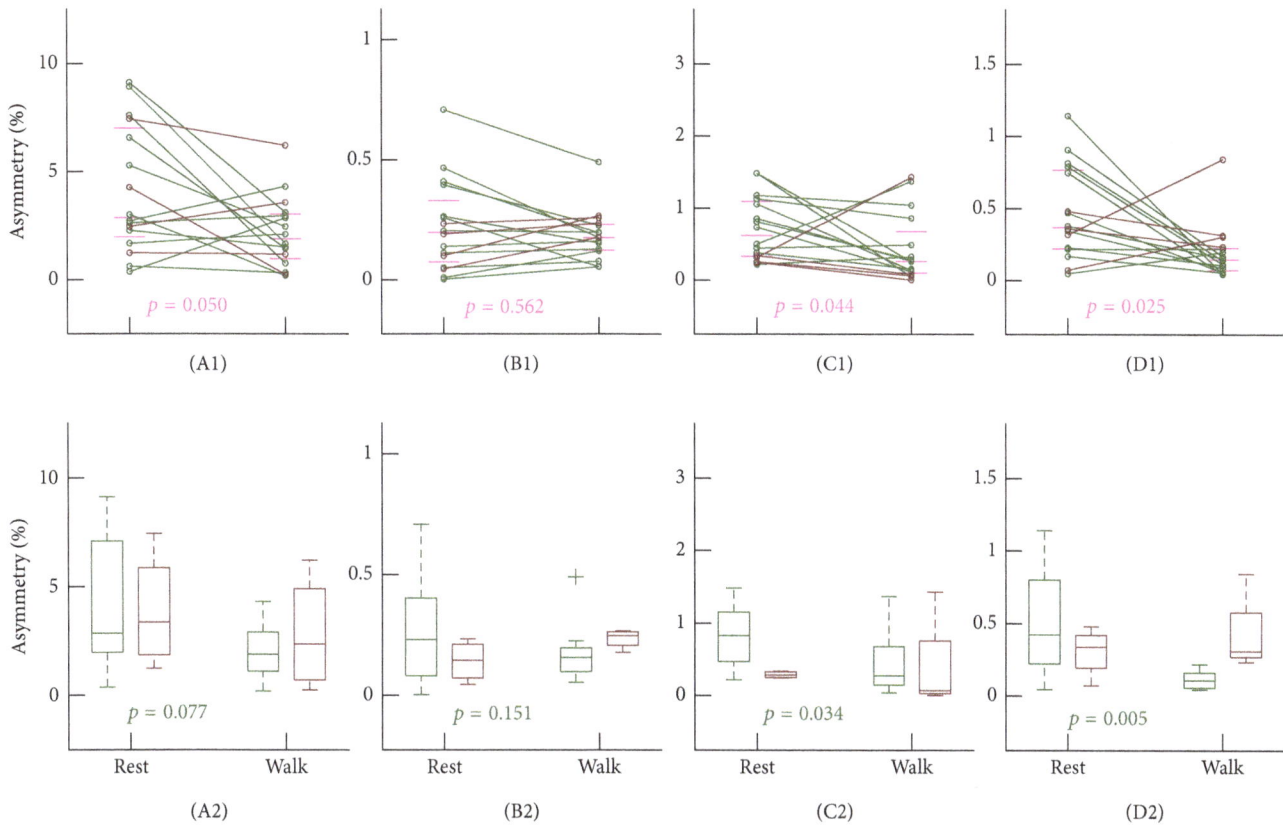

FIGURE 4: The asymmetries of short-term heart rate variability after wavelet detrending. In order to show the changes, results from the same individual were connected by lines. Horizontal bars indicate the median and [1st, 3rd] quartiles. p values were from Wilcoxon signed-rank test of each pair. ((A1) and (A2)) ΔPI; ((B1) and (B2)) ΔGI; ((C1) and (C2)) ΔSI; ((D1) and (D2)) ΔAI. *Rest*: results under resting seated position; *Walk*: results during regular walking. 13 individuals show reduction from *Rest* to *Walk* in (A1), 12 individuals show reduction from *Rest* to *Walk* in (C1), and 12 individuals show reduction from *Rest* to *Walk* in (D1). Results from males and from females are marked in different colors (male: green; female: brown). Lower panels summarize the box plots (that show from top to bottom the max, 3rd quartile, median, 1st quartile, and min) for males and females, separately. Outliers, if there are any, are marked by "+."

on treadmill based on raw HRV data. Based on wavelet-detrended data, reduced PI, SI, and AI were documented while GI still indicated no significant changes. It has been hypothesized that short-term HRA possesses a dominant contribution of vagal activity [9, 12]. Thus, the reduced PI observed from both raw HRV and detrended HRV data may underline the belief that vagal tone is withdrawn during low-intensity exercise [17, 31, 32]. However, none of the remaining three metrics, that is, GI, SI, and AI, showed significant changes based on raw HRV data, suggesting a possible lack of sensitivity to vagal withdrawal. Furthermore, SI and AI indicated significant decreases during walking using detrended HRV data, suggesting that, in addition to short-term HRA, SI and AI may also capture long-term HRA that confounds the changes of short-term HRA even though the contribution of long-term component in 5 min ECG data is low. GI was almost unchanged after detrending, implying that GI, a second-dimensional metric that relies on the distances, may capture mostly long-term HRA. We note that even with significant observations, the changing directions of these metrics with regular walking in several individuals are totally opposite (see Figures 3 and 4). Different changing directions may reflect different autonomic responses across

individuals to the walking stimuli. The difference may come from different exercise habits, different levels of college study stress, or even autonomic disorders [33]. This information will be collected in our future studies in order to uncover what leads to the differences.

Consistently, all our results still held when using data of male subjects. However, with only four females, we could not reliably perform any statistical analyses. Besides, the changing directions of HRA from resting to walking conditions seemed not consistent. Together, they limited our ability to conclude anything for female subjects. In a previous study, an interesting sex difference in HRA in particularly younger subjects has been reported [34]. Further studies are thus warranted to examine whether the effect of regular walking on HRA differs across sexes. In addition, participants in the current study were all quite young. How age influences the effect of regular walking is yet another concern that requires further elucidations.

Our results also show consistency with some published work. For example, there are studies that observed decreased HRA during acute mental stress (i.e., Stroop and arithmetic test) [35] and aerobic exercise [36], both corresponding to an autonomic balance shift towards sympathetic predominance or vagal withdrawal. However, in the study that applied acute mental stress [35], GI was found to better reflect vagal withdrawal than PI did, which is different from what we observed. This difference may partially due to different data lengths used (i.e., 6 min in the mentioned study versus 5 min in ours). And another possible reason might be that we calculated the absolute difference of the actual HRA metrics and 50 (see Section 2.5, and more discussions regarding this can be found in the next paragraph). In a different study, the same group (i.e., the group of the mental stress study) also showed that HRA increased significantly during orthostasis and that GI was more sensitive to the stimulus [37]. HRV of ~15 min was used in that study. The increased HRA during orthostasis based on this relatively long data might reflect mainly the sympathetic activation, and the better performance of GI could thus be understandable as our results before and after detrending provide a hint that GI may be more sensitive to the sympathetic modulation and thus the long-term HRA. What is interesting is that the changing directions of short- and long-term HRA during vagal withdrawal or sympathetic activation are completely opposite which is worth further elucidations. An increase in HRA has also been observed with respiratory maneuver (e.g., inspiration/expiration = 2 : 1 or 1 : 1) [38]. Three 4.5 s metronome breathing patterns (1 : 1, 2 : 1, and normal pattern ~1 : 2) were administered for each participant while ECGs were recorded for 5 min at each breathing pattern. However, in that study no significant differences in traditional HRV parameters (such as power of higher frequency—the marker for vagal activity) were found. Further examinations to clearly figure out what led to the observed HRA changes are thus still required and this also limits the direct comparison between our study and the other three studies reviewed above, that is, [35–37], which attribute HRA changes mainly to autonomic responses.

It is worth noting that we used the absolute difference of an HRA metric to 50 as the index of asymmetric level (see Section 2.5). By calculating the absolute difference, we lost the power to differentiate the contributions of instantaneously accelerated and decelerated patterns. However, in the currently study, we focused mainly on the "asymmetry" phenomenon, which is believed to be existing especially during resting state as reported by many previous studies [3, 12], instead of the unbalanced sympathetic or vagal tones. The calculation of absolute changes provides the possibility of screening more asymmetric patterns out, as stated by a previous study [39]. In addition, the regulation of heart rate is not instantaneous. Instead, it takes a couple of seconds [40], which imparts the importance of measuring the symmetry of changes rather than the exact acceleration or deceleration patterns [39].

Our pilot study also touches a potential important point in short-term HRA analysis—the influence of nonstationary trend. To the best of our knowledge, this has not been considered seriously in previous work. We note that the very low-frequency component of <~0.03 Hz is usually considered nonstationary trend and its removal will hardly affect the beat-to-beat decelerating/accelerating patterns. However, it may affect how much the pattern deviates from symmetric.

Therefore, if an HRA algorithm takes the position of the patterns in the Poincaré plot (either above or below the line of identity) into consideration, the results after trend removal would rarely get affected (such as the case for the metric PI; see Figures 3 and 4). If an algorithm considers the distance or area characteristics, it is possible that a pattern will be considered deviated a little bit more from symmetric before trend removal than from afterwards. This effect will be important when considering long-term asymmetry. In this scenario, a decreased asymmetry (increased symmetry) for the same recording after trend removal would thus be expected when using metrics such as SI and AI, especially for data during walking (which are true when comparing Figures 3 and 4). This also provides a possible explanation that PI decreases significantly during exercise both before and after trend removal while significant changes in SI and AI are only observed after trend removal. Based on our pilot data, nonstationary trend removal is recommended for short-term HRA analysis, and to validate this, definitely further examinations with more participants and different stimulus are warranted.

Recent advances in smart wearables open a new avenue for the monitoring and management of individual's health during daily routine. Perhaps one of the most common wearable devices is the ECG or heart rate monitor that can be used to assess the cardiovascular function and the underlying autonomic control status. A simplest idea in using such devices is to implement the algorithms that are previously developed based on data episodes collected during one time clinic or laboratory visit into continuous data, which provides the opportunity for sporadic, health-related alterations to be picked up, as well as the feasibility to look at the variations of these markers with time throughout a day.

Conflicts of Interest

The authors declare that there are no conflicts of interest regarding the publication of this paper.

Acknowledgments

This work was supported by the Natural Science Foundation of Shandong Province, China (no. BS2012DX019), the National Natural Science Foundation of China (nos. 61601263, 61471223), and the Key Program on Natural Scientific Research from the Department of Education of Anhui Province, China (no. KJ2016A470).

References

[1] E. H. Hon and S. T. Lee, "Electronic evaluations of the fetal heart rate patterns preceding fetal death, further observations," *American Journal of Obstetrics & Gynecology*, vol. 87, pp. 814–826, 1965.

[2] Task Force of the European Society of Cardiology, "Heart rate variability, standards of measurement, physiological interpretation, and clinical use," *Circulation*, vol. 93, pp. 1043–1065, 1996.

[3] M. Costa, A. L. Goldberger, and C.-K. Peng, "Broken asymmetry of the human heartbeat: loss of time irreversibility in aging

and disease," *Physical Review Letters*, vol. 95, no. 19, Article ID 198102, 2005.

[4] M. D. Costa, C.-K. Peng, and A. L. Goldberger, "Multiscale analysis of heart rate dynamics: entropy and time irreversibility measures," *Cardiovascular Engineering*, vol. 8, no. 2, pp. 88–93, 2008.

[5] K. R. Casali, A. G. Casali, N. Montano et al., "Multiple testing strategy for the detection of temporal irreversibility in stationary time series," *Physical Review E: Statistical, Nonlinear, and Soft Matter Physics*, vol. 77, no. 6, Article ID 066204, 2008.

[6] C. Cammarota and E. Rogora, "Time reversal, symbolic series and irreversibility of human heartbeat," *Chaos, Solitons & Fractals*, vol. 32, no. 5, pp. 1649–1654, 2007.

[7] F. Hou, J. Zhuang, C. Bian et al., "Analysis of heartbeat asymmetry based on multi-scale time irreversibility test," *Physica A: Statistical Mechanics and its Applications*, vol. 389, no. 4, pp. 754–760, 2010.

[8] U. R. Acharya, K. P. Joseph, N. Kannathal, C. M. Lim, and J. S. Suri, "Heart rate variability: a review," *Medical & Biological Engineering & Computing*, vol. 44, no. 12, pp. 1031–1051, 2006.

[9] J. Piskorski and P. Guzik, "Compensatory properties of heart rate asymmetry," *Journal of Electrocardiology*, vol. 45, no. 3, pp. 220–224, 2012.

[10] R. Hainsworth, "Physiology of the Cardiac Autonomic System," in *Clinical Guide to Cardiac Autonomic Tests*, M. Malik, Ed., pp. 10–1007, Springer, Dordrecht, Netherlands, 1998.

[11] P. Nicolini, M. M. Ciulla, C. D. Asmundis, F. Magrini, and P. Brugada, "The Prognostic Value of Heart Rate Variability in the Elderly, Changing the Perspective: From Sympathovagal Balance to Chaos Theory," *Pacing and Clinical Electrophysiology*, vol. 35, no. 5, pp. 621–637, 2012.

[12] J. Piskorski and P. Guzik, "Asymmetric properties of long-term and total heart rate variability," *Medical & Biological Engineering & Computing*, vol. 49, no. 11, pp. 1289–1297, 2011.

[13] A. A. Akintola, V. van de Pol, D. Bimmel, A. C. Maan, and D. van Heemst, "Comparative analysis of the equivital EQ02 lifemonitor with holter ambulatory ECG device for continuous measurement of ECG, heart rate, and heart rate variability: A validation study for precision and accuracy," *Frontiers in Physiology*, vol. 7, article no. 391, 2016.

[14] J. Kristiansen, M. Korshøj, J. H. Skotte et al., "Comparison of two systems for long-term heart rate variability monitoring in free-living conditions—a pilot study," *Biomedical Engineering Online*, vol. 10, article 27, 2011.

[15] B. Shi, Y. Zhang, C. Yuan, S. Wang, and P. Li, "Entropy Analysis of Short-Term Heartbeat Interval Time Series during Regular Walking," *Entropy*, vol. 19, no. 10, p. 568, 2017.

[16] C. Karmakar, A. Khandoker, and M. Palaniswami, "Investigating the changes in heart rate asymmetry (HRA) with perturbation of parasympathetic nervous system," *Australasian Physical & Engineering Sciences in Medicine*, vol. 35, no. 4, pp. 465–474, 2012.

[17] S. Boettger, C. Puta, V. K. Yeragani et al., "Heart rate variability, QT variability, and electrodermal activity during exercise," *Medicine & Science in Sports & Exercise*, vol. 42, no. 3, pp. 443–448, 2010.

[18] P. Li, C. Liu, M. Zhang, W. Che, and J. Li, "A Real-Time QRS Complex Detection Method," *Acta Biophysica Sinica*, vol. 27, no. 3, pp. 222–230, 2011.

[19] A. Porta, K. R. Casali, A. G. Casali et al., "Temporal asymmetries of short-term heart period variability are linked to autonomic regulation," *American Journal of Physiology-Regulatory, Integrative and Comparative Physiology*, vol. 295, no. 2, pp. R550–R557, 2008.

[20] P. Guzik, J. Piskorski, T. Krauze, A. Wykretowicz, and H. Wysocki, "Heart rate asymmetry by Poincaré plots of RR intervals," *Biomedizinische Technik. Biomedical Engineering*, vol. 51, no. 4, pp. 272–275, 2006.

[21] C. K. Karmakar, A. H. Khandoker, and M. Palaniswami, "Phase asymmetry of heart rate variability signal," *Physiological Measurement*, vol. 36, no. 2, article no. 303, pp. 303–314, 2015.

[22] C. Yan, P. Li, L. Ji, L. Yao, C. Karmakar, and C. Liu, "Area asymmetry of heart rate variability signal," *Biomedical Engineering Online*, vol. 16, no. 1, 2017.

[23] S. S. Sawilowsky, "Very large and huge effect sizes," *Journal of Modern Applied Statistical Methods*, vol. 8, no. 2, pp. 597–599, 2009.

[24] M. A. Woo, W. G. Stevenson, D. K. Moser, R. B. Trelease, and R. M. Harper, "Patterns of beat-to-beat heart rate variability in advanced heart failure," *American Heart Journal*, vol. 123, no. 3, pp. 704–710, 1992.

[25] P. Guzik, J. Piskorski, K. Awan, T. Krauze, M. Fitzpatrick, and A. Baranchuk, "Obstructive sleep apnea and heart rate asymmetry microstructure during sleep," *Clinical Autonomic Research*, vol. 23, no. 2, pp. 91–100, 2013.

[26] H. V. Huikuri, T. Seppänen, M. J. Koistinen et al., "Abnormalities in beat-to-beat dynamics of heart rate before the spontaneous onset of life-threatening ventricular tachyarrhythmias in patients with prior myocardial infarction," *Circulation*, vol. 93, no. 10, pp. 1836–1844, 1996.

[27] P. K. Stein, P. P. Domitrovich, H. V. Huikuri, and R. E. Kleiger, "Traditional and nonlinear heart rate variability are each independently associated with mortality after myocardial infarction," *Journal of Cardiovascular Electrophysiology*, vol. 16, no. 1, pp. 13–20, 2005.

[28] T. T. Laitio, T. H. Mäkikallio, H. V. Huikuri et al., "Relation of heart rate dynamics to the occurrence of myocardial ischemia after coronary artery bypass grafting," *American Journal of Cardiology*, vol. 89, no. 10, pp. 1176–1181, 2002.

[29] P. Guzik, "Heart rate variability by Poincaré plot and spectral analysis in young healthy subjects and patients with type 1 diabetes," *Folia Cardiol*, vol. 12, pp. suppl D, pp. 64–67, 2005.

[30] P. Guzik, J. Piskorski, P. Barthel et al., "Heart rate deceleration runs for postinfarction risk prediction," *Journal of Electrocardiology*, vol. 45, no. 1, pp. 70–76, 2012.

[31] D. W. White and P. B. Raven, "Autonomic neural control of heart rate during dynamic exercise: revisited," *The Journal of Physiology*, vol. 592, part 12, pp. 2491–2500, 2014.

[32] J. P. Fisher, "Autonomic control of the heart during exercise in humans: Role of skeletal muscle afferents," *Experimental Physiology*, vol. 99, no. 2, pp. 300–305, 2014.

[33] Q. Fu and B. D. Levine, "Exercise and the autonomic nervous system," in *Journal of the Autonomic Nervous System*, vol. 117 of *Handbook of Clinical Neurology*, pp. 147–160, Elsevier, 2013.

[34] A. Voss, R. Schroeder, A. Heitmann, A. Peters, and S. Perz, "Short-term heart rate variability - Influence of gender and age in healthy subjects," *PLoS ONE*, vol. 10, no. 3, Article ID e0118308, 2015.

[35] Z. Visnovcova, M. Mestanik, M. Javorka et al., "Complexity and time asymmetry of heart rate variability are altered in acute mental stress," *Physiological Measurement*, vol. 35, no. 7, pp. 1319–1334, 2014.

[36] B. D. L. C. Torres and J. N. Orellana, "Multiscale time irreversibility of heartbeat at rest and during aerobic exercise," *Cardiovascular Engineering*, vol. 10, no. 1, pp. 1–4, 2010.

[37] L. Chladekova, B. Czippelova, Z. Turianikova et al., "Multiscale time irreversibility of heart rate and blood pressure variability during orthostasis," *Physiological Measurement*, vol. 33, no. 10, article no. 1747, pp. 1747–1756, 2012.

[38] A. Klintworth, Z. Ajtay, A. Paljunite, S. Szabados, and L. Hejjel, "Heart rate asymmetry follows the inspiration/expiration ratio in healthy volunteers," *Physiological Measurement*, vol. 33, no. 10, article 1717, 2012.

[39] A. H. Khandoker, C. Karmakar, M. Brennan, M. Palaniswami, and A. Voss, *Poincaré Plot Methods for Heart Rate Variability Analysis*, Springer US, Boston, MA, USA, 2013.

[40] D. L. Eckberg, "Nonlinearities of the human carotid baroreceptor-cardiac reflex," *Circulation Research*, vol. 47, no. 2, pp. 208–216, 1980.

14

An Intelligent Parkinson's Disease Diagnostic System based on a Chaotic Bacterial Foraging Optimization Enhanced Fuzzy KNN Approach

Zhennao Cai (iD),[1] **Jianhua Gu,**[1] **Caiyun Wen,**[2] **Dong Zhao,**[3] **Chunyu Huang,**[4] **Hui Huang** (iD),[5] **Changfei Tong,**[5] **Jun Li,**[5] **and Huiling Chen** (iD)[5]

[1]*School of Computer Science and Engineering, Northwestern Polytechnical University, Xi'an 710072, China*
[2]*Department of Radiology, The First Affiliated Hospital of Wenzhou Medical University, Wenzhou, Zhejiang 325035, China*
[3]*College of Computer Science and Technology, Changchun Normal University, Changchun 130032, China*
[4]*College of Computer Science and Technology, Changchun University of Science Technology, Changchun 130032, China*
[5]*College of Mathematics, Physics and Electronic Information Engineering, Wenzhou University, Wenzhou, Zhejiang 325035, China*

Correspondence should be addressed to Huiling Chen; chenhuiling.jlu@gmail.com

Academic Editor: Dingchang Zheng

Parkinson's disease (PD) is a common neurodegenerative disease, which has attracted more and more attention. Many artificial intelligence methods have been used for the diagnosis of PD. In this study, an enhanced fuzzy k-nearest neighbor (FKNN) method for the early detection of PD based upon vocal measurements was developed. The proposed method, an evolutionary instance-based learning approach termed CBFO-FKNN, was developed by coupling the chaotic bacterial foraging optimization with Gauss mutation (CBFO) approach with FKNN. The integration of the CBFO technique efficiently resolved the parameter tuning issues of the FKNN. The effectiveness of the proposed CBFO-FKNN was rigorously compared to those of the PD datasets in terms of classification accuracy, sensitivity, specificity, and AUC (area under the receiver operating characteristic curve). The simulation results indicated the proposed approach outperformed the other five FKNN models based on BFO, particle swarm optimization, Genetic algorithms, fruit fly optimization, and firefly algorithm, as well as three advanced machine learning methods including support vector machine (SVM), SVM with local learning-based feature selection, and kernel extreme learning machine in a 10-fold cross-validation scheme. The method presented in this paper has a very good prospect, which will bring great convenience to the clinicians to make a better decision in the clinical diagnosis.

1. Introduction

Parkinson's disease (PD), a degenerative disorder of the central nervous system, is the second most common neurodegenerative disease [1]. The number of people suffering from PD has increased rapidly worldwide [2], especially in developing countries in Asia [3]. Although its underlying cause is unknown, the symptoms associated with PD can be significantly alleviated if detected in the early stages of illness [4–6]. PD is characterized by tremors, rigidity, slowed movement, motor symptom asymmetry, and impaired posture [7, 8]. Research has shown phonation and speech disorders are also common among PD patients [9]. In fact, phonation and speech disorders can appear in PD patients as many as five years before being clinically diagnosed with the illness [10]. The voice disorders associated with PD include dysphonia, impairment in vocal fold vibration, and dysarthria, disability in correctly articulating speech phonemes [11, 12]. Little et al. [13] first attempted to identify PD patients with dysphonic indicators using a combination of support vector machines (SVM), efficient learning machines, and the feature selection approach. The study results indicated that the proposed method efficiently identified PD patients with only four dysphonic features.

Inspired by the results obtained by Little et al. [13], many other researchers conducted studies on the use of machine learning techniques to diagnose PD patients on the same dataset (hereafter Oxford dataset). In [14], Das made a comparison of classification score for diagnosis of PD between artificial neural networks (ANN), DMneural, and Regression and Decision Trees. The ANN classifier yielded the best results of 92.9%. In [15], AStröm et al. designed a parallel feed-forward neural network system and yielded an improvement of 8.4% on PD classification. In [16], Sakar et al. proposed a method that combined SVM and feature selection using mutual information to detect PD and obtained a classification accuracy of 92.75%. In [17], a PD detection method developed by Li et al. using an SVM and a fuzzy-based nonlinear transformation method yielded a maximum classification accuracy of 93.47%. In another study, Shahbaba et al. [18] compared the classification accuracies of a nonlinear model based on a combination of the Dirichlet processes, multinomial logit models, decision trees, and support vector machines, which yielded the highest classification score of 87.7%. In [19], Psorakis et al. put forward novel convergence methods and model improvements for multiclass mRVMs. The improved model achieved an accuracy of 89.47%. In [20], Guo et al. proposed a PD detection method with a maximum classification accuracy of 93.1% by combination of genetic programming and the expectation maximization algorithm (GP-EM). In [21], Luukka used a similarity classifier and a feature selection method using fuzzy entropy measures to detect PD, and a mean classification accuracy of 85.03% is achieved. In [22], Ozcift et al. presented rotation forest ensemble classifiers with feature selection using the correlation method to identify PD patients; the proposed model yielded a highest classification accuracy of 87.13%. In [23], Spadoto et al. used a combination of evolutionary-based techniques and the Optimum-Path Forest (OPF) classifier to detect PD with a maximum classification accuracy of 84.01%. In [24], Polat integrated fuzzy C-means clustering-based feature weighting (FCMFW) into a KNN classifier, which yielded a PD classification accuracy of 97.93%. In [25], Chen et al. combined a fuzzy k-nearest neighbor classifier (FKNN) with the principle component analysis (PCA-FKNN) method to detect PD; the proposed diagnostic system yielded a maximum classification accuracy of 96.07%. In [26], Zuo et al. developed an PSO-enhanced FKNN based PD diagnostic system with a mean classification accuracy of 97.47%. In [27–29], Babu et al. proposed a 'projection based learning meta-cognitive radial basis function network (PBL-McRBFN)' approach for the prediction of PD, which obtained an testing accuracy of 96.87% on the gene expression data sets, 99.35% on standard vocal data sets, 84.36% on gait PD data sets, and 82.32% on magnetic resonance images. In [30], the hybrid intelligent system for PD detection was proposed which included several feature preprocessing methods and classification techniques using three supervised classifiers such as least-square SVM, probabilistic neural networks, and general regression neural network; the experimental results gives a maximum classification accuracy of 100% for the PD detection. Furthermore, in [31], Gök et al. developed a rotation forest ensemble KNN classifier with a classification accuracy of 98.46%. In [32], Shen et al. proposed an enhanced SVM based on fruit fly optimization algorithm, and have

achieved 96.90% classification accuracy for diagnosis of PD. In [33], Peker designed a minimum redundancy maximum relevance (mRMR) feature selection algorithm with the complex-valued artificial neural network to diagnosis of PD, and obtained a classification accuracy of 98.12%. In [34], Chen et al. proposed an efficient hybrid kernel extreme learning machine with feature selection approach. The experimental results showed that the proposed method can achieve the highest classification accuracy of 96.47% and mean accuracy of 95.97% over 10 runs of 10-fold CV. In [35], Cai et al. have proposed an optimal support vector machine (SVM) based on bacterial foraging optimization (BFO) combined with the relief feature selection to predict PD, the experimental results have demonstrated that the proposed framework exhibited excellent classification performance with a superior classification accuracy of 97.42%.

Different from the work of Little et al., Sakar et al. [36] designed voice experiments with sustained vowels, words, and sentences from PD patients and controls. The paper reported that sustained vowels had more PD-discriminative power than the isolated words and short sentences. The study result achieved 77.5% accuracy by using SVM classifier. From then on, several works have been proposed to detect PD using this PD dataset (hereafter Istanbul dataset). Zhang et al. [37] proposed a PD classification algorithm that integrated a multi-edit-nearest-neighbor algorithm with an ensemble learning algorithm. The algorithm achieved higher classification accuracy and stability compared with the other algorithms. Abrol et al. [38] proposed a kernel sparse greedy dictionary algorithm for classification tasks, comparing with kernel K-singular value decomposition algorithm and kernel multilevel dictionary learning algorithm. The method achieved an average classification accuracy of 98.2% and the best accuracy of 99.4% on the Istanbul PD dataset with multiple types of sound recordings. In [39], the authors investigated six classification algorithms, including Adaboost, support vector machines, neural network with multilayer perceptron (MLP) structure, ensemble classifier, K-nearest neighbor, naive Bayes, and presented feature selection algorithms including LASSO, minimal redundancy maximal relevance, relief, and local learning-based feature selection on the Istanbul PD dataset. The paper indicated that applying feature selection methods greatly increased the accuracy of classification. The SVM and KNN classifiers with local learning-based feature selection obtained the optimum prediction ability and execution times.

As shown above, ANN and SVM have been extensively applied to the detection of PD. However, understanding the underlying decision-making processes of ANN and SVM is difficult due to their black-box characteristics. Compared to ANN and SVM, FKNN is much simpler and yield more easily interpretable results. FKNN [40, 41] classifiers, improved versions of traditional k-nearest neighbor (KNN) classifiers, have been studied extensively since first proposed for the use of diagnostic purposes. In recent years, many variant versions of KNNs based on fuzzy sets theory and several extensions have been developed, such as fuzzy rough sets, intuitionistic fuzzy sets, type 2 fuzzy sets, and possibilistic theory based KNN [42]. FKNN allows for the representation of imprecise knowledge via the introduction of fuzzy measures, providing a powerful method of similarity description among instances. In FKNN methods, fuzzy set theories are introduced into KNNs, which assign membership degrees to different classes instead of the distances to their k-nearest neighbors. Thus, each of the instances is assigned a class membership value rather than binary values. When it comes to the voting stage, the highest class membership function value is selected. Then based on these properties, FKNN has been applied to numerous practical problems, such as medical diagnosis problems [25, 43], protein identification and prediction problems [44, 45], bankruptcy prediction problems [46], slope collapse prediction problems [47], and grouting activity prediction problems [48].

The classification performance of an FKNN greatly relies on its tuning parameters, neighborhood size (k), and fuzzy strength (m). Therefore, the two parameters should be precisely determined before applying FKNN to practical problems. Several studies concerning parameter tuning in FKNN have been conducted. In [46], Chen et al. presented the particle swarm optimization (PSO) based method to automatically search for the two tuning parameters of an FKNN. According to the results of the study, the proposed method could be effectively and efficiently applied to bankruptcy prediction problems. More recently, Cheng et al. [48] developed a differential evolution optimization approach to determine the most appropriate tuning parameters of an FKNN and successfully applied to grouting activity prediction problems in the construction industry. Later, Cheng et al. [47] proposed using firefly algorithm to tune the hyperparameters of the FKNN model. The FKNN model was then applied to slop collapse prediction problems. The experiment results indicated that the developed method outperformed other common algorithms. The bacterial foraging optimization (BFO) method [49], a relatively new swarm-intelligence algorithm, mimics the cooperative foraging behavior of several bacteria on a multidimensional continuous search space and, therefore, effectively balances exploration and exploitation events. Since its introduction, BFO has been subtly introduced to real-world optimization problems [50–55], such as optimal controller design problems [49], stock market index prediction problems [56], automatic circle detection problems involving digital images [57], harmonic estimation problems [58], active power filter design problems [59], and especially the parameter optimization of machine learning methods [60–63]. In [60], BFO was introduced to wavelet neural network training and applied successfully to load forecasting. In [61], an improved BFO algorithm was proposed to fine-tune the parameters of fuzzy support vector machines to identify the fatigue status of the electromyography signal. The experimental results have shown that the proposed method is an effective tool for diagnosis of fatigue status. In [62], BFO was proposed to learn the structure of Bayesian networks. The experimental results verify that the proposed BFO algorithm is a viable alternative to learn the structures of Bayesian networks and is also highly competitive compared to state-of-the-art algorithms. In [63], BFO was employed to optimize the

training parameters appeared in adaptive neuro-fuzzy inference system for speed control of matrix converter- (MC-) fed brushless direct current (BLDC) motor. The simulation results have reported that the BFO approach is much superior to the other nature-inspired algorithms. In [64], a chaotic local search based BFO (CLS-BFO) was proposed, which introduced the DE operator and the chaotic search operator into the chemotaxis step of the original BFO.

Inspired from the above works, in this paper, the BFO method was integrated with FKNN for the maximum classification performance. In order to further improve the diversity of the bacteria swarm, chaos theory combination with the Gaussian mutation was introduced in BFO. Then, the resulting CBFO-FKNN model was applied to the detection of PD. In our previous work, we have applied BFO in the classification of speech signals for PD diagnosis [35]. In this work, we have further improved the BFO by embedding the chaotic theory and Gauss mutation and combined with the effective FKNN classifier. In order to validate the effectiveness of the proposed CBFO-FKNN approach, FKNN based on five other meta-heuristic algorithms including original BFO, particle swarm optimization (PSO), genetic algorithms (GA), fruit fly optimization (FOA), and firefly algorithm (FA) was implemented for strict comparison. In addition, advanced machine learning methods, including the support vector machine (SVM), kernel based extreme learning machine (KELM) methods, and SVM with local learning-based feature selection (LOGO) [65] (LOGO-SVM), were compared with the proposed CBFO-FKNN model in terms of classification accuracy (ACC), area under the receiver operating characteristic curve (AUC), sensitivity, and specificity. The experimental results show that the proposed CBFO-FKNN approach has exhibited high ACC, AUC, sensitivity, and specificity on both datasets. This work is a fully extended version of our previously published conference paper [66] and that further improved method has been provided.

The main contributions of this study are as follows:

(a) First, we introduce chaos theory and Gaussian mutation enhanced BFO to adaptively determine the two key parameters of FKNN, which aided the FKNN classifier in more efficiently achieving the maximum classification performance, more stable and robust when compared to five other bio-inspired algorithms-based FKNN models and other advanced machine learning methods such as SVM and KELM.

(b) The resulting model, CBFO-FKNN, is introduced to discriminate the persons with PD from the healthy ones on the two PD datasets of UCI machine learning repository. It is promising to serve as a computer-aided decision-making tool for early detection of PD.

The remainder of this paper is structured as follows. In Section 2, background information regarding FKNN, BFO, chaos theory, and Gaussian mutation is presented. The implementation of the proposed methodology is explained in Section 3. In Section 4, the experimental design is described in detail. The experimental results and a discussion are presented in Section 5. Finally, Section 6 concludes the paper.

2. Background Information

2.1. Fuzzy k-Nearest Neighbor (FKNN). In this section, a brief description of FKNN is provided. A detailed description of FKNN can be referred to in [41]. In FKNN, the fuzzy membership values of samples are assigned to different categories as follows:

$$u_i(x) = \frac{\sum_{j=1}^{K} u_{ij} \left(1/\left\|x - x_j\right\|^{2/(m-1)}\right)}{\sum_{j=1}^{K} \left(1/\left\|x - x_j\right\|^{2/(m-1)}\right)} \tag{1}$$

where $i=1,2,\dots C$, $j=1,2,\dots,K$, C represents the number of classes, and K means the number of nearest neighbors. The fuzzy strength parameter (m) is used to determine how heavily the distance is weighted when calculating each neighbor's contribution to the membership value. $m \in (1,\infty)$. $\left\|x - x_j\right\|$ is usually selected as the value of m. In addition, the Euclidean distance, the distance between x and its jth nearest neighbor x_j, is usually selected as the distance metric. Furthermore, u_{ij} denotes the degree of membership of the pattern x_j from the training set to class i among the k-nearest neighbors of x. In this study, the constrained fuzzy membership approach was adopted in that the k-nearest neighbors of each training pattern (i.e., x_k) were determined, and the membership of x_k in each class was assigned as

$$u_{ij}(x_k) = \begin{cases} 0.51 + \left(\dfrac{n_j}{K}\right) * 0.49, & \text{if } j = i \\ \left(\dfrac{n_j}{K}\right) * 0.49, & \text{if } j \neq i. \end{cases} \tag{2}$$

The value of n_j denotes the number of neighbors belonging to j^{th} class. The membership values calculated using (2) should satisfy the following equations:

$$\sum_{I=1}^{C} \mu_{ij} = 1,$$

$$j = 1, 2, \cdots, n, \; C \text{ is the number of classes} \tag{3}$$

$$0 < \sum_{j=1}^{n} u_{ij} < n, \quad u_{ij} \in [0,1].$$

After calculating all of the membership values of a query sample, it is assigned to the class with which it has the highest degree of membership, i.e.,

$$C(x) = \arg \max_{i=1}^{C} (u_i(x)) \tag{4}$$

2.2. Bacterial Foraging Optimization (BFO). The bacterial foraging algorithm (BFO) is a novel nature-inspired optimization algorithm proposed by Passino in 2002 [49]. The BFO simulates the mechanism of approaching or moving away while sensing the concentration of peripheral substances in bacterial foraging process. This method contains four basic behaviors: chemotaxis, swarming, reproduction, and elimination-dispersal.

2.2.1. Chemotaxis. The chemotaxis behavior simulates two different positional shifts of *E. coli* bacterium that depend on the rotation of the flagellum, namely, tumbling and moving. The tumbling refers to looking for new directions and the moving refers to keeping the direction going. The specific operation is as follows: first, a unit step is moved in a certain random direction. If the fitness value of the new position is more suitable than the previous one, it will continue to move in that direction; if the fitness value of the new position is not better than before, the tumble operation is performed and moves in another random direction. When the maximum number of attempts is reached, the chemotaxis step is stopped. The chemotaxis step to operate is indicated by the following:

$$\theta^i(j+1,k,l) = \theta^i(j,k,l) + C(i) * dct_i$$

$$dct_i = \frac{\Delta(i)}{\sqrt{\Delta^T(i)\Delta(i)}} \tag{5}$$

where $\theta^i(j,k,l)$ is the position of the ith bacterium. The j, k, and l, respectively, indicate the number of bacterial individuals to complete the chemotaxis, reproduction, and elimination-dispersal. $C(i)$ is the chemotaxis step length for the ith bacteria to move. Δ is the random vector between [-1, 1].

2.2.2. Swarming. In the process of foraging, the bacterial community can adjust the gravitation and repulsion between the cell and the cell, so that the bacteria in the case of aggregation characteristics and maintain their relatively independent position. The gravitation causes the bacteria to clump together, and the repulsion forces the bacteria to disperse in a relatively independent position to obtain food.

2.2.3. Reproduction. In the reproduction operation of BFO algorithm, the algorithm accumulates the fitness values of all the positions that the bacterial individual passes through in the chemotaxis operation and arranges the bacteria in descending order. Then the first half of the bacteria divides themselves into two bacteria by binary fission, and the other half die. As a result, the new reproduced bacterial individual has the same foraging ability as the original individual, and the population size of bacterial is always constant.

2.2.4. Elimination-Dispersal. After the algorithm has been reproduced for several generations, the bacteria will undergo elimination-dispersal at a given probability *Ped*, and the selected bacteria will be randomly redistributed to new positions. Specifically, if a bacterial individual in the bacterial community satisfies the probability *Ped* of elimination-dispersal, the individual loses the original position of foraging and randomly selects a new position in the solution space, thereby promoting the search of the global optimal solution.

2.3. Chaotic Mapping. Chaos, as a widespread nonlinear phenomenon in nature, has the characteristics of randomness, ergodicity, sensitivity to initial conditions and so on [67]. Due to the characteristics of ergodicity and randomness, chaotic motions can traverse all the states in a certain range according to their own laws without repetition. Therefore, if we use chaos variables to search optimally, we will undoubtedly have more advantages than random search. Chaos ergodicity features can be used to optimize the search and avoid falling into the local minima; therefore, chaos optimization search method has become a novel optimization technique. Chaotic sequences generated by different mappings can be used such as logistic map, sine map, singer map, sinusoidal map, and tent map. In this paper, several chaotic maps were tried and the best one was chosen to combine with the BFO algorithm. According to the preliminary experiment, logistic map has achieved the best results. Thus, the chaotic sequences are generated by using logistic map as follows:

$$x_{i+1} = ux_i \left(1 - x_i\right) \tag{6}$$

u is the control parameter and let $u = 4$. When $u = 4$, the logistic mapping comes into a thorough chaotic state. Let $x_i \in (0, 1)$ and $x_i \neq 0.25, 0.5, 0.75$.

The initial bacterial population θ is mapped to the chaotic sequence that has been generated according to (6), resulting in a corresponding chaotic bacterial population pch.

$$pch = x_i * \theta \tag{7}$$

2.4. Gaussian Mutation. The Gaussian mutation operation has been derived from the Gaussian normal distribution and has demonstrated its effectiveness with application to evolutionary search [68]. This theory was referred to as classical evolutionary programming (CEP).The Gaussian mutations have been used to exploit the searching capabilities of ABC [69], PSO [70], and DE [71]. Also, Gaussian mutation is more likely to create a new offspring near the original parent because of its narrow tail. Due to this, the search equation will take smaller steps allowing for every corner of the search space to be explored in a much better way. Hence it is expected to provide relatively faster convergence. The Gaussian density function is given by

$$f_{gaussian(0,\sigma^2)}\left(\alpha\right) = \frac{1}{\sqrt{2\pi\sigma^2}} e^{-\alpha^2/2\sigma^2} \tag{8}$$

where σ^2 is the variance for each member of the population.

3. Proposed CBFO-FKNN Model

In this section, we described the new evolutionary FKNN model based on the CBFO strategy. The two key parameters of FKNN were automatically tuned based on the CBFO strategy. As shown in Figure 1, the proposed methodology has two main parts, including the inner parameter optimization procedure and outer performance evaluation procedure. The main objective of the inner parameter optimization procedure was to optimize the parameter neighborhood size (k) and fuzzy strength parameter (m) by using the CBFO technique via a 5-fold cross-validation (CV). Then, the obtained best values of (k, m) were input into the FKNN prediction model in order to perform the PD diagnostic

TABLE 1: Description of the Oxford PD data set.

Label	Feature
S1	MDVP:Fo(Hz)
S2	MDVP:Fhi(Hz)
S3	MDVP:Flo(Hz)
S4	MDVP:Jitter(%)
S5	MDVP:Jitter(Abs)
S6	MDVP:RAP
S7	MDVP:PPQ
S8	Jitter:DDP
S9	MDVP:Shimmer
S10	MDVP:Shimmer(dB)
S11	Shimmer:APQ3
S12	Shimmer:APQ5
S13	MDVP:APQ
S14	Shimmer:DDA
S15	NHR
S16	HNR
S17	RPDE
S18	D2
S19	DFA
S20	Spread1
S21	Spread2
S22	PPE

classification task in the outer loop via the 10-fold CV. The classification error rate was used as the fitness function.

$$fitness = \frac{\left(\sum_{i=1}^{K} testError_i\right)}{k} \tag{9}$$

where $testError_i$ means the average test error of the FKNN classifier.

The main steps conducted by the CBFO strategy are described in detail as shown in Algorithm 1.

4. Experimental Design

4.1. Oxford Parkinson's Disease Data. The Oxford Parkinson's disease data set was donated by Little et al. [13], abbreviation as Oxford dataset. The data set was used to discriminate patients with PD from healthy controls via the detection of differences in vowel sounds. Various biomedical voice measurements were collected from 31 subjects. 23 of them are patients with PD, and 8 of them are healthy controls. The subjects ranged from 46 to 85 years of age. Each subject provided an average of six sustained vowel "ahh..." phonations, ranging from 1 to 36 seconds in length [13], yielding 195 total samples. Each recording was subjected to different measurements, yielding 22 real-value features. Table 1 lists these 22 vocal features and their statistical parameters.

4.2. Istanbul Parkinson's Disease Data. The second data set in this study was deposited by Sakar et al. [36] from Istanbul, Turkey, abbreviation as Istanbul dataset. It contained multiple types of sound recordings, including sustained vowels,

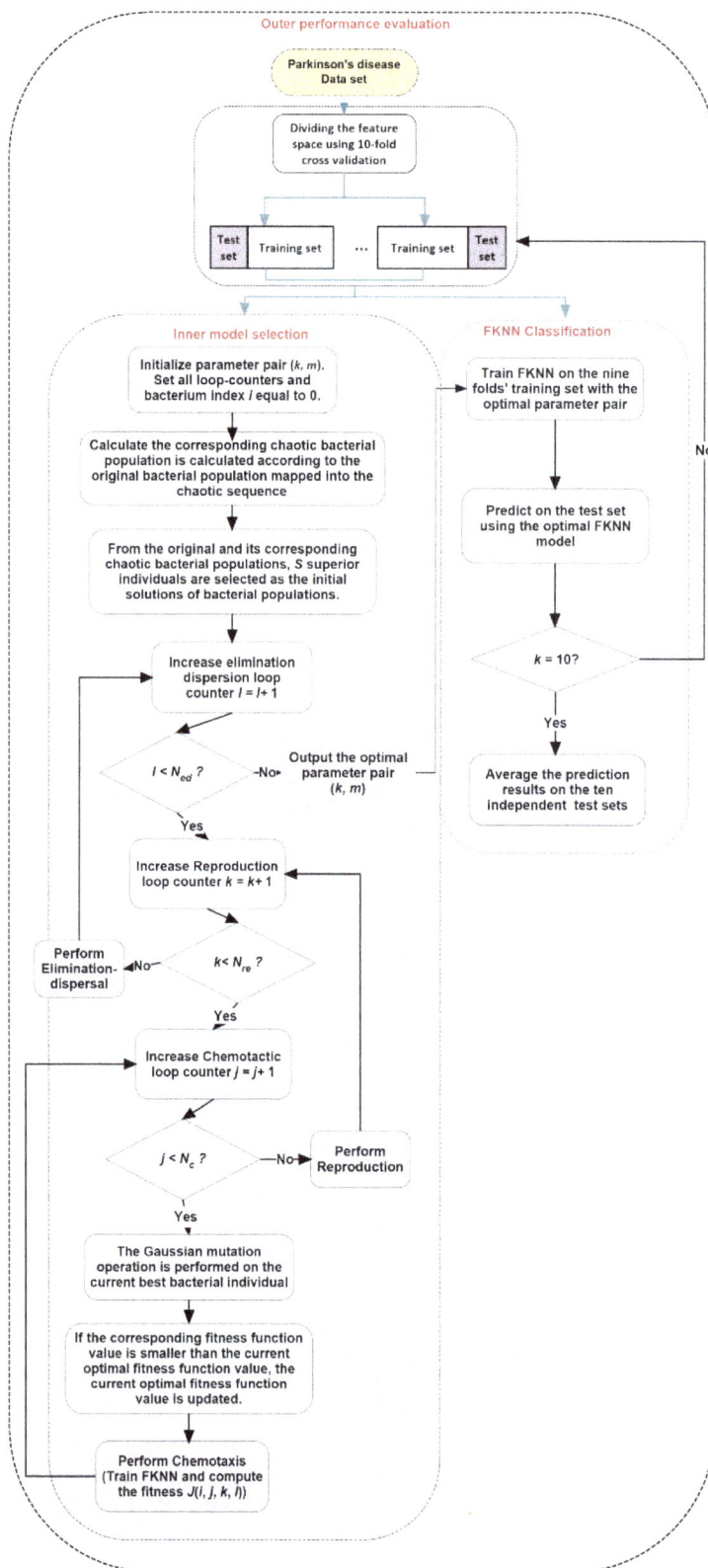

FIGURE 1: Flowchart of the proposed CBFO-FKNN diagnostic system.

Begin

   Step 1: Parameter Initialization. *Initialize the number of dimensions in the search space p, the swarm size of the population S, the number of chemotactic steps Nc, the swimming length Ns, the number of reproduction steps Nre, the number of elimination-dispersal events Ned, the elimination-dispersal probability Ped, the size of the step C(i) taken in the random direction specified by the tumble.*

   Step 2: Population Initialization. *Calculate chaotic sequence according to Eq. (6). The corresponding chaotic bacterial population is calculated according to the original bacterial population mapped into the chaotic sequence according to Eq. (7). From the original and its corresponding chaotic bacterial populations, S superior individuals are selected as the initial solutions of bacterial populations.*

   Step 3: *for ell=1:Ned   /*Elimination and dispersal loop*/*
     *for K=1:Nre   /*Reproduction loop*/*
       for j=1:Nc   / chemotaxis loop*/*
         Intertime=Intertime+1;   / represent the number of iterations*/*
         for i=1:s
          */*fobj represents calculating the fitness of the ith bacterium at the jth chemotactic, Kth reproductive, and lth elimination-dispersal steps.*/*
          J(i,j,K,ell)=fobj(P(:,i,j,K,ell));
          / Jlast stores this value since a cost better than a run may be identified.*/*
          Jlast=J(i,j,K,ell);
          / gbest(1,:) stores the current optimal bacterial individual.*/*
        gbest(1,:):=P(:,i,j,K,ell);
          Tumble according to Eq.(5)
          /* Swim (for bacteria that seem to be headed in the right direction)*/
          m=0;   / Initialize counter for swim length*/*
          while m<Ns
           m=m+1;
           if J(i,j+1,K,ell)<Jlast
            / Jlast stores this value since a cost better than a run may be identified.*/*
            Jlast=J(i,j+1,K,ell);
            Tumble according Eq.(5)
            if *Jlast<Gbest*
             / Gbest stores the current optimal fitness function value.*/*
             Gbest = Jlast;
             gbest(1,:):=P(:,i,j+1,K,ell);
           End
           else
          m=Ns;
           End
           Gaussian mutation operation
           Moth_pos_m_gaus=gbest(1,:)(1+randn(1));*
           Moth_fitness_m_gaus=fobj(Moth_pos_m_gaus);
           Moth_fitness_s=fobj(gbest(1,:));
           Moth_fitness_comb=[Moth_fitness_m_gaus,Moth_fitness_s];
           [~,mm]=min(Moth_fitness_comb);
           if *mm==1*
            gbest(1,:)=Moth_pos_m_gaus;
           end
           fitnessGbest = fobj(gbest(1,:));
           if *fitnessGbest<Gbest*
            Gbest = fitnessGbest;
           end
          End
        End   */*Go to next bacterium*/*
       End   */*Go to the next chemotactic*/*
       */*Reproduction*/*
       Jhealth=sum(J(:,:,K,ell),2);   / Set the health of each of the S bacteria*/*
       *[Jhealth, sortind]=sort(Jhealth);   /*Sorts the nutrient concentration in order of ascending*/*
       / Rearrange the bacterial population*/*
       P(:,:,1,K+1,ell)=P(:,sortind,Nc+1,K,ell);
       */*Split the bacteria (reproduction)*/*
     for i=1:Sr

ALGORITHM 1: Continued.

```
              /* The least fit do not reproduce, the most fit ones split into two identical copies */
              P(:,i+Sr,1,K+1,ell)=P(:,i,1,K+1,ell);
          End
      End   /* Go to next reproduction */
      /* Elimination-Dispersal */
      for m=1:s
          if Ped>rand   /* randomly generates a new individual anywhere in the solution space. */
              Reinitialize bacteria m
          End
      End
  End   /* Go to next Elimination-Dispersal */
End
```

ALGORITHM 1: The steps of CBFO.

numbers, words, and short sentences from 68 subjects. Specifically, the training data collected from 40 persons including 20 patients with PD ranging from 43 to 77 and 20 healthy persons ranging from 45 to 83, while testing data was collected from 28 different patients with PD ranging 39 and 79. In this study, we selected only 3 types of sustained vowel recordings /a/, /o/, and /u/, with similar data type to the Oxford PD dataset. We merged them together and produced a database which contains total 288 sustained vowels samples and the analyses were made on these samples. As shown in Table 2, a group of 26 linear and time-frequency based features are extracted for each voice sample.

4.3. Experimental Setup. The experiment was performed on a platform of Windows 7 operating system with an Intel (R) Xeon (R) CPU E5-2660 v3 @ 2.6 GHz and 16GB of RAM. The CBFO-FKNN, BFO-FKNN, PSO-FKNN, GA-FKNN, FOA-FKNN, FA-FKNN, SVM, and KELM classification models were implemented with MATLAB 2014b. The LIBSVM package [72] was used for the SVM classification. The algorithm available at http://www3.ntu.edu.sg/home/egbhuang was used for the KELM classification. The CBFO-FKNN method was implemented from scratch. The data was scaled into a range of $[0, 1]$ before each classification was conducted.

The parameters C and γ in $K(x, x_i) = \exp(-\gamma \|x - x_i\|^2)$ used during the SVM and KELM classifications were determined via the grid search method; the search ranges were defined as $C \in \{2^{-5}, 2^{-3}, \dots, 2^{15}\}$ and $\gamma \in \{2^{-15}, 2^{-13}, \dots, 2^5\}$. A population swarm size of 8, chemotactic step number of 25, swimming length of 4, reproduction step number of 3, elimination-dispersal event number of 2, and elimination-dispersal probability of 0.25 were selected for the CBFO-FKNN. The chemotaxis step value was established through trial and error, as shown in the experimental results section. The initial parameters of the other four meta-heuristic algorithms involved in training FKNN are chosen by trial and error as reported in Table 3.

4.4. Data Classification. A stratified k-fold CV [73] was used to validate the performance of the proposed approach and other comparative models. In most studies, k is given the value of 10. During each step, 90% of the samples are used

TABLE 2: Description of the Istanbul PD data set.

Label	Feature
S1	Jitter(local)
S2	Jitter(local, absolute)
S3	Jitter(rap)
S4	Jitter(ppq5)
S5	Jitter(ddp)
S6	Number of pulses
S7	Number of periods
S8	Mean period
S9	Standard dev. of period
S10	Shimmer(local)
S11	Shimmer(local, dB)
S12	Shimmer(apq3)
S13	Shimmer(apq5)
S14	Shimmer(apq11)
S15	Shimmer(dda)
S16	Fraction of locally unvoiced frames
S17	Number of voice breaks
S18	Degree of voice breaks
S19	Median pitch
S20	Mean pitch
S21	Standard deviation
S22	Minimum pitch
S23	Maximum pitch
S24	Autocorrelation
S25	Noise-to-Harmonic
S26	Harmonic-to-Noise

to form a training set, and the remaining samples are used as the test set. Then, the average of the results of all 10 trials is computed. The advantage of this method is that all of the test sets remain independent, ensuring reliable results.

A nested stratified 10-fold CV, which has been widely used in previous research, was used for the purposes of this study [74]. The classification performance evaluation was conducted in the outer loop. Since a 10-fold CV was used in the outer loop, the classifiers were evaluated in one

TABLE 3: Parameter setting of other optimizers involved in training FKNN.

Parameters	GA	PSO	FA	FOA
Population size	8	8	8	8
Max iteration	250	250	250	250
Search space	$[2^{-8}, 2^8]$	$[2^{-8}, 2^8]$	$[2^{-8}, 2^8]$	$[2^{-8}, 2^8]$
Crossover rate	0.8	-	-	-
Mutation rate	0.05	-	-	-
Acceleration constants	-	2	-	-
Inertia weight	-	1	-	-
Differential weight			-	-
Alpha	-	-	0.5	-
Beta	-	-	0.2	-
Gamma	-	-	1	-
ax	-	-	-	20
bx	-	-	-	10
ay	-	-	-	20
by	-	-	-	10

independent fold of data, and the other nine folds of data were left for training. The parameter optimization process was performed in the inner loop. Since a 5-fold CV was used in the inner loop, the CBFO-FKNN searched for the optimal values of k and m, and the SVM and KELM searched for the optimal values of C and γ in the remaining nine folds of data. The nine folds of data were further split into one fold of data for the performance evaluation, and four folds of data were left for training.

4.5. Evaluation Criteria. ACC, AUC, sensitivity, and specificity were taken to evaluate the performance of different models. These measurements are defined as

$$ACC = \frac{TP + TN}{(TP + FP + FN + TN)} \times 100\% \qquad (10)$$

$$Sensitivity = \frac{TP}{(TP + FN)} \times 100\% \qquad (11)$$

$$Specificity = \frac{TN}{(FP + TN)} \times 100\% \qquad (12)$$

where TP is the number of true positives, FN means the number of false negatives, TN represents the true negatives, and FP is the false positives. AUC [75] is the area under the ROC curve.

5. Experimental Results and Discussion

5.1. Benchmark Function Validation. In order to test the performance of the proposed algorithm CBFO, 23 benchmark functions which include unimodal, multimodal, and fixed-dimension multimodal were used to do experiments. These functions are listed in Tables 4–6 where Dim represents the dimension, Range is the search space, and $f_{\min}$ is the best value.

In order to verify the validity of the proposed algorithm, the original BFO, Firefly Algorithm(FA)[76], Flower Pollination Algorithm (FPA)[77], Bat Algorithm (BA)[78], Dragonfly Algorithm (DA)[79], Particle Swarm Optimization (PSO)[80], and the improved BFO called PSOBFO were compared on these issues. The parameters of the above algorithm are set according to their original papers, and the specific parameter values are set as shown in Table 7. In order to ensure that the results obtained are not biased, 30 independent experiments are performed. In all experiments, the number of population size is set to 50 and the maximum number of iterations is set to 500.

Tables 8–10 show average results (Avg), standard deviation (Stdv), and overall ranks for different algorithms dealing with F1-23 issues. It should be noted that the ranking is based on the average result (Avg) of 30 independent experiments for each problem. In order to visually compare the convergence performance of our proposed algorithm and other algorithms, Figures 2–4 use the logarithmic scale diagram to reflect the convergence behaviors. In Figures 2–4, we only select typical function convergence curves from unimodal functions, multimodal functions, and fixed-dimension multimodal functions, respectively. The results of the unimodal F1-F7 are shown in Table 8. As shown, the optimization effect of CBFO in F1, F2, F3, and F4 is the same as the improved PSOBFO, but the performance is improved compared with the original BFO. Moreover, From the ranking results, it can be concluded that, compared with other algorithms, CBFO is the best solution to solve the problems of F1-F7.

With respect to the convergence trends described in Figure 2, it can be observed that the proposed CBFO is capable of testifying a very fast convergence and it can be superior to all other methods in dealing with F1, F2, F3, F4, F5, and F7. For F1, F2, F3, and F4, the CBFO has converged so fast during few searching steps compared to other algorithms. In particular, when dealing with cases F1, F2, F3, and F4, the trend converges rapidly after 250 iterations.

The calculated results for multimodal F8-F13 are tabulated in Table 9. It is observed that CBFO has attained the exact optimal solutions for 30-dimension problems F8 and F12 in all 30 runs. From the results for F9, F10, F11, and F13 problems, it can be agreed that the CBFO yields very competitive solutions compared to the PSOBFO. However, based on rankings, the CBFO is the best overall technique and the overall ranks show that the BFO, FA, BA, PSO, FPA, and DA algorithms are in the next places, respectively.

According to the corresponding convergence trend recorded in Figure 3, the relative superiority of the proposed CBFO in settling F8, F11, and F12 test problems can be recognized. In tackling F11, the CBFO can dominate all its competitors in tackling F11 only during few iterations. On the other hand, methods such as FPA, BA, DA, and PSO still cannot improve the quality of solutions in solving F11 throughout more steps.

The results for F14 to F23 are tabulated in Table 10. The results in Table 10 reveal that the CBFO is the best algorithm and can outperform all other methods in dealing with F15 problems. In F16, F17, and F19, it can be seen that

TABLE 4: Unimodal benchmark functions.

Function	Dim	Range	$f_{\min}$
$f_1(x) = \sum_{i=1}^{n} x_i^2$	30	[-100, 100]	0
$f_2(x) = \sum_{i=1}^{n} |x_i| + \prod_{i=1}^{n} |x_i|$	30	[-10, 10]	0
$f_3(x) = \sum_{i=1}^{n} \left(\sum_{j-1}^{i} x_j \right)^2$	30	[-100, 100]	0
$f_4(x) = \max_i \{|x_i|, \ 1 \le i \le n\}$	30	[-100, 100]	0
$f_5(x) = \sum_{i=1}^{n-1} [100(x_{i+1} - x_i^2)^2 + (x_i - 1)^2]$	30	[-30, 30]	0
$f_6(x) = \sum_{i=1}^{n} ([x_i + 0.5])^2$	30	[-100, 100]	0
$f_7(x) = \sum_{i=1}^{n} ix_i^4 + random[0,1)$	30	[-1.28, 1.28]	0

TABLE 5: Multimodal benchmark functions.

Function	Dim	Range	$f_{\min}$
$f_8(x) = \sum_{i=1}^{n} -x_i \sin\left(\sqrt{|x_i|}\right)$	30	[-500,500]	$-418.9829*5$
$f_9(x) = \sum_{i=1}^{n} \left[x_i^2 - 10\cos(2\pi x_i) + 10 \right]$	30	[-5.12,5.12]	0
$f_{10}(x) = -20\exp\left(-0.2\sqrt{\frac{1}{n}\sum_{i=1}^{n} x_i^2}\right) - \exp\left(\frac{1}{n}\sum_{i=1}^{n}\cos(2\pi x_i)\right) + 20 + e$	30	[-32,32]	0
$f_{11}(x) = \frac{1}{4000}\sum_{i=1}^{n} x_i^2 - \prod_{i=1}^{n}\cos\left(\frac{x_i}{\sqrt{i}}\right) + 1$	30	[-600,600]	0
$f_{12}(x) = \frac{\pi}{n}\left\{ 10\sin(\pi y_1) + \sum_{i=1}^{n-1} (y_i - 1)^2 \left[1 + 10\sin^2(\pi y_{i+1}) \right] + (y_n - 1)^2 \right\}$ $+ \sum_{i=1}^{n} u(x_i, 10, 100, 4)$	30	[-50,50]	0
$y_i = 1 + \dfrac{x_i + 1}{4} u(x_i, a, k, m) \begin{cases} k(x_i - a) & x_i > a \\ 0 & -a < x_i < a \\ k(x_i - a) & x_i < -a \end{cases}$			
$f_{13}(x) = 0.1\left\{ \sin^2(3\pi x_1) + \sum_{i=1}^{n}(x_i - 1)]^2 \left[1 + \sin^2(3\pi x_i + 1) \right] + (x_n - 1)^2 \left[1 + \sin^2(2\pi x_n) \right] \right\}$ $+ \sum_{i=1}^{n} u(x_i, 5, 100, 4)$	30	[-50,50]	0

the optimization effect of all the algorithms is not much different. In dealing with F20 case, the CBFO's performance is improved compared to original BFO and the improved PSOBFO. Especially in solving F18, the proposed algorithm is much better than the improved PSOBFO. From Figure 4, we can see that the convergence speed of the CBFO is better than other algorithms in dealing with F15, F18, F19, and F20. For F15, it surpasses all methods.

In order to investigate significant differences of obtained results for the CBFO over other competitors, the Wilcoxon rank-sum test [81] at 5% significance level was also employed in this paper. The p values of comparisons are reported in Tables 11–13. In each table, each p value which is not lower than 0.05 is shown in bold face. It shows that the differences are not significant.

The p values are also provided in Table 11 for F1-F7. Referring to the p values of the Wilcoxon test in Table 11, it is verified that the proposed algorithm is statistically meaningful. The reason is that all p values are less than 0.05 except PSOBFO in F1, F2, F3, and F4. According to the p values in Table 12, all values are less than 0.05 except PSOBFO in F11 problem. Hence, it can be approved that the results of the CBFO are statistically improved compared to the other methods. As can be seen from the p value in Table 13, the CBFO algorithm is significantly better than the PSOBFO, FPA, BA, and PSO for F14-F23.

TABLE 6: Fixed-dimension multimodal benchmark functions.

Function	Dim	Range	f_{min}
$f_{14}(x) = \left(\dfrac{1}{500} + \sum\limits_{j=1}^{25} \dfrac{1}{j + \sum_{i=1}^{2}(x_i - a_{ij})^6} \right)^{-1}$	2	[-65,65]	1
$f_{15}(x) = \sum\limits_{i=1}^{11} \left[a_i - \dfrac{x_1(b_i^2 + b_i x_2)}{b_i^2 + b_i x_3 + x_4} \right]^2$	4	[-5, 5]	0.00030
$f_{16}(x) = 4x_1^2 - 2.1x_1^4 + \dfrac{1}{3}x_1^6 + x_1 x_2 - 4x_2^2 + 4x_2^4$	2	[-5,5]	-1.0316
$f_{17}(x) = \left(x_2 - \dfrac{5.1}{4\pi^2}x_1^2 + \dfrac{5}{\pi}x_1 - 6 \right)^2 + 10\left(1 - \dfrac{1}{8\pi}\right)\cos x_1 + 10$	2	[-5,5]	0.398
$f_{18}(x) = \left[1 + (x_1 + x_2 + 1)^2 (19 - 14x_1 + 3x_1^2 - 14x_2 + 6x_1 x_2 + 3x_2^2) \right]$ $\times \left[30 + (2x_1 - 3x_2)^2\ times\ (18 - 32x_1 + 12x_1^2 + 48x_2 - 36x_1 x_2 + 27x_2^2) \right]$	2	[-2,2]	3
$f_{19}(x) = -\sum\limits_{i=1}^{4} c_i \exp\left(-\sum\limits_{j=1}^{3} a_{ij}(x_j - p_{ij})^2 \right)$	3	[1,3]	-3.86
$f_{20}(x) = -\sum\limits_{i=1}^{4} c_i \exp\left(-\sum\limits_{j=1}^{6} a_{ij}(x_j - p_{ij})^2 \right)$	6	[0,1]	-3.32
$f_{21}(x) = -\sum\limits_{i=1}^{5} \left[(X - a_i)(X - a_i)^{\mathrm{T}} + c_i \right]^{-1}$	4	[0,10]	-10.1532
$f_{22}(x) = -\sum\limits_{i=1}^{7} \left[(X - a_i)(X - a_i)^{\mathrm{T}} + c_i \right]^{-1}$	4	[0,10]	-10.4028
$f_{23}(x) = -\sum\limits_{i=1}^{10} \left[(X - a_i)(X - a_i)^{\mathrm{T}} + c_i \right]^{-1}$	4	[0,10]	-10.5363

TABLE 7: Parameters setting for the involved algorithms.

Method	Population size	Maximum generation	Other parameters
BFO	50	500	$\Delta \in [-1, 1]$
BA	50	500	$Q\ Frequency \in [0\ 2]$; $A\ Loudness$: 0.5; $r\ Pulse\ rate$: 0.5
DA	50	500	$w \in [0.9\ 0.2]$; $s = 0.1$; $a = 0.1$; $c = 0.7$; $f = 1$; $e = 1$
FA	50	500	$\beta_0 = 1$; $\alpha \in [0\ 1]$; $\gamma = 1$
FPA	50	500	$switch\ probability\ p = 0.8$; $\lambda = 1.5$
PSO	50	500	$inertial\ weight = 1$; $c_1 = 2$; $c_2 = 2$
PSOBFO	50	500	$inertial\ weight = 1$; $c_1 = 1.2$; $c_2 = 0.5$; $\Delta \in [-1, 1]$

The results demonstrate that the utilized chaotic mapping strategy and Gaussian mutation in the CBFO technique have improved the efficacy of the classical BFO, in a significant manner. On the one hand, applying the chaotic mapping strategy to the bacterial population initialization process can speed up the initial exploration of the algorithm. On the other hand, adding Gaussian mutation to the current best bacterial individual in the iterative process helps to jump out of the local optimum. In conclusion, the proposed CBFO can make a better balance between explorative and exploitative trends using the embedded strategies.

5.2. Results on the Parkinson's Disease. Many studies have demonstrated that the performance of BFO can be affected heavily by the chemotaxis step size $C(i)$. Therefore, we have also investigated the effects of $C(i)$ on the performance of the CBFO-FKNN. Table 14 displays the detailed results of CBFO-FKNN model with different values of $C(i)$ on the two datasets. In the table, the mean results and their standard deviations (in parentheses) are listed. As shown, the CBFO-FKNN

model performed best with an average accuracy of 96.97%, an AUC of 0.9781, a sensitivity of 96.87%, and a specificity of 98.75% when $C(i) = 0.1$ on the Oxford dataset and an average accuracy of 83.68%, an AUC of 0.6513, a sensitivity of 96.92%, and a specificity of 33.33% when $C(i) = 0.2$ on the Istanbul dataset. Furthermore, the CBFO-FKNN approach also yielded the most reliable results with the minimum standard deviation when $C(i) = 0.1$ and $C(i) = 0.2$ on the Oxford dataset and Istanbul dataset, respectively. Therefore, values of 0.1 and 0.2 were selected as the parameter value of $C(i)$ for CBFO-FKNN on the two datasets, respectively, in the subsequent experimental analysis.

The ACC, AUC, sensitivity, specificity, and optimal (k, m) pair values of each fold obtained via the CBFO-FKNN model with $C(i) = 0.1$ and $C(i) = 0.2$ on the Oxford dataset and Istanbul dataset are shown in Tables 15 and 16, respectively. As shown, each fold possessed a different parameter pair (k, m) since the parameters for each set of fold data were automatically determined via the CBFO method. With the optimal parameter pair, the FKNN yielded different optimal

TABLE 8: Results of unimodal benchmark functions (F1-F7).

F		CBFO	PSOBFO	BFO	FA	FPA	BA	DA	PSO
F1	Avg	0	0	8.73E-03	9.84E-03	1.45E+03	1.70E+01	2.15E+03	1.45E+02
	Stdv	0	0	3.85E-03	3.20E-03	4.07E+02	2.09E+00	1.13E+03	1.56E+01
	Rank	1	1	3	4	7	5	8	6
F2	Avg	0	0	3.55E-01	3.88E-01	4.59E+01	3.32E+01	1.53E+01	1.65E+02
	Stdv	0	0	7.44E-02	8.27E-02	1.49E+01	3.35E+01	6.54E+00	2.87E+02
	Rank	1	1	3	4	7	6	5	8
F3	Avg	0	0	4.96E-12	2.59E+03	1.99E+03	1.15E+02	1.46E+04	5.96E+02
	Stdv	0	0	8.97E-12	8.38E+02	4.84E+02	3.68E+01	8.91E+03	1.57E+02
	Rank	1	1	3	7	6	4	8	5
F4	Avg	0	0	3.24E-02	8.43E-02	2.58E+01	3.78E+00	2.95E+01	4.94E+00
	Stdv	0	0	5.99E-03	1.60E-02	3.96E+00	3.02E+00	8.22E+00	4.34E-01
	Rank	1	1	3	4	7	5	8	6
F5	Avg	2.90E+01	0	6.55E+04	2.33E+02	2.57E+05	4.48E+03	4.96E+05	1.77E+05
	Stdv	2.62E-02	0	NA	4.30E+02	1.88E+05	1.24E+03	6.46E+05	4.95E+04
	Rank	2	1	5	3	7	4	8	6
F6	Avg	1.34E-01	3.71E-01	2.11E+03	1.14E-02	1.53E+03	1.70E+01	2.06E+03	1.39E+02
	Stdv	1.76E-02	5.99E-02	1.15E+04	4.71E-03	4.23E+02	2.51E+00	1.52E+03	1.67E+01
	Rank	2	3	8	1	6	4	7	5
F7	Avg	3.62E-04	4.88E-03	3.77E-03	1.08E-02	4.60E-01	1.89E+01	6.92E-01	1.05E+02
	Stdv	3.21E-04	3.44E-03	3.33E-03	2.79E-03	1.42E-01	2.00E+01	3.79E-01	2.44E+01
	Rank	1	3	2	4	5	7	6	8
Sum of ranks		9	11	27	27	45	35	50	44
Average rank		1.2857	1.5714	3.8571	3.8571	6.4286	5	7.1429	6.2857
Overall rank		1	2	3	3	7	5	8	6

TABLE 9: Results of multimodal benchmark functions (F8-F13).

F		CBFO	PSOBFO	BFO	FA	FPA	BA	DA	PSO
F8	Avg	-3.47E+04	-2.55E+03	-2.47E+03	-6.55E+03	-7.58E+03	-7.45E+03	-5.44E+03	-7.05E+03
	Stdv	1.79E+04	5.80E+02	5.25E+02	6.70E+02	2.12E+02	6.56E+02	5.55E+02	5.98E+02
	Rank	1	7	8	5	2	3	6	4
F9	Avg	-2.89E+02	-2.90E+02	-2.88E+02	3.37E+01	1.44E+02	2.73E+02	1.71E+02	3.78E+02
	Stdv	2.98E-01	0	8.61E-01	1.13E+01	1.68E+01	3.08E+01	4.15E+01	2.46E+01
	Rank	2	1	3	4	5	7	6	8
F10	Avg	-9.66E+12	-1.07E+13	-9.08E+12	5.47E-02	1.31E+01	5.56E+00	1.02E+01	8.71E+00
	Stdv	3.21E+11	3.97E-03	7.34E+11	1.31E-02	1.59E+00	3.77E+00	2.15E+00	3.94E-01
	Rank	2	1	3	4	8	5	7	6
F11	Avg	0	0	4.99E-03	6.53E-03	1.49E+01	6.35E-01	1.65E+01	1.04E+00
	Stdv	0	0	3.18E-03	2.63E-03	3.38E+00	6.31E-02	8.41E+00	6.33E-03
	Rank	1	1	3	4	7	5	8	6
F12	Avg	1.34E-11	1.27E-08	3.04E-10	2.49E-04	1.16E+02	1.33E+01	7.90E+04	5.49E+00
	Stdv	3.46E-11	2.02E-08	5.97E-10	1.06E-04	4.75E+02	4.93E+00	4.26E+05	9.04E-01
	Rank	1	3	2	4	7	6	8	5
F13	Avg	4.20E-02	9.92E-02	9.92E-02	3.18E-03	6.18E+04	2.77E+00	4.46E+05	2.90E+01
	Stdv	4.64E-02	2.52E-08	4.17E-10	2.53E-03	9.34E+04	4.37E-01	7.19E+05	6.58E+00
	Rank	2	3	3	1	7	5	8	6
Sum of ranks		9	16	22	22	36	31	43	35
Average rank		1.5000	2.6667	3.6667	3.6667	6.0000	5.1667	7.1667	5.8333
Overall rank		1	2	3	3	7	5	8	6

TABLE 10: Results of fixed-dimension multimodal benchmark functions (F14-F23).

F		CBFO	PSOBFO	BFO	FA	FPA	BA	DA	PSO
F14	Avg	9.83E+00	3.11E+00	2.96E+00	1.82E+00	1.04E+00	4.53E+00	1.30E+00	4.41E+00
	Stdv	4.51E+00	1.71E+00	2.22E+00	8.42E-01	1.56E-01	3.91E+00	6.96E-01	3.20E+00
	Rank	8	5	4	3	1	7	2	6
F15	Avg	4.33E-04	9.49E-04	6.24E-04	2.85E-03	7.44E-04	8.29E-03	3.73E-03	1.41E-03
	Stdv	1.65E-04	3.00E-04	2.25E-04	4.71E-03	1.41E-04	1.35E-02	5.95E-03	4.04E-04
	Rank	1	4	2	6	3	8	7	5
F16	Avg	-1.03E+00	-1.03E+00	-1.03E+00	-1.03E+00	-1.03E+00	-1.03E+00	-1.03E+00	-1.03E+00
	Stdv	5.23E-06	1.60E-04	7.96E-06	3.36E-09	2.55E-08	8.94E-04	3.47E-06	2.49E-03
	Rank	1	1	1	1	1	1	1	1
F17	Avg	3.98E-01	3.98E-01	3.98E-01	3.98E-01	3.98E-01	3.98E-01	3.98E-01	3.99E-01
	Stdv	2.24E-06	4.80E-05	2.02E-06	1.76E-09	6.28E-09	5.45E-04	1.84E-07	1.65E-03
	Rank	1	1	1	1	1	1	1	1
F18	Avg	3.00E+00	3.01E+00	3.00E+00	3.00E+00	3.00E+00	3.10E+00	3.00E+00	3.24E+00
	Stdv	2.00E-04	6.53E-03	3.13E-04	2.59E-08	1.60E-06	8.65E-02	6.09E-07	3.61E-01
	Rank	1	6	1	1	1	6	1	8
F19	Avg	-3.86E+00	-3.86E+00	-3.86E+00	-3.86E+00	-3.86E+00	-3.83E+00	-3.86E+00	-3.84E+00
	Stdv	4.86E-04	4.56E-03	5.87E-04	1.03E-09	2.38E-06	2.49E-02	1.16E-03	2.10E-02
	Rank	1	1	1	1	1	8	1	7
F20	Avg	-3.29E+00	-3.24E+00	-3.27E+00	-3.28E+00	-3.31E+00	-2.89E+00	-3.25E+00	-2.71E+00
	Stdv	2.41E-02	2.38E-02	2.48E-02	6.10E-02	6.06E-03	1.31E-01	1.01E-01	3.54E-01
	Rank	2	6	4	3	1	7	5	8
F21	Avg	-6.03E+00	-1.01E+01	-9.80E+00	-7.92E+00	-1.01E+01	-4.64E+00	-6.61E+00	-3.67E+00
	Stdv	9.74E-01	4.27E-02	1.28E+00	3.47E+00	1.30E-01	2.43E+00	2.62E+00	1.31E+00
	Rank	6	1	3	4	1	7	5	8
F22	Avg	-6.45E+00	-1.01E+01	-1.02E+01	-9.89E+00	-1.02E+01	-5.03E+00	-7.35E+00	-4.33E+00
	Stdv	1.22E+00	9.60E-01	9.61E-01	1.94E+00	4.87E-01	2.93E+00	2.98E+00	1.67E+00
	Rank	6	3	1	4	1	7	5	8
F23	Avg	-6.91E+00	-9.73E+00	-9.98E+00	-1.05E+01	-1.02E+01	-5.36E+00	-6.35E+00	-4.42E+00
	Stdv	1.30E+00	1.82E+00	1.63E+00	1.07E-06	4.94E-01	2.90E+00	3.36E+00	1.33E+00
	Rank	5	4	3	1	2	7	6	8
Sum of ranks		32	32	21	25	13	59	34	60
Average rank		3.2	3.2	2.1	2.5	1.3	5.9	3.4	6
Overall rank		4	4	2	3	1	7	6	8

TABLE 11: The calculated p-values from the functions (F1-F7) for the CBFO versus other optimizers.

Problem	PSOBFO	BFO	FA	FPA	BA	DA	PSO
F1	1	1.73E-06	1.73E-06	1.73E-06	1.73E-06	1.73E-06	1.73E-06
F2	1	1.73E-06	1.73E-06	1.73E-06	1.73E-06	1.73E-06	1.73E-06
F3	1	1.73E-06	1.73E-06	1.73E-06	1.73E-06	1.73E-06	1.73E-06
F4	1	1.73E-06	1.73E-06	1.73E-06	1.73E-06	1.73E-06	1.73E-06
F5	1.73E-06	1.73E-06	6.04E-03	1.73E-06	1.73E-06	1.73E-06	1.73E-06
F6	1.73E-06	1.73E-06	1.73E-06	1.73E-06	1.73E-06	1.73E-06	1.73E-06
F7	1.92E-06	3.52E-06	1.73E-06	1.73E-06	1.73E-06	1.73E-06	1.73E-06

classification performance values in each fold. This was attributed to the adaptive tuning of the two parameters by the CBFO based on the specific distribution of each data set.

In order to investigate the convergence behavior of the proposed CBFO-FKNN method, the classification error rate versus the number of iterations was recorded. For simplicity, herein we take the Oxford dataset for example. Figures 5(a)–5(d) display the learning curves of the CBFO-FKNN for folds 1, 3, 5, and 7 in the 10-fold CV, respectively. As shown, all four fitness curves of CBFO converged into a global optimum in fewer than 20 iterations. The fitness curves gradually improved from iterations 1 through 20 but

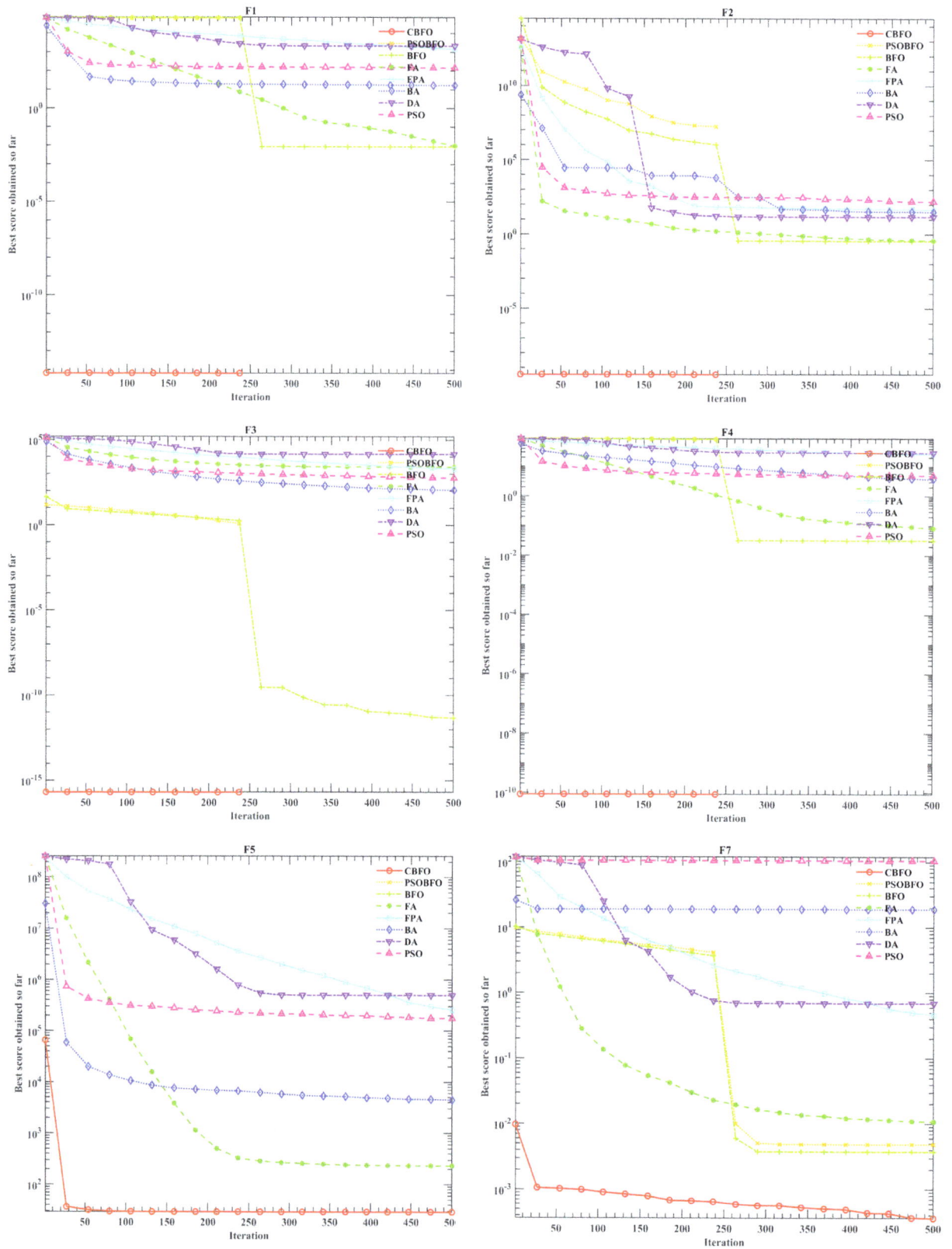

FIGURE 2: Convergence curves of unimodal functions.

TABLE 12: The calculated p-values from the functions (F8-F13) for the CBFO versus other optimizers.

Problem	PSOBFO	BFO	FA	FPA	BA	DA	PSO
F8	1.73E-06	1.73E-06	1.73E-06	1.92E-06	1.73E-06	1.73E-06	1.92E-06
F9	1.73E-06	6.89E-05	1.73E-06	1.73E-06	1.73E-06	1.73E-06	1.73E-06
F10	1.73E-06	4.90E-04	1.73E-06	1.73E-06	1.73E-06	1.73E-06	1.73E-06
F11	1	1.73E-06	1.73E-06	1.73E-06	1.73E-06	1.73E-06	1.73E-06
F12	3.52E-06	5.79E-05	1.73E-06	1.73E-06	1.73E-06	1.73E-06	1.73E-06
F13	1.73E-06	1.92E-06	3.61E-03	1.73E-06	1.73E-06	1.73E-06	1.73E-06

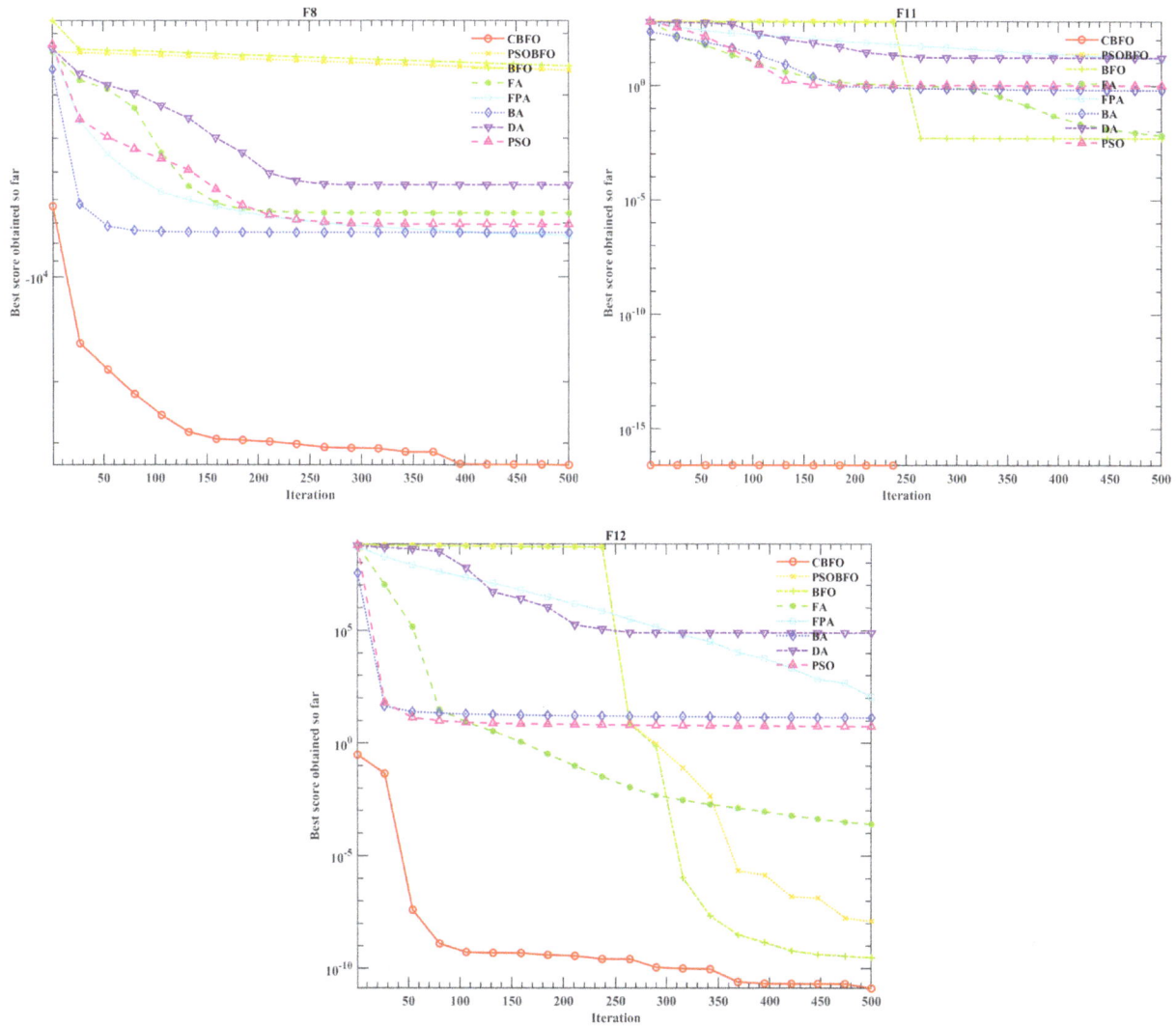

FIGURE 3: Convergence curves of multimodal functions.

exhibited no significant improvements after iteration 20. The fitness curves ceased after 50 iterations (the maximum number of iterations). The error rates of the fitness curves decreased rapidly at the beginning of the evolutionary process and continued to decrease slowly after a certain number of iterations. During the latter part of the evolutionary process, the fitness curves remained stable until the stopping criteria,

the maximum number of iterations, were satisfied. Thus, the proposed CBFO-FKNN model efficiently converged toward the global optima.

To validate the effectiveness of the proposed method, the CBFO-FKNN model was compared to five other meta-heuristic algorithms-based FKNN models as well as three other advanced machine learning approaches including

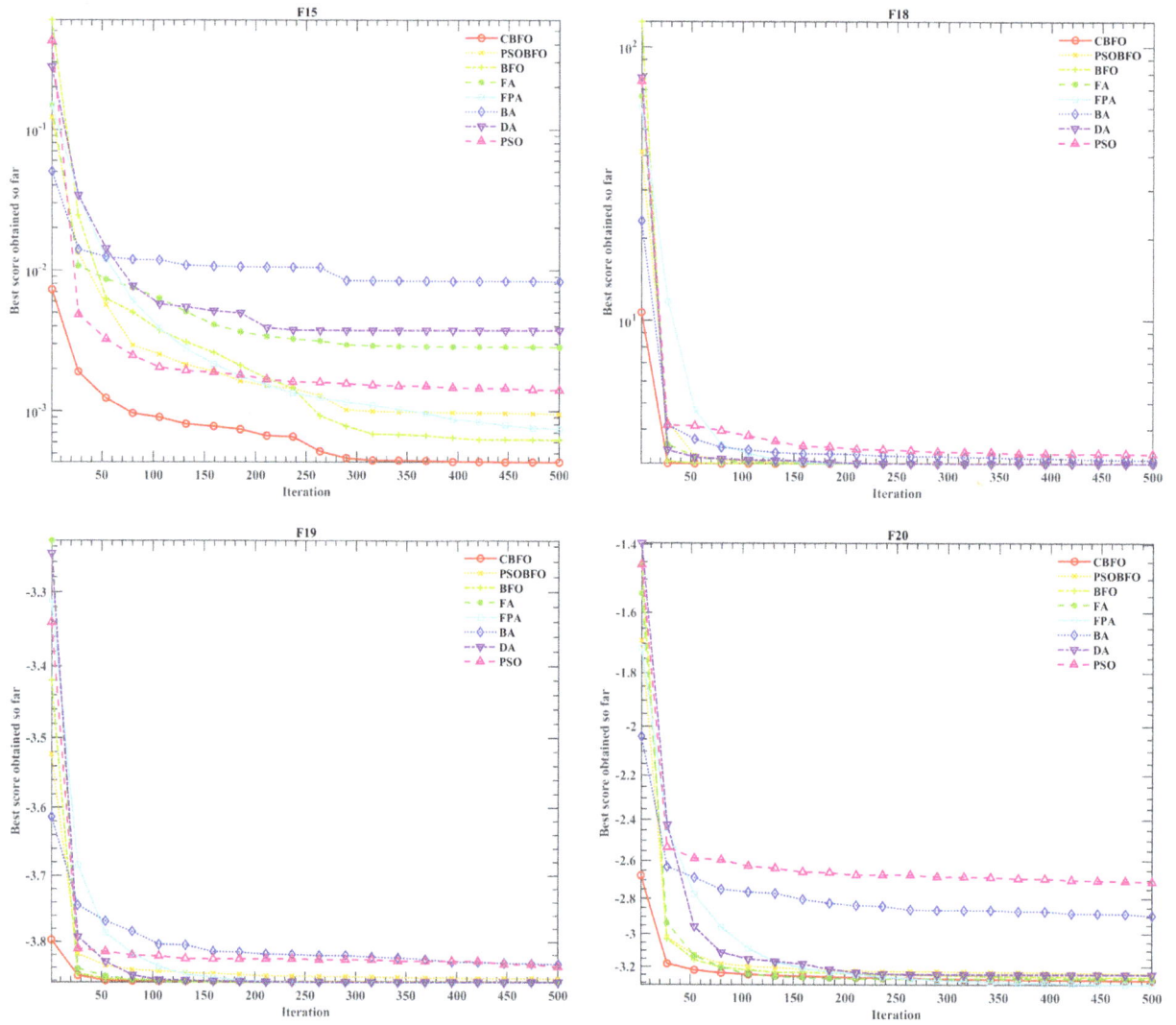

FIGURE 4: Convergence curves based on fixed-dimension multimodal functions.

TABLE 13: The calculated p-values from the functions (F14-F23) for the CBFO versus other optimizers.

Problem	PSOBFO	BFO	FA	FPA	BA	DA	PSO
F14	6.34E-06	6.98E-06	5.22E-06	3.18E-06	2.22E-04	1.73E-06	1.06E-04
F15	3.88E-06	8.31E-04	1.73E-06	1.24E-05	1.92E-06	4.29E-06	1.92E-06
F16	2.35E-06	**7.50E-01**	1.73E-06	1.73E-06	1.73E-06	1.97E-05	1.73E-06
F17	1.92E-06	**3.60E-01**	1.73E-06	1.73E-06	1.73E-06	2.60E-06	1.73E-06
F18	2.35E-06	**8.45E-01**	1.73E-06	1.73E-06	1.73E-06	1.73E-06	1.73E-06
F19	1.92E-06	**8.22E-02**	1.73E-06	1.73E-06	1.73E-06	8.19E-05	1.73E-06
F20	3.41E-05	8.94E-04	**6.44E-01**	2.60E-06	1.73E-06	**3.82E-01**	1.73E-06
F21	1.73E-06	2.13E-06	4.99E-03	1.73E-06	8.22E-03	**7.04E-01**	6.34E-06
F22	3.88E-06	2.60E-06	1.64E-05	1.73E-06	1.85E-02	**1.85E-01**	8.92E-05
F23	1.24E-05	2.60E-05	1.73E-06	1.73E-06	1.96E-02	**4.05E-01**	1.02E-05

TABLE 14: Detailed results of CBFO-FKNN with different values of $C(i)$ on the two datasets.

$C(i)$	Oxford dataset				Istanbul dataset			
	ACC	AUC	Sen	Spec	ACC	AUC	Sen	Spec
0.05	0.9542	0.9417	0.9666	0.9167	0.8230	0.6180	0.9694	0.2667
	(0.0370)	(0.0774)	(0.0356)	(0.1620)	(0.0636)	(0.1150)	(0.0413)	(0.2108)
0.1	**0.9697**	**0.9781**	**0.9687**	**0.9875**	0.8054	0.5946	0.9559	0.2333
	(0.0351)	**(0.0253)**	**(0.0432)**	**(0.0395)**	(0.0414)	(0.0746)	(0.0297)	(0.1405)
0.15	0.9489	0.9479	0.9358	0.9600	0.8155	0.6074	0.9648	0.2500
	(0.0629)	(0.0609)	(0.1158)	(0.0843)	(0.0669)	(0.1204)	(0.0450)	(0.2257)
0.2	0.9589	0.9466	0.9600	0.9333	**0.8368**	**0.6512**	**0.9691**	**0.3333**
	(0.0469)	(0.0860)	(0.0555)	(0.1610)	**(0.0283)**	**(0.0698)**	**(0.0360)**	**(0.1571)**
0.25	0.9587	0.9459	0.9669	0.9250	0.8257	0.6385	0.9603	0.3167
	(0.0536)	(0.0901)	(0.0459)	(0.1687)	(0.0770)	(0.1560)	(0.0328)	(0.2987)
0.3	0.9639	0.9689	0.9670	0.9708	0.8090	0.6165	0.9478	0.2833
	(0.0352)	(0.0308)	(0.0454)	(0.0623)	(0.0439)	(0.1112)	(0.0534)	(0.2491)

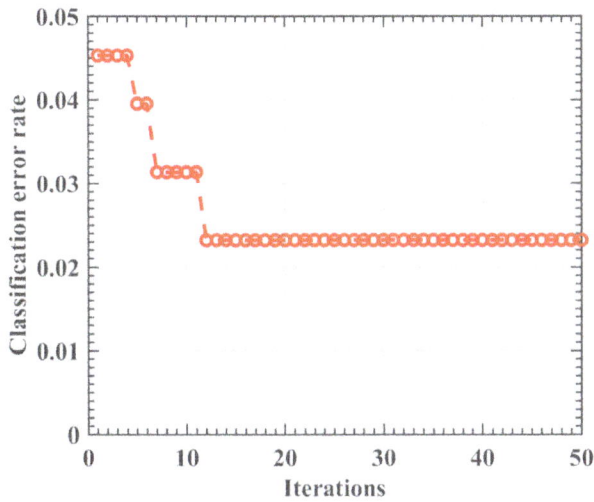

(a)

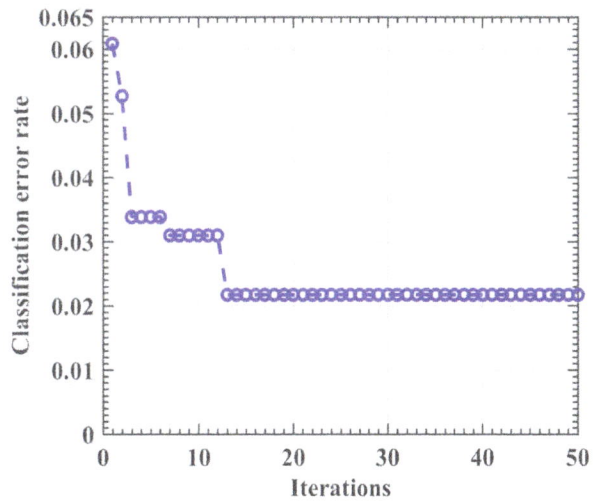

(b)

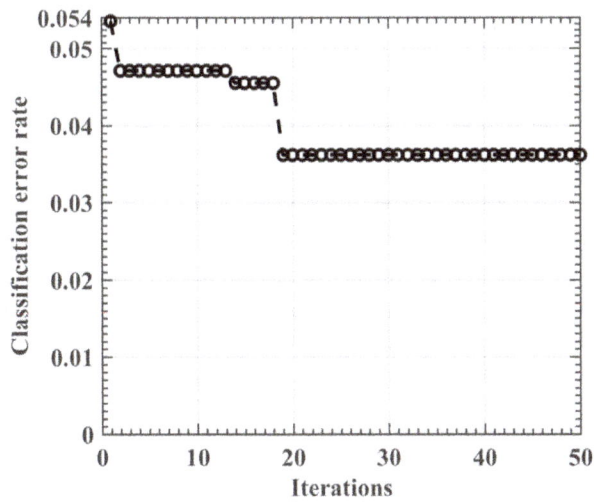

(c)

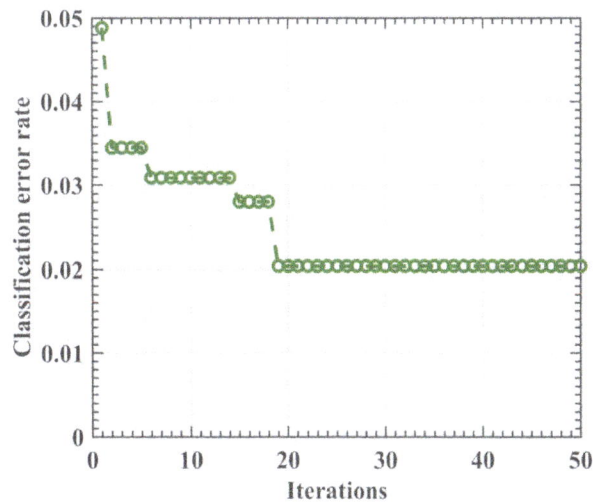

(d)

FIGURE 5: Learning curves of CBFO for fold 2 (a), fold 4 (b), fold 6 (c), and fold 8 (d) during the training stage.

TABLE 15: Detailed classification results of CBFO-FKNN on the Oxford dataset.

Fold	CBFO-FKNN					
No.	ACC	AUC	Sen	Spec	k	m
1	0.9474	0.9667	0.9333	1.0000	1	1.77
2	1.0000	1.0000	1.0000	1.0000	1	2.94
3	0.9500	0.9688	0.9375	1.0000	1	3.92
4	0.9500	0.9375	1.0000	0.8750	1	6.89
5	0.9500	0.9667	0.9333	1.0000	1	9.33
6	0.9000	0.9412	0.8824	1.0000	1	7.26
7	1.0000	1.0000	1.0000	1.0000	1	9.21
8	1.0000	1.0000	1.0000	1.0000	1	7.61
9	1.0000	1.0000	1.0000	1.0000	1	8.95
10	1.0000	1.0000	1.0000	1.0000	1	7.25
Mean	**0.9697**	**0.9781**	**0.9687**	**0.9875**	**1**	**6.51**

TABLE 16: Detailed classification results of CBFO-FKNN on the Istanbul dataset.

Fold	CBFO-FKNN					
No.	ACC	AUC	Sen	Spec	k	m
1	0.8571	0.7273	0.9545	0.5000	3	4.80
2	0.8276	0.5833	1.0000	0.1667	3	3.70
3	0.8276	0.7065	0.9130	0.5000	3	7.30
4	0.8276	0.5833	1.0000	0.1667	3	4.16
5	0.8966	0.7500	1.0000	0.5000	3	9.40
6	0.7931	0.6232	0.9130	0.3333	3	2.50
7	0.8621	0.7283	0.9565	0.5000	3	9.70
8	0.8276	0.5833	1.0000	0.1667	3	4.30
9	0.8276	0.5833	1.0000	0.1667	3	8.20
10	0.8214	0.6439	0.9545	0.3333	3	7.04
Mean	**0.8368**	**0.6513**	**0.9692**	**0.3333**	**3**	**6.11**

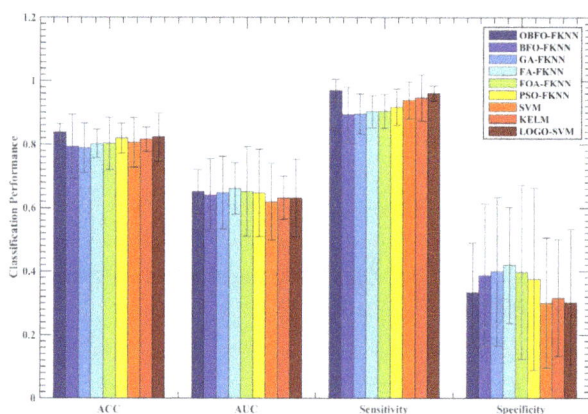

FIGURE 7: Comparison results obtained on the Istanbul dataset by the nine methods.

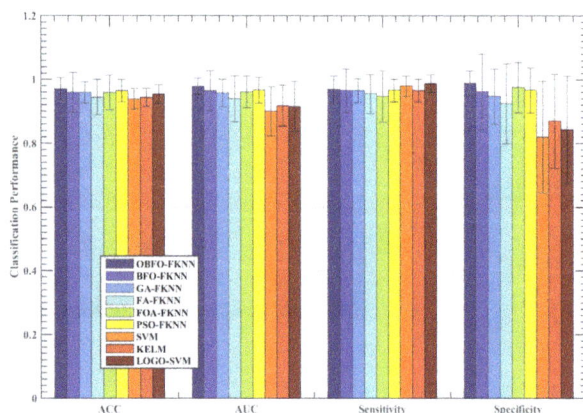

FIGURE 6: Comparison results obtained on the Oxford dataset by the nine methods.

SVM, KELM, and SVM with local learning-based feature selection (LOGO-SVM). As shown in Figure 6, the CBFO-FKNN method performed better than other competitors in terms of ACC, AUC, and sensitivity on the Oxford dataset. We can see that the CBFO-FKNN method yields the highest average ACC value of 96.97%, followed by PSO-FKNN, LOGO-SVM, KELM, SVM, FOA-FKNN, FA-FKNN, and BFO-FKNN. GA-FKNN has got the worst result among the all methods. On the AUC metric, OBF-FKNN obtained similar results with FA-FKNN, followed by FOA-FKNN, GA-FKNN, PSO-FKNN, BFO-FKNN, KELM, and LOGO-SVM, and SVM has got the worst result. On the sensitivity metric, CBFO-FKNN has achieved obvious advantages, LOGO-FKNN ranked second, followed by KELM, SVM, PSO-FKNN, FOA-FKNN, FA-FKNN, and GA-FKNN. BFO-FKNN has got the worst performance. On the specificity metric, FA-FKNN achieved the maximum results, GA-FKNN and FOA-FKNN have achieved similar results, which ranked second, followed by BFO-FKNN, PSO-FKNN, CBFO-FKNN, and SVM. KELM and LOGO-SVM have obtained similar results, both of which got the worst performance. Regarding the Istanbul dataset, CBFO-FKNN produced the highest result with the ACC of 83.68%, while the LOGO-SVM and PSO-FKNN method yields the second best average ACC value as shown in Figure 7, followed by

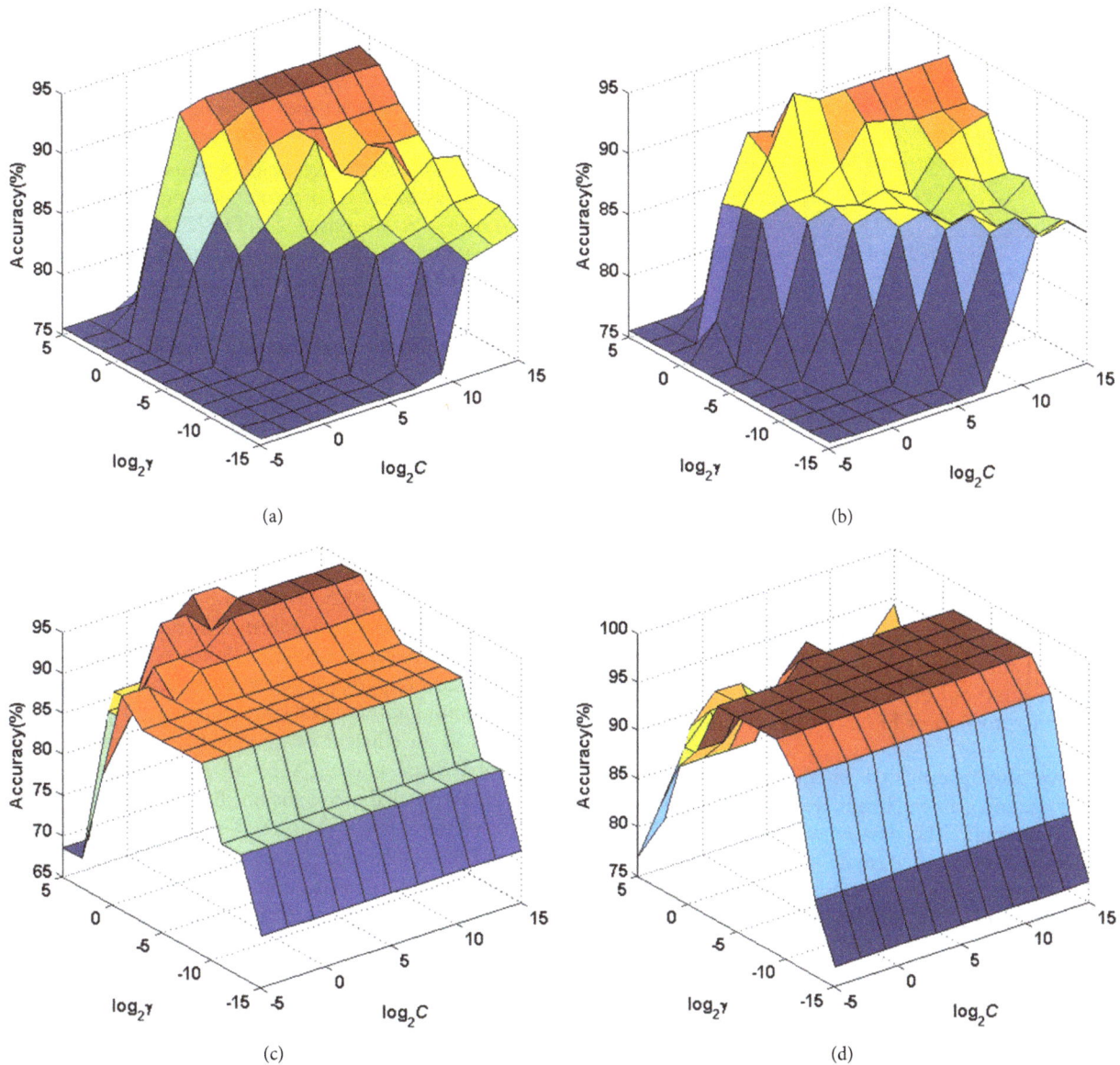

(a)

(b)

(c)

(d)

FIGURE 8: Training accuracy surfaces of SVM and KELM via the grid search method on the Oxford dataset. (a) Fold 2 for SVM. (b) Fold 4 for SVM on the data. (c) Fold 6 for KELM on the data. (d) Fold 8 for SVM on the data.

KELM, SVM, FOA-FKNN, FA-FKNN, BFO-FKNN, and GA-FKNN. From Figures 6 and 7, we can also find that the CBFO-FKNN can yield a smaller or comparative standard deviation than the other counterparts in terms of the four performance metrics on the both datasets. Additionally, we can find that the SVM with local learning-based feature selection can improve the performance of the two datasets. It indicates that there are some irrelevant features or redundant features in these two datasets. It should be noted that the LOGO method was used for feature selection, all the features were ranked by the LOGO, then all the feature subsets were evaluated incrementally, and finally the feature subset achieved the best accuracy was chosen as the one in the experiment.

According to the results, the superior performance of the proposed CBFO-FKNN indicates that the proposed method was the most robust tool for detection of PD among the nine methods. The main reason may lie in that the OBL mechanism greatly improves the diversity of the population and increases the probability of BFO escaping from the local optimum. Thus, it gets more chances to find the optimal neighborhood size and fuzzy strength values by the CBFO, which aided the FKNN classifier in more efficiently achieving the maximum classification performance. Figure 8 displays the surface of training classification accuracies achieved by the SVM and KELM methods for several folds of the training data via the grid search strategy on the Oxford dataset.

TABLE 17: The confusion matrix obtained by CBFO-FKNN via 10-fold CV for each group.

Male	Predicted PD	Predicted health
Actual PD	97	3
Actual health	2	16
Female	Predicted PD	Predicted health
Actual PD	44	3
Actual health	2	28
Old	Predicted PD	Predicted health
Actual PD	87	4
Actual health	0	18
Young	Predicted PD	Predicted health
Actual PD	56	0
Actual health	0	30

Through the experimental process, we can find the original BFO is more prone to overfitting; this paper introduces chaotic initialization, enriches the diversity of the initial population, and improves the convergence speed of the population as well; in addition, this paper also introduced Gaussian mutation strategy for enhancing the ability of the algorithm to jump out of local optimum, so as to alleviate the overfitting problem of FKNN in the process of classification.

We have also investigated whether the diagnosis was affected by age and gender. Herein, we have taken the Oxford dataset for example. The dataset was divided by the age (old or young) and gender (male or female), respectively. Regarding the age, we have chosen the mean age of 65.8 years as the dividing point. The samples in the old group are more than 65.8, and the samples in the young group are less than 65.8. Therefore, we can obtain four groups of data including male group, female group, old group, and young group. The classification results of the four groups in terms of confusion matrix are displayed in Table 17. As shown, we can find that either in the male group or in the female group 3 PD samples were wrongly classified as healthy ones, and 2 healthy samples were misjudged as PD ones. It indicates that the gender has little impact on the diagnostic results. In the old group, we can find that 4 PD samples were wrongly identified as healthy ones. However, none of the samples were misjudged in the young group. It suggests that the speech samples in the old group are much easier to be wrongly predicted than those in the young group.

To further investigate the impact of gender and age on the diagnosis results. We have further divided the samples into male group and female group on the premise of young and old age and old group and young group on the premise of male and female, respectively. So we can obtain 8 groups as shown in Table 18, and the detailed classification results are displayed in terms of confusion matrix. As shown, we can find that the probability of the sample being misclassified is closer in the old group and young group on the premise of male and female. It can be also observed that there was no sample being wrongly predicted in male and female groups on the premise of young persons, while there was one sample being wrongly predicted in male and female groups on the premise of old persons, respectively. We can arrive at the conclusion that the presbyphonic may play a confounding role in the female and male dysphonic set, and the results of diagnosis were less affected by gender.

The classification accuracies of other methods applied to the diagnosis of PD are presented for comparison in Table 19. As shown, the proposed CBFO-FKNN method achieved relatively high classification accuracy and, therefore, it could be used as an effective diagnostic tool.

6. Conclusions and Future Work

In this study, we have proposed a novel evolutionary instance-based approach based on a chaotic BFO and applied it to differentiating the PD from the healthy people. In the proposed methodology, the chaos theory enhanced BFO strategy was used to automatically determine the two key parameters, thereby utilizing the FKNN to its fullest potential. The results suggested that the proposed CBFO-FKNN approach outperformed five other FKNN models based on nature-inspired methods and three commonly used advanced machine learning methods including SVM, LOGO-SVM, and KELM, in terms of various performance metrics. In addition, the simulation results indicated that the proposed CBFO-FKNN could be used as an efficient computer-aided diagnostic tool for clinical decision-making. Through the experimental analysis, we can arrive at the conclusion that the presbyphonic may play a confounding role in the female and male dysphonic set, and the results of diagnosis were less affected by gender. Additionally, the speech samples in the old group are much easier to be wrongly predicted than those in the young group.

In future studies, the proposed method will be implemented in a distributed environment in order to further boost its PD diagnostic efficacy. Additionally, implementing the feature selection using CBFO strategy to further boost the performance of the proposed method is another future work. Finally, due to the small vocal datasets of PD, we will generalize the proposed method to much larger datasets in the future.

Conflicts of Interest

The authors declare that there are no conflicts of interest regarding the publication of article.

Acknowledgments

This research is supported by the National Natural Science Foundation of China (61702376 and 61402337). This research is also funded by Zhejiang Provincial Natural Science Foundation of China (LY17F020012, LY14F020035, LQ13F020011, and LQ13G010007) and Science and Technology Plan Project of Wenzhou of China (ZG2017019, H20110003, Y20160070, and Y20160469).

TABLE 18: The confusion matrix obtained by CBFO-FKNN for each group with precondition.

		Predicted PD	Predicted health
Old	**Male**	**Predicted PD**	**Predicted health**
	Actual PD	62	1
	Actual health	0	6
	Female	**Predicted PD**	**Predicted health**
	Actual PD	27	1
	Actual health	0	12
Young	**Male**	**Predicted PD**	**Predicted health**
	Actual PD	37	0
	Actual health	0	12
	Female	**Predicted PD**	**Predicted health**
	Actual PD	19	0
	Actual health	0	18
Male	**Old**	**Predicted PD**	**Predicted health**
	Actual PD	61	2
	Actual health	0	6
	Young	**Predicted PD**	**Predicted health**
	Actual PD	35	2
	Actual health	0	12
Female	**Old**	**Predicted PD**	**Predicted health**
	Actual PD	27	1
	Actual health	0	12
	Young	**Predicted PD**	**Predicted health**
	Actual PD	19	0
	Actual health	0	18

TABLE 19: Comparison of the classification accuracies of various methods.

Study	Method	Accuracy (%)
Little et al. (2009)	Pre-selection filter + Exhaustive search + SVM	91.4(bootstrap with 50 replicates)
Shahbaba et al. (2009)	Dirichlet process mixtures	87.7(5-fold CV)
Das (2010)	ANN	92. (hold-out)
Sakar et al. (2010)	Mutual information based feature selection + SVM	92.75(bootstrap with 50 replicates)
Psorakis et al. (2010)	Improved mRVMs	89.47(10-fold CV)
Guo et al. (2010)	GP-EM	93.1(10-fold CV)
Ozcift et al. (2011)	CFS-RF	87.1(10-fold CV)
Li et al. (2011)	Fuzzy-based non-linear transformation + SVM	93.47(hold-out)
Luukka (2011)	Fuzzy entropy measures + Similarity classifier	85.03(hold-out)
Spadoto et al. (2011)	Particle swarm optimization + OPF	73.53(hold-out)
	Harmony search + OPF	84.01(hold-out)
	Gravitational search algorithm + OPF	84.01(hold-out)
AStröm et al. (2011)	Parallel NN	91.20(hold-out)
Chen et al.(2013)	PCA-FKNN	96.07(10-fold CV)
Babu et al. (2013)	projection based learning for meta-cognitive radial basis function network (PBL-McRBFN)	99.35% (hold-out)
Hariharan et al. (2014)	integration of feature weighting method, feature selection method and classifiers	100%(10-fold CV)
Cai et al. (2017)	support vector machine (SVM) based on bacterial foraging optimization (BFO)	97.42%(10-fold CV)
This Study	CBFO-FKNN	97.89%(10-fold CV)

References

[1] L. M. de Lau and M. M. Breteler, "Epidemiology of Parkinson's disease," *The Lancet Neurology*, vol. 5, no. 6, pp. 525–535, 2006.

[2] S. K. van den Eeden, C. M. Tanner, A. L. Bernstein et al., "Incidence of Parkinson's disease: variation by age, gender, and race/ethnicity," *American Journal of Epidemiology*, vol. 157, no. 11, pp. 1015–1022, 2003.

[3] E. R. Dorsey, R. Constantinescu, J. P. Thompson et al., "Projected number of people with Parkinson disease in the most populous nations, 2005 through 2030," *Neurology*, vol. 68, no. 5, pp. 384–386, 2007.

[4] N. Singh, V. Pillay, and Y. E. Choonara, "Advances in the treatment of Parkinson's disease," *Progress in Neurobiology*, vol. 81, no. 1, pp. 29–44, 2007.

[5] B. T. Harel, M. S. Cannizzaro, H. Cohen, N. Reilly, and P. J. Snyder, "Acoustic characteristics of Parkinsonian speech: A potential biomarker of early disease progression and treatment," *Journal of Neurolinguistics*, vol. 17, no. 6, pp. 439–453, 2004.

[6] J. Rusz, R. Cmejla, H. Ruzickova, and E. Ruzicka, "Quantitative acoustic measurements for characterization of speech and voice disorders in early untreated Parkinson's disease," *The Journal of the Acoustical Society of America*, vol. 129, no. 1, pp. 350–367, 2011.

[7] J. Jankovic, "Parkinsons disease: clinical features and diagnosis," *Journal of Neurology, Neurosurgery & Psychiatry*, vol. 79, pp. 368–376, 2008.

[8] J. Massano and K. P. Bhatia, "Clinical approach to Parkinson's disease: features, diagnosis, and principles of management," *Cold Spring Harbor Perspectives in Medicine*, vol. 2, no. 6, Article ID a008870, 2012.

[9] A. K. Ho, R. Iansek, C. Marigliani, J. L. Bradshaw, and S. Gates, "Speech impairment in a large sample of patients with Parkinson's disease," *Behavioural Neurology*, vol. 11, no. 3, pp. 131–137, 1998.

[10] B. Harel, M. Cannizzaro, and P. J. Snyder, "Variability in fundamental frequency during speech in prodromal and incipient Parkinson's disease: A longitudinal case study," *Brain and Cognition*, vol. 56, no. 1, pp. 24–29, 2004.

[11] R. J. Baken and R. F. Orlikoff, *Clinical Measurement of Speech and Voice*, Singular Publishing Group, San Diego, CA, USA, 2nd edition, 2000.

[12] L. Brabenec, J. Mekyska, Z. Galaz, and I. Rektorova, "Speech disorders in Parkinson's disease: early diagnostics and effects of medication and brain stimulation," *Journal of Neural Transmission*, vol. 124, no. 3, pp. 303–334, 2017.

[13] M. A. Little, P. E. McSharry, E. J. Hunter, J. Spielman, and L. O. Ramig, "Suitability of dysphonia measurements for telemonitoring of Parkinson's disease," *IEEE Transactions on Biomedical Engineering*, vol. 56, no. 4, pp. 1015–1022, 2009.

[14] R. Das, "A comparison of multiple classification methods for diagnosis of Parkinson disease," *Expert Systems with Applications*, vol. 37, no. 2, pp. 1568–1572, 2010.

[15] F. Åström and R. Koker, "A parallel neural network approach to prediction of Parkinson's Disease," *Expert Systems with Applications*, vol. 38, no. 10, pp. 12470–12474, 2011.

[16] C. O. Sakar and O. Kursun, "Telediagnosis of parkinson's disease using measurements of dysphonia," *Journal of Medical Systems*, vol. 34, no. 4, pp. 591–599, 2010.

[17] D.-C. Li, C.-W. Liu, and S. C. Hu, "A fuzzy-based data transformation for feature extraction to increase classification performance with small medical data sets," *Artificial Intelligence in Medicine*, vol. 52, no. 1, pp. 45–52, 2011.

[18] B. Shahbaba and R. Neal, "Nonlinear models using Dirichlet process mixtures," *Journal of Machine Learning Research*, vol. 10, pp. 1829–1850, 2009.

[19] I. Psorakis, T. Damoulas, and M. A. Girolami, "Multiclass relevance vector machines: sparsity and accuracy," *IEEE Transactions on Neural Networks and Learning Systems*, vol. 21, no. 10, pp. 1588–1598, 2010.

[20] P. F. Guo, P. Bhattacharya, and N. Kharma, "Advances in Detecting Parkinsons Disease," *Medical Biometrics*, pp. 306–314, 2010.

[21] P. Luukka, "Feature selection using fuzzy entropy measures with similarity classifier," *Expert Systems with Applications*, vol. 38, no. 4, pp. 4600–4607, 2011.

[22] A. Ozcift and A. Gulten, "Classifier ensemble construction with rotation forest to improve medical diagnosis performance of machine learning algorithms," *Computer Methods and Programs in Biomedicine*, vol. 104, no. 3, pp. 443–451, 2011.

[23] A. A. Spadoto, R. C. Guido, F. L. Carnevali, A. F. Pagnin, A. X. Falcão, and J. P. Papa, "Improving Parkinson's disease identification through evolutionary-based feature selection," *Conference proceedings: IEEE Engineering in Medicine and Biology Society*, vol. 2011, pp. 7857–7860, 2011.

[24] K. Polat, "Classification of Parkinson's disease using feature weighting method on the basis of fuzzy C-means clustering," *International Journal of Systems Science*, vol. 43, no. 4, pp. 597–609, 2012.

[25] H.-L. Chen, C.-C. Huang, X.-G. Yu et al., "An efficient diagnosis system for detection of Parkinson's disease using fuzzy k-nearest neighbor approach," *Expert Systems with Applications*, vol. 40, no. 1, pp. 263–271, 2013.

[26] W.-L. Zuo, Z.-Y. Wang, T. Liu, and H.-L. Chen, "Effective detection of Parkinson's disease using an adaptive fuzzy k-nearest neighbor approach," *Biomedical Signal Processing and Control*, vol. 8, no. 4, pp. 364–373, 2013.

[27] G. Sateesh Babu and S. Suresh, "Parkinson's disease prediction using gene expression- A projection based learning meta-cognitive neural classifier approach," *Expert Systems with Applications*, vol. 40, no. 5, pp. 1519–1529, 2013.

[28] G. S. Babu, S. Suresh, and B. S. Mahanand, "A novel PBL-McRBFN-RFE approach for identification of critical brain regions responsible for Parkinson's disease," *Expert Systems with Applications*, vol. 41, no. 2, pp. 478–488, 2014.

[29] G. Sateesh Babu, S. Suresh, K. Uma Sangumathi, and H. J. Kim, "A Projection Based Learning Meta-cognitive RBF Network Classifier for Effective Diagnosis of Parkinson's Disease," in *Advances in Neural Networks – ISNN 2012*, vol. 7368 of *Lecture Notes in Computer Science*, pp. 611–620, Springer, Berlin, Germany, 2012.

[30] M. Hariharan, K. Polat, and R. Sindhu, "A new hybrid intelligent system for accurate detection of Parkinson's disease," *Computer Methods and Programs in Biomedicine*, vol. 113, no. 3, pp. 904–913, 2014.

[31] M. Gök, "An ensemble of k-nearest neighbours algorithm for detection of Parkinson's disease," *International Journal of Systems Science*, vol. 46, no. 6, pp. 1108–1112, 2015.

[32] L. Shen, H. Chen, Z. Yu et al., "Evolving support vector machines using fruit fly optimization for medical data classification," *Knowledge-Based Systems*, vol. 96, pp. 61–75, 2016.

[33] M. Peker, B. Şen, and D. Delen, "Computer-aided diagnosis of Parkinson's disease using complex-valued neural networks and mRMR feature selection algorithm," *Journal of Healthcare Engineering*, vol. 6, no. 3, pp. 281–302, 2015.

[34] H.-L. Chen, G. Wang, C. Ma, Z.-N. Cai, W.-B. Liu, and S.-J. Wang, "An efficient hybrid kernel extreme learning machine approach for early diagnosis of Parkinson's disease," *Neurocomputing*, vol. 184, no. 4745, pp. 131–144, 2016.

[35] Z. Cai, J. Gu, and H.-L. Chen, "A New Hybrid Intelligent Framework for Predicting Parkinson's Disease," *IEEE Access*, vol. 5, pp. 17188–17200, 2017.

[36] B. E. Sakar, M. E. Isenkul, C. O. Sakar et al., "Collection and analysis of a Parkinson speech dataset with multiple types of sound recordings," *IEEE Journal of Biomedical and Health Informatics*, vol. 17, no. 4, pp. 828–834, 2013.

[37] H. Zhang, L. Yang, Y. Liu et al., "Classification of Parkinson's disease utilizing multi-edit nearest-neighbor and ensemble learning algorithms with speech samples," *Biomedical Engineering Online*, vol. 15, no. 1, 2016.

[38] V. Abrol, P. Sharma, and A. K. Sao, "Greedy dictionary learning for kernel sparse representation based classifier," *Pattern Recognition Letters*, vol. 78, pp. 64–69, 2016.

[39] İ. Cantürk and F. Karabiber, "A Machine Learning System for the Diagnosis of Parkinson's Disease from Speech Signals and Its Application to Multiple Speech Signal Types," *Arabian Journal for Science and Engineering*, vol. 41, no. 12, pp. 5049–5059, 2016.

[40] A. Jóźwik, "A learning scheme for a fuzzy k-NN rule," *Pattern Recognition Letters*, vol. 1, no. 5-6, pp. 287–289, 1983.

[41] J. M. Keller, M. R. Gray, and J. A. Givens, "A fuzzy K-nearest neighbor algorithm," *IEEE Transactions on Systems, Man, and Cybernetics*, vol. SMC-15, no. 4, pp. 580–585, 1985.

[42] J. Derrac, S. García, and F. Herrera, "Fuzzy nearest neighbor algorithms: Taxonomy, experimental analysis and prospects," *Information Sciences*, vol. 260, pp. 98–119, 2014.

[43] D.-Y. Liu, H.-L. Chen, B. Yang, X.-E. Lv, L.-N. Li, and J. Liu, "Design of an enhanced Fuzzy k-nearest neighbor classifier based computer aided diagnostic system for thyroid disease," *Journal of Medical Systems*, vol. 36, no. 5, pp. 3243–3254, 2012.

[44] J. Sim, S.-Y. Kim, and J. Lee, "Prediction of protein solvent accessibility using fuzzy k-nearest neighbor method," *Bioinformatics*, vol. 21, no. 12, pp. 2844–2849, 2005.

[45] Y. Huang and Y. Li, "Prediction of protein subcellular locations using fuzzy k-NN method," *Bioinformatics*, vol. 20, no. 1, pp. 21–28, 2004.

[46] H.-L. Chen, B. Yang, G. Wang et al., "A novel bankruptcy prediction model based on an adaptive fuzzy k-nearest neighbor method," *Knowledge-Based Systems*, vol. 24, no. 8, pp. 1348–1359, 2011.

[47] M.-Y. Cheng and N.-D. Hoang, "A Swarm-Optimized Fuzzy Instance-based Learning approach for predicting slope collapses in mountain roads," *Knowledge-Based Systems*, vol. 76, pp. 256–263, 2015.

[48] M.-Y. Cheng and N.-D. Hoang, "Groutability estimation of grouting processes with microfine cements using an evolutionary instance-based learning approach," *Journal of Computing in Civil Engineering*, vol. 28, no. 4, Article ID 04014014, 2014.

[49] K. M. Passino, "Biomimicry of bacterial foraging for distributed optimization and control," *IEEE Control Systems Magazine*, vol. 22, no. 3, pp. 52–67, 2002.

[50] L. Liu, L. Shan, Y. Dai, C. Liu, and Z. Qi, "A Modified Quantum Bacterial Foraging Algorithm for Parameters Identification of Fractional-Order System," *IEEE Access*, vol. 6, pp. 6610–6619, 2018.

[51] B. Hernandez-Ocana, O. Chavez-Bosquez, J. Hernandez-Torruco, J. Canul-Reich, and P. Pozos-Parra, "Bacterial Foraging Optimization Algorithm for Menu Planning," *IEEE Access*, vol. 6, pp. 8619–8629, 2018.

[52] A. M. Othman and H. A. Gabbar, "Enhanced microgrid dynamic performance using a modulated power filter based on enhanced bacterial foraging optimization," *Energies*, vol. 10, no. 6, 2017.

[53] S. S. Chouhan, A. Kaul, U. P. Singh, and S. Jain, "Bacterial Foraging Optimization Based Radial Basis Function Neural Network (BRBFNN) for Identification and Classification of Plant Leaf Diseases: An Automatic Approach Towards Plant Pathology," *IEEE Access*, vol. 6, pp. 8852–8863, 2018.

[54] B. Turanoğlu and G. Akkaya, "A new hybrid heuristic algorithm based on bacterial foraging optimization for the dynamic facility layout problem," *Expert Systems with Applications*, vol. 98, pp. 93–104, 2018.

[55] X. Lv, H. Chen, Q. Zhang, X. Li, H. Huang, and G. Wang, "An improved bacterial-foraging optimization-based machine learning framework for predicting the severity of somatization disorder," *Algorithms*, vol. 11, no. 2, article 17, 2018.

[56] R. Majhi, G. Panda, B. Majhi, and G. Sahoo, "Efficient prediction of stock market indices using adaptive bacterial foraging optimization (ABFO) and BFO based techniques," *Expert Systems with Applications*, vol. 36, no. 6, pp. 10097–10104, 2009.

[57] S. Dasgupta, S. Das, A. Biswas, and A. Abraham, "Automatic circle detection on digital images with an adaptive bacterial foraging algorithm," *Soft Computing*, vol. 14, no. 11, pp. 1151–1164, 2010.

[58] S. Mishra, "A hybrid least square-fuzzy bacterial foraging strategy for harmonic estimation," *IEEE Transactions on Evolutionary Computation*, vol. 9, no. 1, pp. 61–73, 2005.

[59] S. Mishra and C. N. Bhende, "Bacterial foraging technique-based optimized active power filter for load compensation," *IEEE Transactions on Power Delivery*, vol. 22, no. 1, pp. 457–465, 2007.

[60] M. Ulagammai, P. Venkatesh, P. S. Kannan, and N. Prasad Padhy, "Application of bacterial foraging technique trained artificial and wavelet neural networks in load forecasting," *Neurocomputing*, vol. 70, no. 16-18, pp. 2659–2667, 2007.

[61] Q. Wu, J. F. Mao, C. F. Wei et al., "Hybrid BF-PSO and fuzzy support vector machine for diagnosis of fatigue status using EMG signal features," *Neurocomputing*, vol. 173, pp. 483–500, 2016.

[62] C. Yang, J. Ji, J. Liu, J. Liu, and B. Yin, "Structural learning of Bayesian networks by bacterial foraging optimization," *International Journal of Approximate Reasoning*, vol. 69, pp. 147–167, 2016.

[63] T. S. Sivarani, S. Joseph Jawhar, C. Agees Kumar, and K. Prem Kumar, "Novel bacterial foraging-based ANFIS for speed control of matrix converter-fed industrial BLDC motors operated under low speed and high torque," *Neural Computing and Applications*, pp. 1–24, 2016.

[64] F. Zhao, Y. Liu, Z. Shao, X. Jiang, C. Zhang, and J. Wang, "A chaotic local search based bacterial foraging algorithm and its application to a permutation flow-shop scheduling problem," *International Journal of Computer Integrated Manufacturing*, vol. 29, no. 9, pp. 962–981, 2016.

[65] Y. Sun, S. Todorovic, and S. Goodison, "Local-learning-based feature selection for high-dimensional data analysis," *IEEE*

Transactions on Pattern Analysis and Machine Intelligence, vol. 32, no. 9, pp. 1610–1626, 2010.

[66] H. Chen, J. Lu, Q. Li, C. Lou, D. Pan, and Z. Yu, "A New Evolutionary Fuzzy Instance-Based Learning Approach: Application for Detection of Parkinson's Disease," in *Advances in Swarm and Computational Intelligence*, Y. Tan, Y. Shi, F. Buarque et al., Eds., vol. 9141 of *Lecture Notes in Computer Science*, pp. 42–50, Springer International Publishing, 2015.

[67] T. Kapitaniak, "Continuous control and synchronization in chaotic systems," *Chaos, Solitons & Fractals*, vol. 6, no. C, pp. 237–244, 1995.

[68] T. Bäck and H.-P. Schwefel, "An overview of evolutionary algorithms for parameter optimization," *Evolutionary Computation*, vol. 1, no. 1, pp. 1–23, 1993.

[69] X. Cheng and M. Jiang, "An improved artificial bee colony algorithm based on Gaussian mutation and chaos disturbance," *Lecture Notes in Computer Science*, vol. 7331, no. 1, pp. 326–333, 2012.

[70] N. Higashi and H. Iba, "Particle swarm optimization with Gaussian mutation," in *Proceedings of the 2003 IEEE Swarm Intelligence Symposium, SIS 2003*, pp. 72–79, April 2003.

[71] C. Jena, M. Basu, and C. K. Panigrahi, "Differential evolution with Gaussian mutation for combined heat and power economic dispatch," *Soft Computing*, vol. 20, no. 2, pp. 681–688, 2016.

[72] C. Chang and C. Lin, "LIBSVM: a Library for support vector machines," *ACM Transactions on Intelligent Systems and Technology*, vol. 2, no. 3, article 27, 2011.

[73] S. L. Salzberg, "On comparing classifiers: pitfalls to avoid and a recommended approach," *Data Mining and Knowledge Discovery*, vol. 1, no. 3, pp. 317–328, 1997.

[74] A. Statnikov, I. Tsamardinos, Y. Dosbayev, and C. F. Aliferis, "GEMS: a system for automated cancer diagnosis and biomarker discovery from microarray gene expression data," *International Journal of Medical Informatics*, vol. 74, no. 7-8, pp. 491–503, 2005.

[75] T. Fawcett, "ROC graphs: Notes and practical considerations for researchers," *Machine Learning*, vol. 31, pp. 1–38, 2004.

[76] A. H. Gandomi, X.-S. Yang, S. Talatahari, and A. H. Alavi, "Firefly algorithm with chaos," *Communications in Nonlinear Science and Numerical Simulation*, vol. 18, no. 1, pp. 89–98, 2013.

[77] X. S. Yang, "Flower pollination algorithm for global optimization," in *Unconventional Computation and Natural Computation*, vol. 7445 of *Lecture Notes in Computer Science*, pp. 240–249, Springer, Berlin, Germany, 2012.

[78] X.-S. Yang, "A new metaheuristic bat-inspired Algorithm," *Studies in Computational Intelligence*, vol. 284, pp. 65–74, 2010.

[79] S. Mirjalili, "Dragonfly algorithm: a new meta-heuristic optimization technique for solving single-objective, discrete, and multi-objective problems," *Neural Computing and Applications*, vol. 27, pp. 1053–1073, 2016.

[80] J. Kennedy and R. Eberhart, "Particle swarm optimization," in *Proceedings of the IEEE International Conference on Neural Networks*, pp. 1942–1948, Perth, Australia, December 1995.

[81] J. Derrac, S. García, D. Molina, and F. Herrera, "A practical tutorial on the use of nonparametric statistical tests as a methodology for comparing evolutionary and swarm intelligence algorithms," *Swarm and Evolutionary Computation*, vol. 1, no. 1, pp. 3–18, 2011.

15

The Scatter Search based Algorithm for Beam Angle Optimization in Intensity-Modulated Radiation Therapy

Ali Ghanbarzadeh [iD],[1] **Majid Pouladian** [iD],[2] **Ali Shabestani Monfared,**[3] **and Seied Rabi Mahdavi**[4]

[1]*Department of Medical Radiation Engineering, Tehran Science and Research Branch, Islamic Azad University, Tehran, Iran*
[2]*Department of Biomedical Engineering, Tehran Science and Research Branch, Islamic Azad University, Tehran, Iran*
[3]*Cancer Research Center, Medical Physics Department, Babol University of Medical Sciences, Babol, Iran*
[4]*Radiobiology Research Center, Department of Medical Physics, Iran University of Medical Sciences, Tehran, Iran*

Correspondence should be addressed to Majid Pouladian; pouladian@srbiau.ac.ir

Academic Editor: John Mitchell

This article introduces a new framework for beam angle optimization (BAO) in intensity-modulated radiation therapy (IMRT) using the Scatter Search Based Algorithm. The potential benefits of plans employing the coplanar optimized beam sets are also examined. In the proposed beam angle selection algorithm, the problem is solved in two steps. Initially, the gantry angles are selected using the Scatter Search Based Algorithm, which is a global optimization method. Then, for each beam configuration, the intensity profile is calculated by the conjugate gradient method to score each beam angle set chosen. A simulated phantom case with obvious optimal beam angles was used to benchmark the validity of the presented algorithm. Two clinical cases (TG-119 phantom and prostate cases) were examined to prepare a dose volume histogram (DVH) and determine the dose distribution to evaluate efficiency of the algorithm. A clinical plan with the optimized beam configuration was compared with an equiangular plan to determine the efficiency of the proposed algorithm. The BAO plans yielded significant improvements in the DVHs and dose distributions compared to the equispaced coplanar beams for each case. The proposed algorithm showed its potential to effectively select the beam direction for IMRT inverse planning at different tumor sites.

1. Introduction

Intensity-modulated radiation therapy (IMRT) is an advanced form of the state-of-the-art three-dimensional conformal radiation treatment that improves therapeutic ratios. In IMRT, the radiation beam is modulated by a multileaf collimator. Intensity-modulated beams from different directions are irradiated to achieve a higher degree of uniform dosage for the planning target volume (PTV) and to decrease the dose as much as possible to the organs at risk (OAR) [1]. Conventionally, IMRT treatment planning starts with beam angle selection and is followed by determination of the intensity profiles for preselected beams using an inverse planning method [2, 3].

Currently, in many locations, beam angle selection for IMRT treatment planning is done simply by choosing equiangular spaced beams or through time-consuming trial and error based on the experience of the treatment planners. These methods provide little chance for arriving at the optimal beam configuration because the total dose distribution is affected by the complexity of the profile intensities from every beam direction [4–6].

Selection of the optimal beam direction significantly improves the quality of IMRT treatment both for tumor coverage and in OAR sparing [4, 5, 7–11]. Briefly, determining the optimum beam configuration is a combinatorial optimization problem, in which the best angle configuration is obtained from the results of subproblem solving such as fluence map optimization (FMO) [12]. FMO optimizes the intensity profile for each selected beam angle to ensure that the resulting treatment plan meets the prescribed dose distribution and clinical criteria [13–15].

Beam angle optimization (BAO) is a computationally intensive problem for a number of reasons. First, the search space of the solutions is huge, requiring enumeration of all possible beam orientation combinations. For example, when choosing 4 angles out of 36 candidate beam angles, $C_4^{36} = 58905$ possible combinations exist. Second, any change in a beam configuration requires recalculation and reoptimization of intensity maps, itself a time-consuming process. Third, many local minima (maxima) will appear in the objective function [15–18].

The complexity of the beam angle problem has prompted a wide body of research on automatization of the process in two past decades. There are two important methodologies for solving the beam selection problem. The first is the scoring method, where scores are assigned to beam angles based on the different beam angle ranking functions, the beam-eye view [19], geometric algorithms [20], and dosimetric information [21, 22]. When beams with higher scores are selected, the intensity of each beamlet can be obtained by FMO. This kind of algorithm is very efficient computationally because the interdependence of the multiple modulated beams is neglected during beam angle selection. There is no guarantee, however, that the beam set is optimal because beam selection in this method is not based on the optimal response of FMO and the interplay between the beam sets [4, 19].

The second method is beam configuration based on the objective function value of the FMO which measures plan quality. This framework is very time-consuming because the FMO problem must be solved for each beam configuration to obtain the optimal objective function value. If the function becomes trapped in the multiple local minima of the problem, it may lead to a suboptimal solution [17, 18]. Metaheuristic and stochastic algorithms have been used to escape from the local minimum to obtain a global optimum and the problem can be solved efficiently using simulated annealing [4–7, 23], genetic [23–26], particle swarm optimization [27], pattern search [28], and branch and prune algorithms [29].

Due to the multiple local optimal solutions and nonconvex nature of the BAO, the current study chose the Scatter Search Based Algorithm as the optimization technique as a rapid method to reach the global optimum. The Scatter Search (ScS) method is an optimization derivative-free algorithm based on the sparse grid numerical integration. This algorithm is suitable for a pure and mixed integer nonlinear objective function for which calculation of the gradient is impossible and evaluation of its value is time-consuming [30].

The present study was undertaken to investigate beam angle selection by a new framework. This is the first time that the Scatter Search Algorithm has been incorporated with FMO to search along a discrete-angle candidate pool to find the optimal angle set. The performance of the selected beam angle selection framework was verified using a simulated box phantom with obvious optimal beam angles. The plan quality was compared with a typical equispaced beam selection treatment plan for a TG-119 phantom and a prostate case.

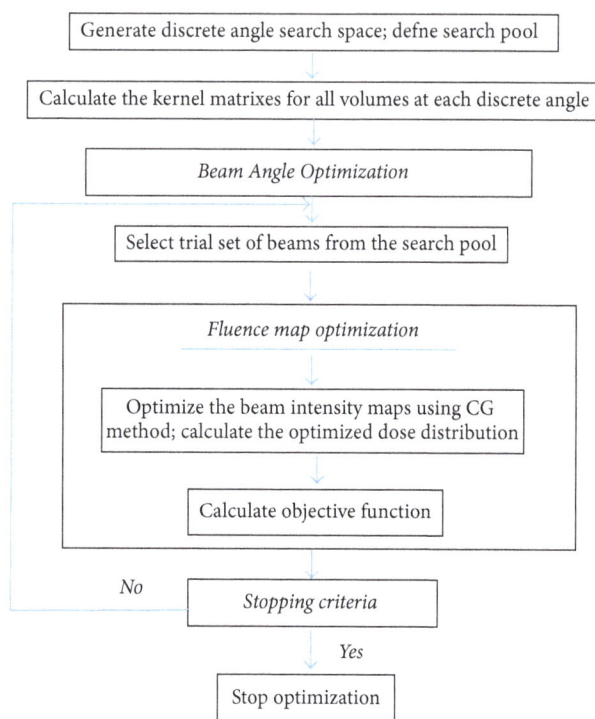

FIGURE 1: Flowchart of beam angle selection algorithm.

2. Materials and Methods

The goal was to find a set of beam directions and corresponding beamlet intensities that could produce the desired conformal dose distribution. The proposed beam angle selection algorithms use two optimization loops. First, for beam orientation selection, the BAO algorithm suggests a small set of beam orientations denoted by θ among a beam candidate pool denoted as Θ. Second, the beam intensity map is fluence-optimized to determine the corresponding dose distribution inside the body volume. This dose distribution is used to evaluate the performance of the trial solution using the value of the objective function ($F(\theta)$). The beam intensity maps are first optimized. Details of the algorithm are provided in a flowchart in Figure 1.

2.1. BAO Problem Formulation. The angle search space in this study covered an entire $360°$ coplanar gantry angle that is divided into equally spaced directions. It is set to $10°$ for the simulated case and $5°$ for other cases and the collimator angle and coach angle are kept fixed. The combinations of these discrete angles are referred to as trial angles [25].

Let Θ be a set of candidate angles that contain the combination of n coplanar beams defined as $\Theta = (\theta_1, \theta_2, \ldots, \theta_N)$ in which N is the total number of feasible beam orientations. Each beam configuration (θ_i) is made up of n coplanar beam directions $\theta = (b_1, b_2, \ldots, b_n)$ and each beam angle b_i is divided into $1 \times 1 \, \text{cm}^2$ beamlets on the isocenter plane along the irradiation. The beamlet intensities of angle b_i are $\vec{x}_i = (x_1, x_2, \ldots, x_k)$. In FMO, the weights (intensities) of the rays are optimized. Once the optimized intensity maps are determined, the corresponding objective function of the current beam configuration can be calculated. The BAO problem can be stated mathematically as

$$\min \quad F(\theta_i)$$
$$\text{subject to} \quad \theta_i \in \Theta. \tag{1}$$

Objective function $F(\theta_i)$ is the optimal FMO value resulting from the angle set specified by $(b_1, b_2, \ldots, b_n)$ in the FMO problem and is formulated such that the lower objective function values correspond to improved solutions. During optimization, the algorithm provides candidate starting points for any gradient-based local solver. This process is called Scatter Search. The gradient-based local solver seeks the answer with the best fitness value near the sparse starting points [31].

2.2. FMO Problem Formulation.

In the FMO formulation, each beam angle can be treated as hundreds of smaller beamlets, each of which having its own radiation intensity (called a fluence). The modulation of these fluences for the beamlets in a set of beams allows for precise control of radiation delivery to the patient. To accelerate each iteration of dose calculation, a strategy similar to that reported by Djajaputra et al. [6] was used, in which the dose deposited in voxel i by an IMRT beam is given by $D_i = \sum K_{im} x_m$, where x_m is the weight for the mth beamlet. Kernel K_{im} is the "dose kernel" or "dose matrix" deposited by each beamlet j at unit intensity K_{ij} for each voxel i in structure s.

Several types of objective functions exist and are implemented in clinical IMRT optimization problems. A quadratic objective function of the difference between the actual and desired dose as introduced by Oelfke and Bortfeld [32] was used to find the ideal fluence modulation $\vec{x} = (x_1, x_2, \ldots, x_n)$ for a given N_{ray} beam ensemble θ_i. The parameter notations are shown in Notations.

The FMO problem for a given set of beams θ is as follows:

$$\min \quad F\left(\vec{x}\right)$$

$$= \sum_{i=1}^{\text{NT}_{\text{PTV}}} p_i \left(D_i\left(\vec{x}\right) - D_i^{\text{pres}}\right)^2 \tag{2}$$

$$+ \sum_{j=1}^{N_{\text{OAR}}} \sum_{i=1}^{\text{NT}_j} p_i \left\lfloor D_i\left(\vec{x}\right) - D_i^{\text{max}}\right\rfloor_+^2$$

$$\text{subject to} \quad D_i\left(\vec{x}\right) = \sum_{m=1}^{N_{\text{ray}}} K_{im} \cdot \vec{x}_m, \tag{3}$$

$$\vec{x}_m \geq 0. \tag{4}$$

The positive operator ensures that only violated constraints contribute to the objective function; that is, $\lfloor x \rfloor_+ = x$ for $x > 0$ and $\lfloor x \rfloor_+ = 0$; otherwise, negative weights of beamlets will not be acceptable in the optimization. A hard constraint was thus defined, which will not violate (4). The final objective value shows a difference between the desired and calculated

dose distribution which denotes the quality of the beam angle sets.

Optimization aims to minimize the dose difference between the prescribed and calculated dose distributions. A conjugate gradient (CG) algorithm is used to solve the FMO problem in the proposed framework. CGs are beneficial from the computational standpoints. The problem may be trapped in local minima, because CG is a local search method [27, 33], but several investigators have demonstrated that those minima are very close to one another and the resulting treatment plans are almost the same [17, 18, 33].

2.3. The Scatter Search Based Method.

The investigation algorithm attempts to find the global solution by starting a local solver from multiple start points in search space. The algorithm uses multiple start points to sample multiple basins of attraction [31, 34].

The Scatter Search Based Algorithm performs the following steps:

(1) The Scatter Search based Algorithm runs a local solver (in MATLAB, fmincon is this local solver) from the start point which was given the problem structure. If this run converges, algorithm records the start point and the end point for an initial estimate on the radius of a basin of attraction.

(2) Generate trial points.

The proposed algorithm uses the Scatter Search Algorithm to generate a set of trial points that are potential start points.

Scatter Search (ScS) is a population-based metaheuristic algorithm that operates on a set of solutions called the reference set or population. Reference set is generated from a population of solution. Then, in the improvement procedure, the solutions in this reference set are combined to get starting solutions, whose result may update the reference set and even the population of solutions from iteration to iteration. ScS is an evolutionary algorithm (EA) because it builds, maintains, and evolves a set of solutions throughout the search. In contrast to other evolutionary methods like genetic algorithms (GA), in Scatter Search the selection of the parents is made using a deterministic method called Subset Generation Method but, in GA, parents are chosen following a random sampling scheme [35, 36]. Implementation of Scatter Search is based on the following steps:

o Generate a starting set of solution vectors by heuristic processes designed for the problem considered and designate a subset of the best vectors to be reference solutions.

o The trial solution improves to transform into enhanced trial solution.

o The reference set updates based on the best of solutions found. Solutions are ranked according to their quality or their diversity.

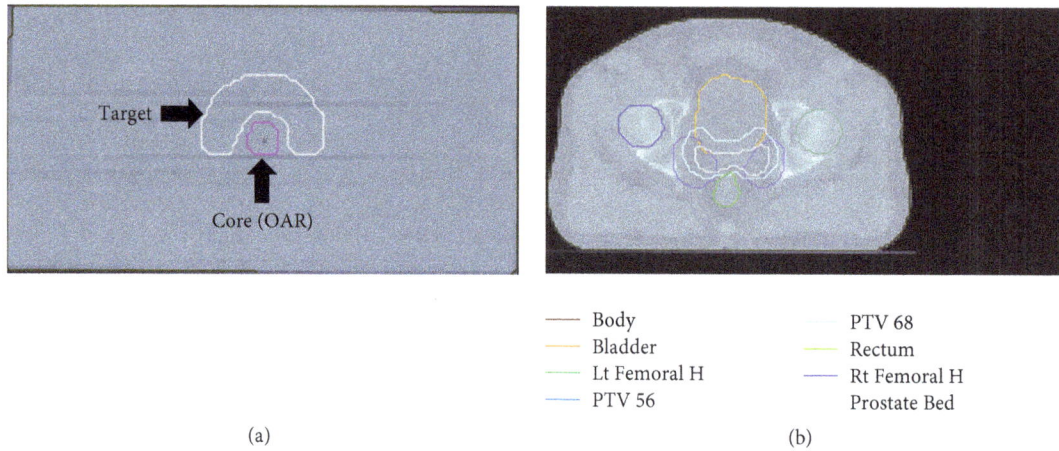

— Body   PTV 68
— Bladder   Rectum
— Lt Femoral H   — Rt Femoral H
— PTV 56   Prostate Bed

(a)   (b)

FIGURE 2: Axial view CT and structures for both cases using CORT dataset: (a) TG-119 phantom; (b) prostate.

o Linear combinations of subsets of the current reference solutions generate a new combined solution and new reference set.

o A collection of the best solutions are starting points for new heuristic processes of step (I). Repeat these steps until reaching a specified iteration limit [36, 37].

(3) The algorithm evaluates the score function of a set of trial points. It then takes the point with the best score and runs local solver from that point. The algorithm removes the set of trial points from its list of points for examination.

(4) Initialize basins and counters: the algorithm heuristic assumption is that basins of attraction are spherical. The initial estimates of basins of attraction for the solution point from $x0$ and the solution point from Stage 1 are spheres centered at the solution points. The radius of each sphere is the distance from the initial point to the solution point. These estimated basins can overlap.

There are two sets of counters associated with the algorithm. Each counter is the number of consecutive trial points that

(i) lie within a basin of attraction, where there is one counter for each basin,

(ii) have score function greater than localSolver-Threshold. For a definition of the score. All counters are initially 0.

(5) Begin main loop.

The Scatter Search Based Algorithm repeatedly examines a remaining trial point from the list and performs the following steps. It continually monitors the time and stops the search if elapsed time exceeds MaxTime seconds.

After reaching MaxTime seconds or running out of trial points, the algorithm creates a vector of Global Optimal Solution objects and orders the elements of the vector by

objective function value, from lowest (best) to highest (worst) [34].

3. Results

The proposed beam angle selection algorithm was tested using simulated and clinical cases. These involved a box phantom to benchmark the framework for finding the best optimal solution along with a TG-119 phantom and a prostate case to compare the plan quality of the optimal angles with equispaced beam angle selection (Figure 2). Beam angle selection algorithms were coded in Matlab R2016R and run on a laptop with Intel Core i7 CPU-6700HQ @ 2.6 GHz with 16 GB of main memory.

Dose volume histogram (DVH) analysis was used to evaluate the quality of proposed treatment plans. Some plan indices that are routinely used to describe a plan are as follows: Dose homogeneity index (HI): analyze the uniformity of dose distribution within the target volume as [38]

$$\text{HI} = \frac{D_5 - D_{95}}{D_p} \times 100, \tag{5}$$

where D_5 and D_{95} are the minimum doses at 5% and 95% of the target volumes, respectively. They denote the maximum and minimum dose of the target, respectively, with D_p denoting the prescribed dose. The ideal value for HI is zero when D_5 and D_{95} are equal [39]. The conformity index (CI) was defined by Van't Riet et al. (1997) as [40]

$$\text{CI} = \text{CI}_1 \cdot \text{CI}_2 = \frac{V_{t,\text{ref}}}{V_t} \cdot \frac{V_{t,\text{ref}}}{V_{\text{ref}}}, \tag{6}$$

where V_t denotes the target volume, $V_{t,\text{ref}}$ denotes the target volume covered by the reference isodose, and V_{ref} denotes the volume covered by the reference isodose. CI ranges from 0 to 1 with the ideal being CI = 1.

CI_1 expresses the fraction of the target volume that receives at least 95% of the prescribed dose. This term is equal to or slightly lower than one for ideal plans. CI_2 indicates how high a dose (greater than 95% of the prescribed dose) is

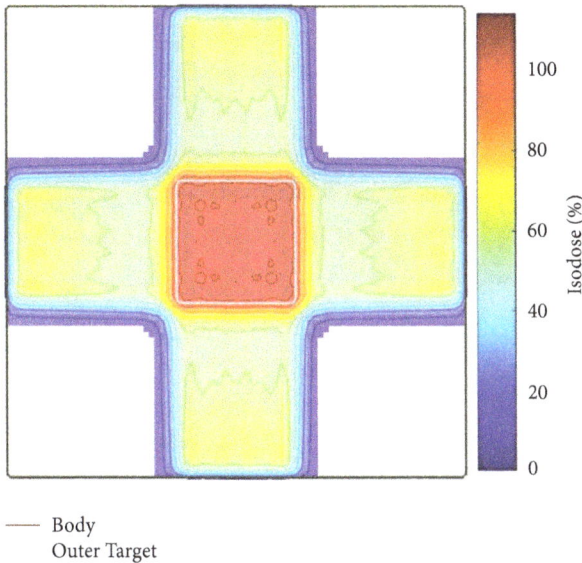

FIGURE 3: Box phantom isodose from optimal angles of 0°, 90°, 180°, and 270°.

— Body
Outer Target

TABLE 1: Comparison of plan quality indices for selection of three angles in TG-119 phantom case.

VOI	Optimal plan	Equiangular plan
Target		
D_5 [Gy]	52.74	54.19
D_{95} [Gy]	44.73	43.3
HI (%)	16.02	21.77
CI	0.478	0.321
Core (OAR)		
Mean dose [Gy]	21.82	24.34
Max. dose [Gy]	32.63	33.95

delivered adjacent to the target volume. A lower value means that the higher dose has spilled around the tumor volume. This term was considerably lower for the optimum plan.

3.1. Simulated Case. The simulated box phantom with defined optimal angles was used to benchmark the BAO algorithm to find the optimal angle set. The simulated case contains a cubic PTV with four obvious optimal beam angles (0°, 90°, 180°, and 270°) [25]. The parameters and the shape of the simulated case are based on the CORT dataset (common optimization for radiation therapy) [41].

The voxel size was set to $0.3 \times 0.3 \times 0.5 \, cm^3$. The beamlet size was set to $1 \times 1 \, cm^2$ on the isocenter plane. The objective function parameters were selected as follows: PTV prescribed dose = 30 Gy, penalty factor of PTV = 1000, body maximum dose = 20 Gy, and body penalty factor = 100. The BAO algorithm was run to find four coplanar 6-MV photon beams.

To the best of our knowledge, the optimal angles of box phantom are equispaced. The starting point of the algorithm and upper and lower bounds of each angle did not include the 0°, 90°, 180°, and 270° beam angles to allow full testing of algorithm performance. The proposed BAO algorithm found the expected optimal angles (i.e., 0°, 90°, 180°, and 270°). The dose distribution of the optimal angles is shown in Figure 3.

3.2. TG-119 Case. The TG-119 phantom with a concave PTV and cylindrical OAR is shown in Figure 2. The simulated TG-119 phantom in the CORT dataset was used. The voxel size was set to $0.3 \times 0.3 \times 0.25 \, cm^3$. The numbers of target voxels and total patient voxels were equal to 7,429 and 599,440, respectively. The objective function parameters were set as follows: prescribed dose to PTV = 50 Gy with a penalty factor of 1000, OAR max dose = 30 Gy with a penalty factor of 300, and body max dose = 30 Gy with a penalty factor of 100. For this case, the BAO algorithm considered three optimal

beam angles (30°, 180°, and 285°) from the coplanar candidate orientations. To show the effectiveness of the algorithm in reaching a better beam orientation, the dose distribution of the optimal plan was compared with equispaced beams as illustrated in Figure 4.

The reason for the fact that comparison of the performance of the algorithm was evaluated with the equispaced beams is because such beams are commonly used in clinical treatment planning and are clinically acceptable [10]. The planning target coverage and OAR sparing of the plans were evaluated with DVH and some of the clinical matrices (e.g., homogeneity and conformity indices).

The DVHs (Figure 5) showed that the OAR received a lower dose in the optimized plan than in the manual plan; furthermore, the uniformity of the dose in PTV was slightly improved in the optimal plan. Table 1 shows that the BAO algorithm produced better-quality treatment plans in terms of target coverage (CI), target dose homogeneity (HI), and OAR sparing (mean and maximum dose of core).

3.3. A Clinical Case: Prostate Tumor. For the prostate case, the CORT dataset was used. In this case, two PTVs with prescribed doses of 56 and 68 Gy were defined, which were surrounded by the OARs of the rectum and bladder (Figure 2). The voxel size was set to $0.3 \times 0.3 \times 0.3 \, cm^3$ and the voxel numbers of the target and patient body in the image were 9491 and 690,373, respectively. The optimization objective function parameters are shown in Table 2.

The seven angles selected by the BAO algorithm were 5°, 50°, 110°, 200°, 225°, 260°, and 320°. It was observed through several runs of the problem that some beam angles in the configuration changed slightly, but the overall objective function value did not change significantly (Figure 6) compared to the DVHs of the sets of seven optimal coplanar beams and seven equispaced beams. The target dose did not change significantly, while the bladder and rectum doses decreased. These plans were optimized using the same dose prescription for the objective function. Figure 7 shows the dose distributions and confirms that the BAO improved the quality of the plan in comparison with the equispaced method. Quality indicator values for both the optimal beam angle treatment plan and the reference plan (equispaced beam selection) are listed in Table 3.

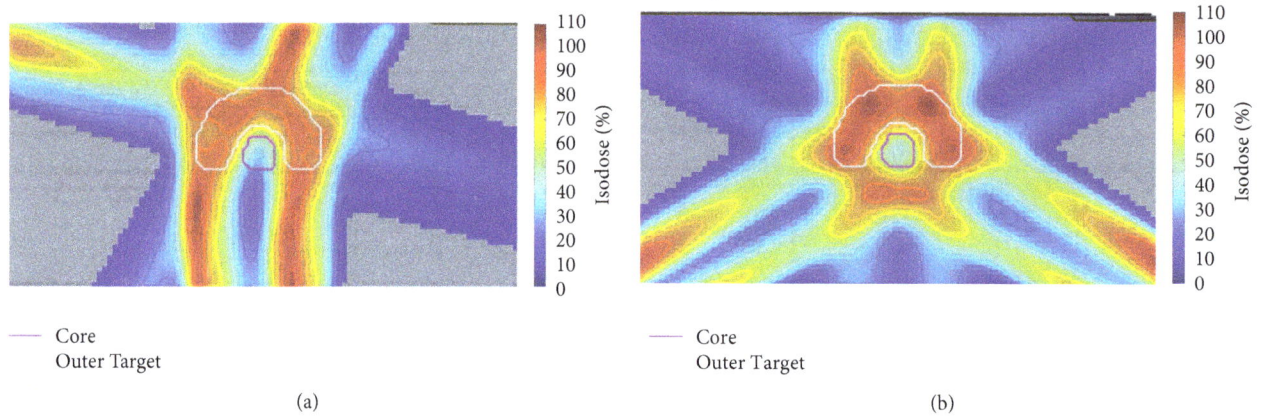

(a)   (b)

FIGURE 4: TG-119 phantom case. Comparison of axial dose distribution obtained in (a) optimal angle set plan (30°, 180°, and 285°) and (b) equiangular plan (0°, 120°, and 240°).

TABLE 2: Objective function parameters for all structures considered for BAO of the prostate case.

VOI	VOI type	Objective function	Penalty	Prescribed dose [Gy]	Mean dose [Gy]	Maximum dose [Gy]
PTV 56	Target	Square deviation	1000	56	- - -	- - -
PTV 68	Target	Square deviation	1000	68	- - -	- - -
Bladder	VOI	Square overdosing	300	- - -	45	- - -
Rectum	VOI	Square overdosing	300	- - - -	45	- - -
Body	VOI	Square overdosing	100	- - -	- - -	70

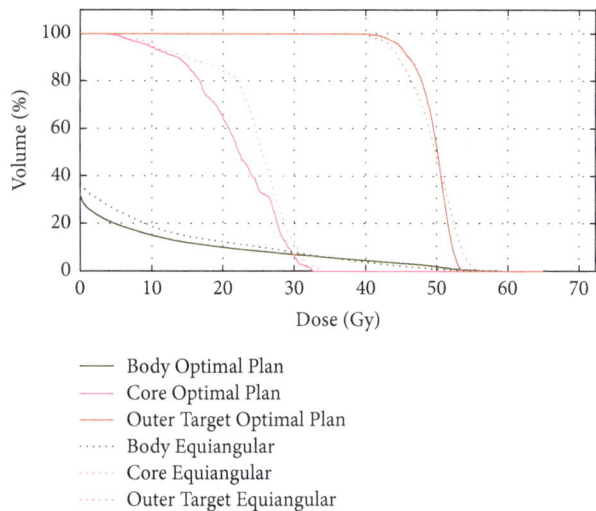

FIGURE 5: DVH comparison for TG-119 phantom case of equiangular and optimal beam angle set plans. Three coplanar 6 MV photon beams were used for both plans.

Comparison of the DVH of the five optimal angles and seven equiangular plans shows that target coverages were similar, but the BAO plans delivered a smaller dose to the bladder and rectum (Figure 8). Figure 7 shows the plan using five beams to achieve the best possible dose distribution with quality as good as or better than a plan with a larger number of equispaced beam angles.

4. Discussions

This paper introduces a Scatter Search Based Algorithm to solve the problem of beam angle selection in IMRT planning. The results of testing on a simulated box phantom showed the ability of the proposed algorithm to reach an optimal coplanar beam configuration, which is the benchmarking framework for receiving optimal beam angles for IMRT treatment planning. As in previously published works in BAO, the proposed framework can improve the quality of plan by choosing the preferable beam orientation, but there is no way to determine whether or not the solutions of BAO are a global optimum or perhaps suboptimal.

The ability of proposed beam angle selection framework to clinically improve complicated IMRT plans (TG-119 phantom and prostate cases) was compared to manual equispaced beams. The DVH, dose distribution, and quality indices of the plans confirmed that the optimum beam angle set improved OAR sparing while guaranteeing target coverage and dose uniformity. Table 1 showed a decrease of approximately 2.52 and 1.32 Gy for mean and maximum core doses (OAR) in the TG-119 case, respectively. Table 3 shows that the mean doses for the bladder and rectum of the optimal plan decreased by 3.22 and 2.03 Gy, respectively, over those of the equiangular plan.

The stochastic and heuristic proposed Scatter Search Based Algorithm for solving the beam angle optimization problem was suitable due to the nonconvex nature of the problem with multiple local minima [15, 16]. The proposed algorithm analyzes feasible solutions by running multiple

TABLE 3: Comparison of plan quality indices for seven-angle selection of prostate case.

VOI	Optimal plan	Equiangular plan
PTV 56 (Target)		
D_5 [Gy]	67.35	67.33
D_{95} [Gy]	54.56	54.55
HI (%)	22.83	22.82
CI	0.4153	0.3548
PTV 68 (target)		
D_5 [Gy]	69.8	70.06
D_{95} [Gy]	63.45	63.44
HI (%)	9.3359	9.7482
CI	0.8243	0.7647
Bladder (OAR)		
Mean dose [Gy]	42.32	45.54
Max. dose [Gy]	71.19	71.45
D_5 [Gy]	68.33	68.78
D_{95} [Gy]	25.39	30.13
Rectum (OAR)		
Mean dose [Gy]	40.92	42.95
Max. dose [Gy]	69.37	69.94
D_5 [Gy]	61.36	60.94
D_{95} [Gy]	15.25	9.89

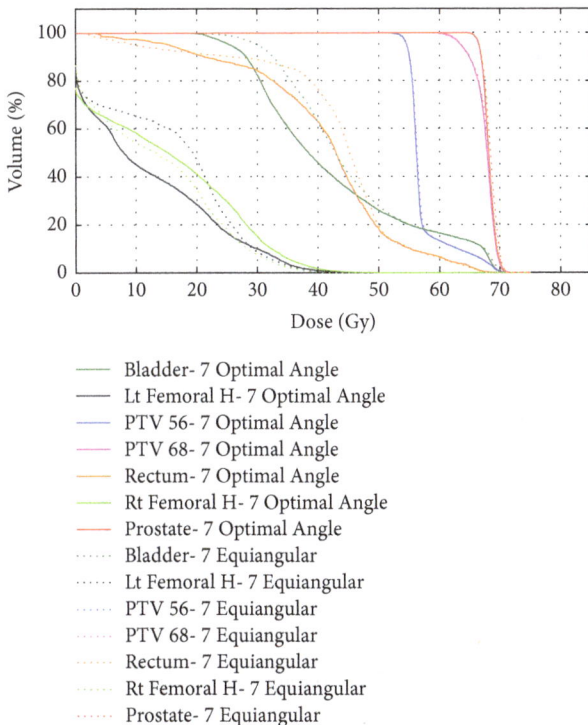

— Bladder- 7 Optimal Angle
— Lt Femoral H- 7 Optimal Angle
— PTV 56- 7 Optimal Angle
— PTV 68- 7 Optimal Angle
— Rectum- 7 Optimal Angle
— Rt Femoral H- 7 Optimal Angle
— Prostate- 7 Optimal Angle
⋯⋯ Bladder- 7 Equiangular
⋯⋯ Lt Femoral H- 7 Equiangular
⋯⋯ PTV 56- 7 Equiangular
⋯⋯ PTV 68- 7 Equiangular
⋯⋯ Rectum- 7 Equiangular
⋯⋯ Rt Femoral H- 7 Equiangular
⋯⋯ Prostate- 7 Equiangular

FIGURE 6: Comparison of DVHs of seven-beam angle selection plan and BAO algorithm plus seven-beam equiangular plan.

starting points selected from the scattered base by a search poll. This allows the algorithm to overcome local minima.

The computation time of the proposed framework increased with control of the main factors that influence beam selection time such as the BAO coupled with FMO, the size of the initial candidate beam configuration, number of targets and OAR voxels, and size of the dose matrix. The algorithm spent the most time finding an intensity map of each beam configuration because the objective function for beam angle optimization was based on the optimal dose distribution obtained from each beam configuration. FMO was used to conjugate the gradient algorithm, which is preferred to other algorithms in many studies because of its faster convergence [33]. The CG, however, is a local search algorithm that can be trapped in the local minima and make suboptimal plans. The dose distribution obtained from the optimal intensity of solving FMO must be calculated by scoring each beam angle set during BAO because the fast gradient algorithm can significantly decrease computing time.

Choosing an optimum number of beams improves the quality of the IMRT treatment plan. In the proposed framework, the number of beams was selected before BAO based on the complexity level of the given case [4, 9]. Moreover, noncoplanar beam angles were not investigated in this study, which may further improve the quality of the plan.

The beam angle discretization resolution was set at 10° for the box phantom case and 5° for the TG-119 and prostate case. Many investigators have discussed the influence of this resolution on the final solution for the BAO algorithm and computation time [6, 42]. To speed up the algorithm, the search space size can be reduced by prior knowledge, such as selection of more beams in favorable directions and vice versa. An alternative method to reduce the feasible beam direction is to discrete the coplanar pool using a reasonable

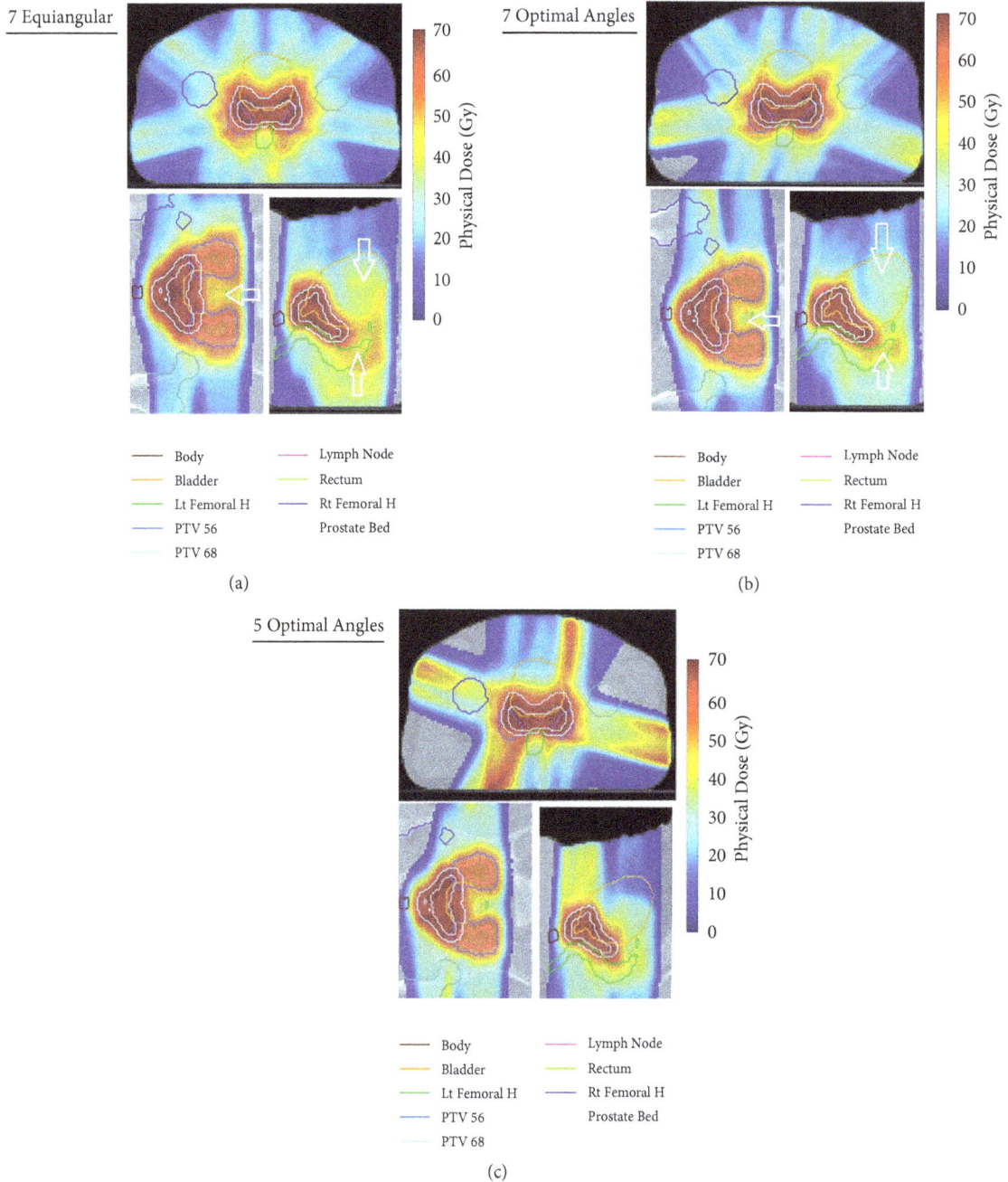

FIGURE 7: Dose distributions for prostate case in axial, coronal, and sagittal views: (a) seven-angle equiangular plan (0°, 50°, 100°, 150°, 200°, 255°, and 305°); (b) seven-angle optimal plan (5°, 50°, 110°, 200°, 225°, 260°, and 320°); (c) five-angle optimal plan (5°, 105°, 185°, 210°, and 290°).

space of, for example, 10 instead of 5, to allow half candidate directions that significantly decrease the number of possible beam configurations.

Figures 7 and 8 showed that a lower number of optimal angles in the plan can reach dose distributions that are as good as plans using a greater number of equispaced orientations. Furthermore, a plan with a small number is more highly desirable from the clinical perspective to limit the volume of normal tissue being irradiated or simplifying treatment delivery to shorten treatment time and hence lower

potential error caused by patient movement during dose delivery [4, 5, 11].

5. Conclusions

The proposed angle selection algorithm is able to provide better beam orientation configurations for IMRT, which will spare OARs and achieve better target volume coverage. The small number of optimized orientations can obtain results

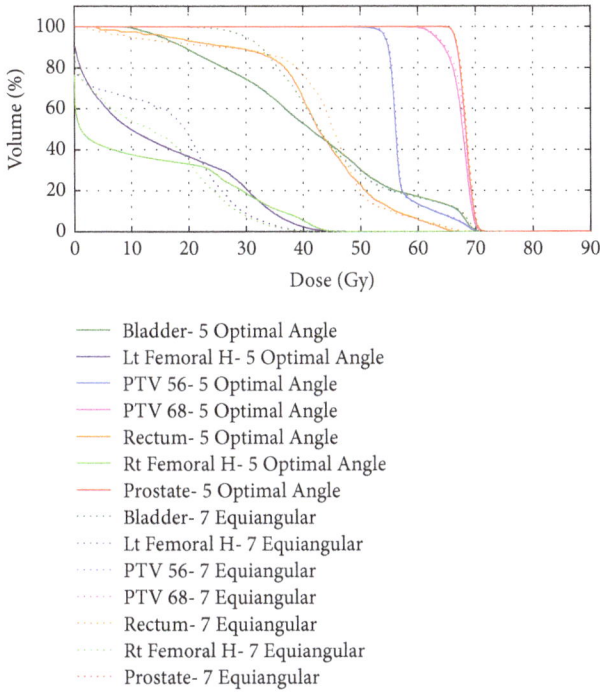

Bladder- 5 Optimal Angle
Lt Femoral H- 5 Optimal Angle
PTV 56- 5 Optimal Angle
PTV 68- 5 Optimal Angle
Rectum- 5 Optimal Angle
Rt Femoral H- 5 Optimal Angle
Prostate- 5 Optimal Angle
Bladder- 7 Equiangular
Lt Femoral H- 7 Equiangular
PTV 56- 7 Equiangular
PTV 68- 7 Equiangular
Rectum- 7 Equiangular
Rt Femoral H- 7 Equiangular
Prostate- 7 Equiangular

FIGURE 8: DVHs for the prostate case. Solid lines denote the five-beam plan generated by BAO algorithm. Dotted lines denote the results of the treatment plan with seven equiangular beams.

similar to plans with a greater number of manual beam directions, which means easier quality assurance and a decrease in treatment time and patient setup error. The main advantage of this method is that the Scatter Search Algorithm fits with the nonconvex nature of the problem and can search all space in a short time to choose the beam angles, which may be very helpful for routine clinical usage. Also, the proposed algorithm can run any IMRT case and can fulfill different clinical desires by changing the parameters of the objective function.

Notations

Notations and Definitions of Parameters Considered for the Objective Function

$\vec{x_m}$:   Intensity of mth ray
p_i: Penalty coefficient in voxel i
$D_i(\vec{x})$:   The calculated dose of the ith point in the volume
D_i^{pres}:   The prescribed dose in the planning target volume
D_i^{max}:   The tolerance dose in organs at risk (OARs)
N_{OAR}:   The total number of the OARs
NT_j: Number of voxels in jth OARs
NT_{PTV}:   Number of voxels in the target
N_{ray}:   The total number of the rays
K_{im}:   The dose deposited to the ith point (voxel) from the mth ray with a unit beamlet weight.

Conflicts of Interest

The authors declare that they have no conflicts of interest.

Acknowledgments

The authors would like to acknowledge the Mehraneh charity radiotherapy center for the pleasant cooperation.

References

[1] S. Webb, *Intensity-Modulated Radiation Therapy*, CRC Press, Boca Raton, Fla, USA, 2001.

[2] S. Webb, "Optimizing the planning of intensity-modulated radiotherapy," *Physics in Medicine and Biology*, vol. 39, no. 12, article no. 007, pp. 2229–2246, 1994.

[3] L. Xing, R. J. Hamilton, D. Spelbring, C. A. Pelizzari, G. T. Y. Chen, and A. L. Boyer, "Fast iterative algorithms for three-dimensional inverse treatment planning," *Medical Physics*, vol. 25, no. 10, pp. 1845–1849, 1998.

[4] J. Stein, R. Mohan, X.-H. Wang et al., "Number and orientations of beams in intensity-modulated radiation treatments," *Medical Physics*, vol. 24, no. 2, pp. 149–160, 1997.

[5] A. B. Pugachev, A. L. Boyer, and L. Xing, "Beam orientation optimization in intensity-modulated radiation treatment planning," *Medical Physics*, vol. 27, no. 6, pp. 1238–1245, 2000.

[6] D. Djajaputra, Q. Wu, Y. Wu, and R. Mohan, "Algorithm and performance of a clinical IMRT beam-angle optimization system," *Physics in Medicine and Biology*, vol. 48, no. 19, pp. 3191–3212, 2003.

[7] A. Pugachev, J. G. Li, A. L. Boyer et al., "Role of beam orientation optimization in intensity-modulated radiation therapy," *International Journal of Radiation Oncology • Biology • Physics*, vol. 50, no. 2, pp. 551–560, 2001.

[8] C. G. Rowbottom, C. M. Nutting, and S. Webb, "Beam-orientation optimization of intensity-modulated radiotherapy: Clinical application to parotid gland tumours," *Radiotherapy & Oncology*, vol. 59, no. 2, pp. 169–177, 2001.

[9] S. Söderström and A. Brahme, "Which is the most suitable number of photon beam portals in coplanar radiation therapy?" *International Journal of Radiation Oncology • Biology • Physics*, vol. 33, no. 1, pp. 151–159, 1995.

[10] E. Schreibmann and L. Xing, "Feasibility study of beam orientation class-solutions for prostate IMRT," *Medical Physics*, vol. 31, no. 10, pp. 2863–2870, 2004.

[11] A. Shukla, S. Kumar, I. Sandhu, A. Oinam, R. Singh, and R. Kapoor, "Dosimetric study of beam angle optimization in intensity-modulated radiation therapy planning," *Journal of Cancer Research and Therapeutics*, vol. 12, no. 2, pp. 1045–1049, 2016.

[12] M. Ehrgott, A. Holder, and J. Reese, "Beam selection in radiotherapy design," *Linear Algebra and its Applications*, vol. 428, no. 5-6, pp. 1272–1312, 2008.

[13] S. K. Das and L. B. Marks, "Selection of coplanar or noncoplanar beams using three-dimensional optimization based on maximum beam separation and minimized nontarget irradiation," *International Journal of Radiation Oncology • Biology • Physics*, vol. 38, no. 3, pp. 643–655, 1997.

[14] E. Schreibmann, M. Lahanas, L. Xing, and D. Baltas, "Multiobjective evolutionary optimization of the number of beams, their orientations and weights for intensity-modulated radiation

therapy," *Physics in Medicine and Biology*, vol. 49, no. 5, pp. 747–770, 2004.

[15] D. Craft, T. Halabi, H. A. Shih, and T. Bortfeld, "An approach for practical multiobjective imrt treatment planning," *International Journal of Radiation Oncology • Biology • Physics*, vol. 69, no. 5, pp. 1600–1607, 2007.

[16] X. Jia, C. Men, Y. Lou, and S. B. Jiang, "Beam orientation optimization for intensity modulated radiation therapy using adaptive l2,1-minimization," *Physics in Medicine and Biology*, vol. 56, no. 19, article no. 004, pp. 6205–6222, 2011.

[17] J. Llacer, J. O. Deasy, T. R. Bortfeld, T. D. Solberg, and C. Promberger, "Absence of multiple local minima effects in intensity modulated optimization with dose-volume constraints," *Physics in Medicine and Biology*, vol. 48, no. 2, pp. 183–210, 2003.

[18] Q. Wu and R. Mohan, "Multiple local minima in IMRT optimization based on dose-volume criteria," *Medical Physics*, vol. 29, no. 7, pp. 1514–1527, 2002.

[19] A. Pugachev and L. Xing, "Pseudo beam's-eye-view as applied to beam orientation selection in intensity-modulated radiation therapy," *International Journal of Radiation Oncology • Biology • Physics*, vol. 51, no. 5, pp. 1361–1370, 2001.

[20] P. S. Potrebko, B. M. C. McCurdy, J. B. Butler, A. S. El-Gubtan, and Z. Nugent, "A simple geometric algorithm to predict optimal starting gantry angles using equiangular-spaced beams for intensity modulated radiation therapy of prostate cancer," *Medical Physics*, vol. 34, no. 10, pp. 3951–3961, 2007.

[21] W. D. D'Souza, R. R. Meyer, and L. Shi, "Selection of beam orientations in intensity-modulated radiation therapy using single-beam indices and integer programming," *Physics in Medicine and Biology*, vol. 49, no. 15, pp. 3465–3481, 2004.

[22] R. Vaitheeswaran, V. K. Sathiya Narayanan, J. R. Bhangle et al., "An algorithm for fast beam angle selection in intensity modulated radiotherapy," *Medical Physics*, vol. 37, no. 12, pp. 6443–6452, 2010.

[23] M. Bangert, P. Ziegenhein, and U. Oelfke, "Characterizing the combinatorial beam angle selection problem," *Physics in Medicine and Biology*, vol. 57, no. 20, article no. 6707, pp. 6707–6723, 2012.

[24] Q. Hou, J. Wang, Y. Chen, and J. M. Galvin, "Beam orientation optimization for IMRT by a hybrid method of the genetic algorithm and the simulated dynamics," *Medical Physics*, vol. 30, no. 9, pp. 2360–2367, 2003.

[25] Y. Li, J. Yao, and D. Yao, "Automatic beam angle selection in IMRT planning using genetic algorithm," *Physics in Medicine and Biology*, vol. 49, no. 10, pp. 1915–1932, 2004.

[26] J. Dias, H. Rocha, B. g. Ferreira, and M. d. Lopes, "A genetic algorithm with neural network fitness function evaluation for IMRT beam angle optimization," *Central European Journal of Operations Research*, vol. 22, no. 3, pp. 431–455, 2014.

[27] Y. Li, D. Yao, J. Yao, and W. Chen, "A particle swarm optimization algorithm for beam angle selection in intensity-modulated radiotherapy planning," *Physics in Medicine and Biology*, vol. 50, no. 15, pp. 3491–3514, 2005.

[28] H. Rocha, J. M. Dias, B. C. Ferreira, and M. C. Lopes, "Beam angle optimization for intensity-modulated radiation therapy using a guided pattern search method," *Physics in Medicine and Biology*, vol. 58, no. 9, pp. 2939–2953, 2013.

[29] G. J. Lim and W. Cao, "A two-phase method for selecting IMRT treatment beam angles: branch-and-prune and local neighborhood search," *European Journal of Operational Research*, vol. 217, no. 3, pp. 609–618, 2012.

[30] L. Dixon, "The global optimization problem: An introduction," *Towards Global Optimiation*, vol. 2, pp. 1–15, 1978.

[31] Z. Ugray, L. Lasdon, J. Plummer, F. Glover, J. Kelly, and R. Martí, "Scatter search and local NLP solvers: a multistart framework for global optimization," *INFORMS Journal on Computing*, vol. 19, no. 3, pp. 328–340, 2007.

[32] U. Oelfke and T. Bortfeld, "Inverse planning for photon and proton beams," *Medical Dosimetry*, vol. 26, no. 2, pp. 113–124, 2001.

[33] X. Zhang, H. Liu, X. Wang, L. Dong, Q. Wu, and R. Mohan, "Speed and convergence properties of gradient algorithms for optimization of IMRT," *Medical Physics*, vol. 31, no. 5, pp. 1141–1152, 2004.

[34] MATLAB., "MATLAB and Global Optimization Toolbox, 2016," https://www.mathworks.com/products/global-optimization.html.

[35] F. Herrera, M. Lozano, and D. Molina, "Continuous scatter search: an analysis of the integration of some combination methods and improvement strategies," *European Journal of Operational Research*, vol. 169, no. 2, pp. 450–476, 2006.

[36] J. A. Egea, E. Vazquez, J. R. Banga, and R. Martí, "Improved scatter search for the global optimization of computationally expensive dynamic models," *Journal of Global Optimization*, vol. 43, no. 2-3, pp. 175–190, 2009.

[37] F. Glover, "A template for scatter search and path relinking," in *Artificial Evolution*, vol. 1363 of *Lecture Notes in Computer Science*, pp. 13–54, Springer, Berlin, Germany, 1998.

[38] T. Kataria, K. Sharma, V. Subramani, K. P. Karrthick, and S. S. Bisht, "Homogeneity Index: an objective tool for assessment of conformal radiation treatments," *Journal of Medical Physics*, vol. 37, no. 4, pp. 207–213, 2012.

[39] Q. Wu, R. Mohan, M. Morris, A. Lauve, and R. Schmidt-Ullrich, "Simultaneous integrated boost intensity-modulated radiotherapy for locally advanced head-and-neck squamous cell carcinomas. I: dosimetric results," *International Journal of Radiation Oncology • Biology • Physics*, vol. 56, no. 2, pp. 573–585, 2003.

[40] A. Van't Riet, A. C. A. Mak, M. A. Moerland, L. H. Elders, and W. Van der Zee, "A conformation number to quantify the degree of conformality in brachytherapy and external beam irradiation: application to the prostate," *International Journal of Radiation Oncology • Biology • Physics*, vol. 37, no. 3, pp. 731–736, 1997.

[41] D. Craft, M. Bangert, T. Long, D. Papp, and J. Unkelbach, "Shared data for intensity modulated radiation therapy (IMRT) optimization research: The CORT dataset," *GigaScience*, vol. 3, no. 1, article no. 37, 2014.

[42] S. Das, T. Cullip, G. Tracton et al., "Beam orientation selection for intensity-modulated radiation therapy based on target equivalent uniform dose maximization," *International Journal of Radiation Oncology • Biology • Physics*, vol. 55, no. 1, pp. 215–224, 2003.

16

Mathematical Analysis of Influenza A Dynamics in the Emergence of Drug Resistance

Caroline W. Kanyiri [ID],[1] **Kimathi Mark,**[2] **and Livingstone Luboobi**[3]

[1]*Department of Mathematics, Pan African University Institute of Basic Sciences, Technology and Innovation, P.O. Box 62000-00200, Nairobi, Kenya*
[2]*Department of Mathematics, Machakos University, P.O. Box 139-90100, Machakos, Kenya*
[3]*Institute of Mathematical Sciences, Strathmore University, P.O. Box 59857-00200, Nairobi, Kenya*

Correspondence should be addressed to Caroline W. Kanyiri; kanyiricarolyne2@gmail.com

Academic Editor: Konstantin Blyuss

Every year, influenza causes high morbidity and mortality especially among the immunocompromised persons worldwide. The emergence of drug resistance has been a major challenge in curbing the spread of influenza. In this paper, a mathematical model is formulated and used to analyze the transmission dynamics of influenza A virus having incorporated the aspect of drug resistance. The qualitative analysis of the model is given in terms of the control reproduction number, R_c. The model equilibria are computed and stability analysis carried out. The model is found to exhibit backward bifurcation prompting the need to lower R_c to a critical value R_c^* for effective disease control. Sensitivity analysis results reveal that vaccine efficacy is the parameter with the most control over the spread of influenza. Numerical simulations reveal that despite vaccination reducing the reproduction number below unity, influenza still persists in the population. Hence, it is essential, in addition to vaccination, to apply other strategies to curb the spread of influenza.

1. Introduction

Influenza is a contagious respiratory illness caused by influenza viruses. There are three major types of flu viruses: types A, B, and C. The majority of human infections are caused by types A and B. Of major concern is influenza A virus which is clinically the most vicious. It is a negative-sense single-stranded RNA virus with eight gene segments. The segmented nature of influenza A virus genome allows the exchange of gene segments between viruses that coinfect the same cell [1]. This process of genetic exchange is termed reassortment. Reassortment leads to sudden changes in viral genetics and to susceptibility in hosts. Influenza A virus has a wide range of susceptible avian hosts and mammalian hosts such as humans, pigs, horses, seals, and mink. In addition, the virus is able to repeatedly switch hosts to infect multiple avian and mammalian species. The unpredictability of influenza A virus evolution and interspecies movement creates continual public health challenges [2].

Influenza A virus constantly mutates and is able to elude the immune system of an individual. It can mutate in two different ways: antigenic shift and antigenic drift. Antigenic shift is an abrupt, major change in the influenza virus which happens occasionally and results in a new subtype that most people have no protection against. Such a shift occurred in the spring of 2009 in Mexico and United States, when H1N1 virus with a new combination of genes emerged to infect people and quickly spread, causing a pandemic [3]. This antigenic shift was as a result of extensive reassortment in swine that brought together genes from avian, swine, and human flu viruses [4]. On the other hand, antigenic drift refers to small changes in the genes of influenza viruses that occur continually as the virus replicates. Over time, these small genetic changes result in new strains which the antibodies can no longer recognize. The changes in the influenza viruses are the main reason why individuals are infected with the flu more than once. The viruses infect the nose, throat, and lungs. They usually are spread through the air when the infected people cough, sneeze, or talk making the surrounding air and surfaces to be temporarily contaminated with infected droplets [5, 6]. People get infected when they inhale the infected droplets. A person might also get flu by touching the surface or object that has flu virus on it and then touching their own mouth, eyes, or possibly their nose [6].

Influenza can be prevented by getting vaccination each year. However, given that the virus mutates rapidly, a vaccine made for one year may not be useful in the following year. In addition, antigenic drift in the virus may occur after the year's vaccine has been formulated, rendering the vaccine less protective, and hence, outbreaks can easily occur especially among high-risk individuals [7]. According to [8], other preventive actions include staying away from people who are sick, covering coughs and sneezes, and frequent handwashing.

Influenza spreads rapidly around the world during seasonal epidemics and pandemics [9]. It has afflicted the human population for centuries. For instance, the 1918 influenza pandemic infected nearly one quarter of the world's population and resulted in the deaths of about 100 million people [10]. Studies show that this pandemic is especially responsible for the high morbidity and mortality among vulnerable groups such as children, the elderly, and patients with underlying health conditions [11]. Within the past one hundred years, there have been four pandemics resulting from the emergence of a novel influenza strain for which the human population possessed little or no immunity. Table 1 gives a brief summary of the four influenza pandemics.

Besides the influenza pandemics, there is an outbreak of influenza every year around the world which results in about three to five million cases of severe illness and about 250,000 to 500,000 deaths [14]. According to a report by Centers for Disease Control and Prevention (CDC), as of December 2017, the estimated number of deaths worldwide resulting from seasonal influenza had risen to between 291,000 and 646,000 [15]. This new estimate was from a collaborative study by CDC and global health partners. In the temperate northern hemisphere (i.e., north of the Tropic of Cancer) and temperate southern hemisphere (i.e., south of the Tropic of Capricorn), influenza has been observed to peak in the winter months [16, 17]. In tropical regions, influenza seasonality is less obvious and epidemics can occur throughout the year and more specifically during the rainy seasons [18]. According to [19], the mortality rates due to this respiratory disease are much higher in Africa than anywhere else in the world. Poor nutritional status, poor access to healthcare including vaccination and antibiotics, and the presence of other, less measurable factors related to poverty in Africa may be additional risk factors for higher mortality rates. WHO Global Influenza Surveillance and Response System (GISRS) monitors the evolution of influenza viruses.

TABLE 1: Summary of influenza pandemics in the past one hundred years.

Pandemic name	Year	Strain	Approximate number of deaths
Spanish flu	1918–1920	H1N1	40–100 million
Asian flu	1957–1958	H2N2	1–2 million
Hong Kong flu	1968–1970	H3N2	0.5–2 million
Swine flu	2009–2010	H1N1	Up to 575,000

Source: [10, 12, 13].

Figures 1 and 2 show the global circulation of influenza viruses from 2016 to week 24 of 2018 [20, 21].

Influenza-attributable mortality varies across the seasons. There is however paucity of published estimates of influenza mortality for low- and middle-income countries. Data from Centers for Disease Control and Prevention (CDC) databases from the 1999–2000 to the 2014–2015 seasons for the U.S. population aged 65 years and above were used to estimate excess deaths per month over that 15-year span [22]. The data are presented in Figure 3.

In addition to pandemics and seasonal epidemics caused by influenza A virus, over the past 20 years, multiple zoonotic influenza A virus outbreaks have occurred causing a great concern to public health [23–26]. For instance, H5N1 influenza virus from avian hosts poses an ongoing threat to human and animal health due to its high mortality rate [26–28]. H7N9 is yet another highly pathogenic subtype of influenza A virus that is of major concern. According to the World Health Organization (WHO), as of January 2018, 1566 laboratory-confirmed cases of human infection with H7N9 virus have been reported in China, including at least 613 deaths [29]. In addition to the ongoing H5N1 and H7N9 influenza A virus outbreaks, other subtypes, such as H5N6, H9N2, H10N8, and H6N1, have sporadically caused serious human infections in China and Taiwan [30–33]. The death toll from influenza is unacceptably high, given that it is preventable. Efforts to combat it must therefore be accelerated. In view of the catastrophic effects of influenza globally, several models have been proposed and analyzed with the aim of shedding more light in the transmission dynamics of influenza, for instance [34–41]. Among the pioneer mathematical models used to describe influenza dynamics is one developed by [38].

Emergence of drug resistance which is a growing menace globally [42] complicates influenza even more [43, 44]. Drug resistance refers to reduction in the effectiveness of a drug in curing a disease. It occurs when microorganisms such as bacteria, viruses, fungi, and parasites change in ways that render the medications used to cure the infections they cause ineffective [45, 46]. The microorganisms are therefore able to survive the treatment. According to [47], epidemics with drug-resistant strains and those with drug-sensitive strains are fundamentally different in their growth and dynamics. Drug-sensitive epidemics are fuelled by only one process, that is, transmission; however, drug-resistant epidemics are fuelled by two processes: transmission and the conversion of treated drug-sensitive infections to drug-resistant infections

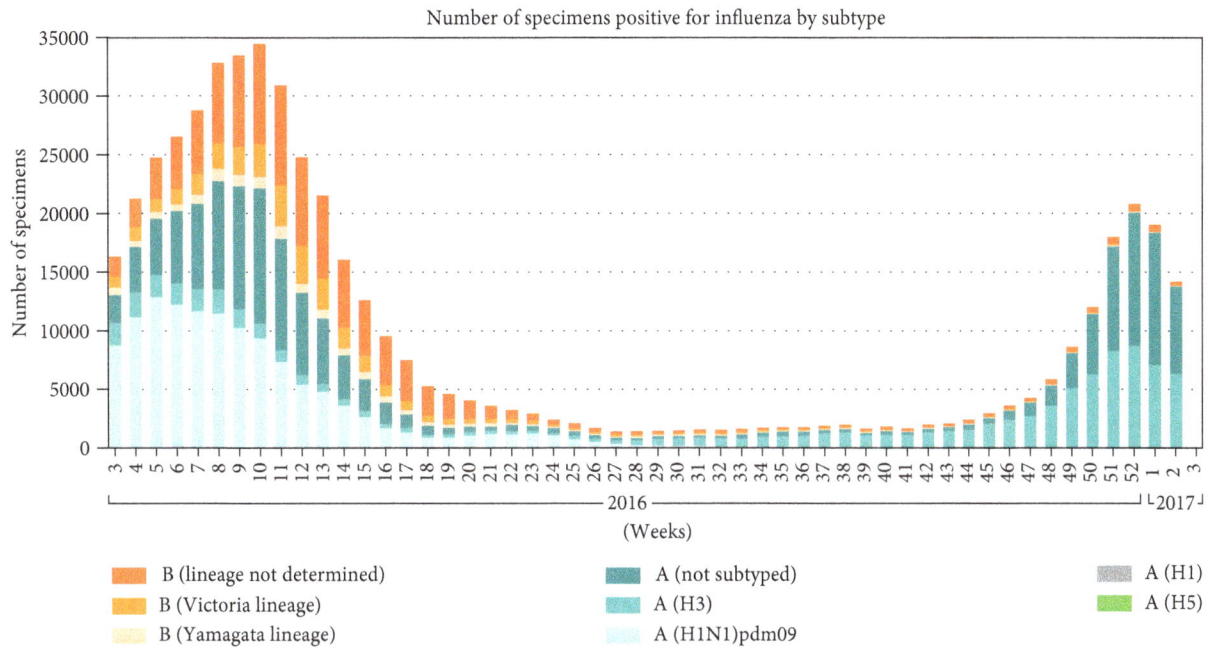

FIGURE 1: Global circulation of influenza viruses from 2016 to 2017.

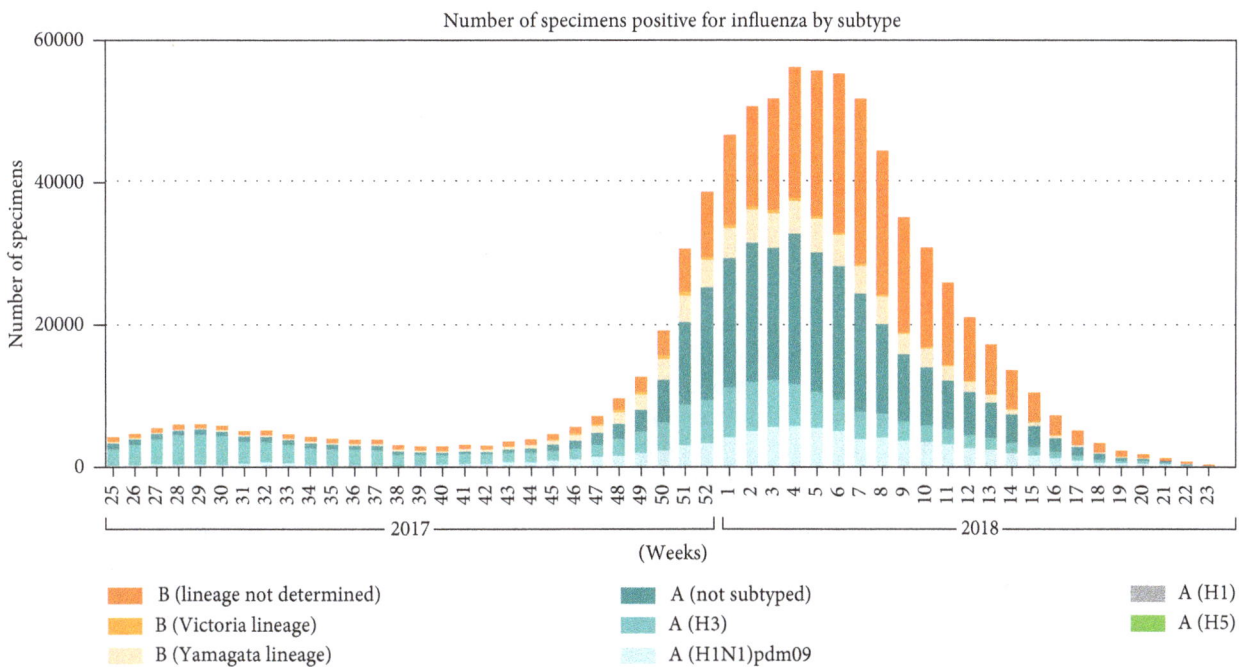

FIGURE 2: Global circulation of influenza viruses from 2017 to week 24 of 2018.

(acquired resistance). Therefore, the rate of increase in drug-resistant infections can be much faster than the rate of increase in drug-sensitive infections. Studies from [48] show that drug resistance is a function of time and treatment rate. In addition, immunosuppression especially in individuals with compromised immune systems contributes to lack of viral clearance often despite antiviral therapy leading to emergence of antiviral resistance [49].

There are two classes of antiviral drugs that are used to treat influenza: adamantanes and neuraminidase inhibitors.

The adamantanes are only effective against influenza A viruses, as they inhibit the M2 protein, which is not coded by influenza B [50]. These drugs are associated with several toxic effects and rapid emergence of drug-resistant strains. The neuraminidase inhibitors interfere with the release of progeny influenza virus from infected host cells, a process that prevents infection of new host cells and thereby halts the spread of infection in the respiratory tract [7]. Since these drugs act at the stage of viral replication, they must be administered as early as possible. According to [51],

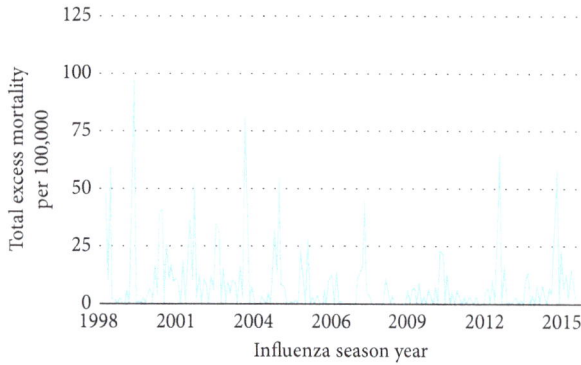

FIGURE 3: Excess mortality due to influenza for the U.S. population aged 65 years and above.

influenza viruses mutate constantly, either from one season to the next or within the course of one flu season. As a flu virus replicates, the genetic makeup may change rendering the virus resistant to one or more of the antiviral drugs used to treat or prevent influenza. Antiviral resistance in influenza may not only emerge during treatment but also sometimes transmit widely to replace wild-type strains in the absence of drug pressure. The transmission of resistant strains is evidenced by the global spread of adamantane-resistant A (H3N2) viruses since 2003, oseltamivir-resistant seasonal A (H1N1) viruses since 2007, and adamantane-resistant pandemic A(H1N1) viruses in 2009, leading to increased challenges in the management of influenza [52]. With the development of drug-resistant influenza viruses, various models have also been formulated in order to understand this phenomenon better. Among them are [53–57].

The morbidity, mortality, and economic burden of influenza cannot be overlooked. With the emerging menace of drug resistance, this burden becomes even more complicated. In order to curb the spread of influenza, there is a dire need to understand among its many aspects, its transmission dynamics especially in light of the drug resistance aspect. In this paper, a mathematical model that illustrates the transmission dynamics of a wild-type influenza strain and the development and transmission of drug-resistant influenza strain is formulated and analyzed.

2. Mathematical Model

2.1. Model Formulation.

The model subdivides the total population into five compartments: Susceptible (S), Vaccinated (V), Infected with Wild-type strain (I_w), Infected with Resistant strain (I_R), and Recovered (R). Individuals in a given compartment are assumed to have similar characteristics. Parameters vary from compartment to compartment but are identical for all individuals in a given compartment. Individuals enter the population at the rate of π, and all recruited individuals are assumed to be susceptible. The Susceptible get infected after effective contact with either the Infected with Wild-type strain or the Infected with Resistant strain. The force of infection is given by either $\lambda_1 = \beta_w I_w$ (Infection by Wild-type strain) or $\lambda_2 = \overline{\beta_r} I_R$ (Infection by Resistant strain), where $\overline{\beta_r} = f(\beta_r, b)$. Parameters β_w and

β_r refer to the transmission rate of wild-type strain and resistant strain, respectively. Parameter b is the rate of developing drug resistance. The susceptible can only be infected by one strain at a time. The rate of vaccination is ϕ. The vaccinated can also become infected with either the wild-type strain or the resistant strain. This depends on the vaccine efficacy. When the vaccine efficacy is 100%, the vaccinated cannot become infected. Individuals who are infected with the wild-type strain are treated and recover at the rate of α, while those who are infected with the resistant strain recover at the rate of α_r. The wild-type strain is assumed to mutate to resistant strain, and hence, those infected with the wild type join those infected with the resistant strain at the rate of b. Individuals with wild-type strain and those with resistant strain suffer disease-induced death at the rates a_w and a_r, respectively. The recovered lose immunity at the rate of ϑ joins the susceptible class. Individuals in all the epidemiological compartments suffer natural death at the rate of μ. The model diagram is given in Figure 4.

2.2. Model Equations.

Given the dynamics described in Figure 4, the following system of nonlinear ordinary differential equations, with nonnegative initial conditions, describes the dynamics of influenza:

$$\frac{dS}{dt} = \pi + \vartheta R - (\phi + \mu + \lambda_1 + \lambda_2)S(t),$$

$$\frac{dV}{dt} = \phi S(t) - ((1-\varepsilon)\lambda_1 + (1-\varepsilon)\lambda_2 + \mu)V(t),$$

$$\frac{dI_w}{dt} = \lambda_1 S(t) + (1-\varepsilon)\lambda_1 V(t) - (b + \mu + a_w + \alpha)I_w(t),$$

$$\frac{dI_R}{dt} = \lambda_2 S(t) + (1-\varepsilon)\lambda_2 V(t) + bI_w(t) - (\mu + \alpha_r + a_r)I_R(t),$$

$$\frac{dR}{dt} = \alpha I_w(t) + \alpha_r I_R(t) - (\vartheta + \mu)R(t),$$

$$(1)$$

where $\lambda_1 = \beta_w I_w$ and $\lambda_2 = \beta_r(1 + b^2)I_R$.

We assume that all the model parameters are positive and the initial conditions of the model system (1) are given by

$$S(0) > 0, \ V(0) \geq 0, \ I_W(0) \geq 0, \ I_R(0) \geq 0, \ R(0) \geq 0. \quad (2)$$

Table 2 gives the description of the various parameters used in the model along with reasonable estimates of their values.

3. Model Analysis

3.1. Basic Properties

3.1.1. Positivity of Solutions.

The model system (1) monitors the changes in human population. It is therefore important to prove that the solutions of system (1) with nonnegative

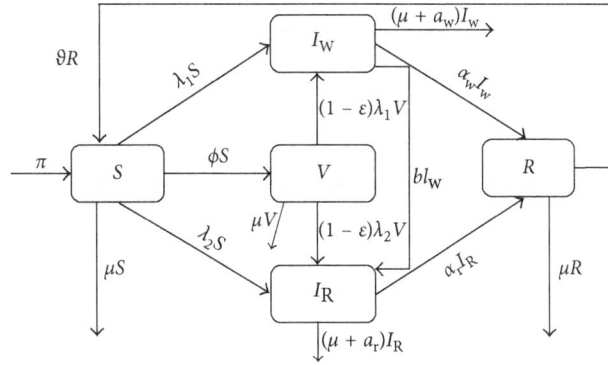

FIGURE 4: Schematic diagram showing population flow between different epidemiological classes.

TABLE 2: Description and values of parameters used.

Parameter	Description	Value	Reference
β_w	Transmission rate of wild-type strain	0.00102 day^{-1}	Estimated
β_r	Transmission rate of resistant strain	0.00026 day^{-1}	Estimated
ε	Vaccine efficacy	0.77	[58]
ϕ	Vaccination rate	0.00027375 day^{-1}	[59]
b	Rate of developing drug resistance	0.118	Estimated
α	Recovery rate for individuals in I_w class	0.1998 day^{-1}	[6]
α_r	Recovery rate for individuals in I_R class	0.0714 day^{-1}	Estimated
ϑ	Rate of losing immunity	0.00833 day^{-1}	[34]
a_w	Death rate due to infection with wild-type strain	0.01	[39]
$\frac{1}{\mu}$	Average human lifespan	70×365 days	Estimated
π	Recruitment rate	0.0381	Estimated
a_r	Death rate due to infection with resistant strain	0.021	Estimated

initial conditions will remain nonnegative for all $t > 0$. Thus, we have the following theorem:

Theorem 1. *Given that the initial conditions of system (1) are $S(0) > 0$, $V(0) \geq 0$, $I_W(0) \geq 0$, $I_R(0) \geq 0$, and $R(0) \geq 0$, the solutions $S(t)$, $V(t)$, $I_w(t)$, $I_R(t)$, and $R(t)$ are non-negative for all $t > 0$.*

Proof. Assume that

$$\widehat{t} = \sup\{t > 0 \ : \ S(t) > 0, \ V(t) > 0, \ I_w(t) > 0,$$
$$I_R(t) > 0, \ R(t) > 0\} \in [0, t]. \tag{3}$$

Thus $\widehat{t} > 0$, and it follows directly from the first equation of system (1) that

$$\frac{dS}{dt} \geq \pi - (\lambda_1 + \lambda_2 + \mu)S. \tag{4}$$

Using the integrating factor method to solve inequality (4), we have

$$\frac{d}{dt}\left\{S(t) \exp\left[\mu t + \int_0^t (\lambda_1(s) + \lambda_2(s))\, ds\right]\right\}$$
$$\geq \pi \exp\left[\mu t + \int_0^t (\lambda_1(s) + \lambda_2(s))\, ds\right]. \tag{5}$$

Integrating both sides yields

$$S(\widehat{t}) \exp\left[\mu \widehat{t} + \int_0^{\widehat{t}} (\lambda_1(s) + \lambda_2(s))\, ds\right]$$
$$\geq \int_0^{\widehat{t}} \pi \exp\left[\mu \widehat{t} + \int_0^{\widehat{t}} (\lambda_1(w) + \lambda_2(w))\, dw\right] d\widehat{t} + C, \tag{6}$$

where C is the constant of integration. Hence,

$$S(\widehat{t}) \geq S(0) \exp\left[-\left(\mu \widehat{t} + \int_0^{\widehat{t}} (\lambda_1(s) + \lambda_2(s))\, ds\right)\right]$$
$$+ \exp\left[-\left(\mu \widehat{t} + \int_0^{\widehat{t}} (\lambda_1(s) + \lambda_2(s))\, ds\right)\right]$$
$$\cdot \left(\int_0^{\widehat{t}} \pi \exp\left[\mu \widehat{t} + \int_0^{\widehat{t}} (\lambda_1(w) + \lambda_2(w))\, dw\right] d\widehat{t}\right) > 0. \tag{7}$$

Hence, $S(\widehat{t}) > 0 \ \forall \ \widehat{t} > 0$.
From the second equation in system (1), we obtain

$$\frac{dV}{dt} \geq -((1 - \varepsilon)\lambda_1 + (1 - \varepsilon)\lambda_2 + \mu)V. \tag{8}$$

Hence,

$$V(\hat{t}) \geq V(0)$$

$$\cdot \exp\left[-\left\{\mu\hat{t} + \int_0^{\hat{t}} (1-\varepsilon)\lambda_1(s) + (1-\varepsilon)\lambda_2(s)\,ds\right\}\right] > 0. \tag{9}$$

Similarly, it can be shown that

$$I_w(\hat{t}) \geq I_w(0)\exp\{-(b + \alpha + a_w + \mu)\hat{t}\} > 0,$$

$$I_R(\hat{t}) \geq I_R(0)\exp\{-(\alpha_r + a_r + \mu)\hat{t}\} > 0, \tag{10}$$

$$R(\hat{t}) \geq R(0)\exp\{-(\vartheta + \mu)\hat{t}\} > 0.$$

Therefore, all the solutions of system (1) with nonnegative initial conditions will remain nonnegative for all time $t > 0$.

3.1.2. Invariant Region.

We show that the total population is bounded for all time $t > 0$. The analysis of system (1) will therefore be analyzed in a region Ω of biological interest. Thus, we have the following theorem on the region that system (1) is restricted to.

Theorem 2. *The feasible region Ω defined by*

$$\Omega = \left\{(S(t),\ V(t),\ I_W(t),\ I_R(t),\ R(t)) \in R_5^+ \mid 0 \leq N\right.$$

$$\left. \leq \max\left\{N(0), \frac{\Pi}{\mu}\right\}\right\}, \tag{11}$$

with initial conditions $S(0) \geq 0$, $V(0) \geq 0$, $I_W(0) \geq 0$, $I_R(0) \geq 0$, and $R(0) \geq 0$, is positively invariant and attracting with respect to system (1) for all $t > 0$.

Proof. Summing up the equations in (1), we obtain that the total population satisfies the following differential equation:

$$\frac{dN(t)}{dt} = \pi - \mu N - a_w I_w - a_r I_R. \tag{12}$$

In the absence of influenza infection, it follows that

$$\frac{dN(t)}{dt} \leq \pi - \mu N. \tag{13}$$

It can easily be seen that

$$N(t) \leq \frac{\Pi}{\mu} + \left(N(0) - \frac{\Pi}{\mu}\right)\exp(-\mu t). \tag{14}$$

From (14), we observe that as $t \to \infty$, $N(t) \to (\Pi/\mu)$. So if $N(0) \leq (\Pi/\mu)$, then $\lim_{t\to\infty}N(t) = (\Pi/\mu)$. On the other hand, if $N(0) > (\Pi/\mu)$, then N will decrease to (Π/μ) as $t \to \infty$. This means that $N(t) \leq \max\{N(0),(\Pi/\mu)\}$.

Therefore, $N(t)$ is bounded above. Subsequently, $S(t)$, $V(t)$, $I_w(t)$, $I_R(t)$, and $R(t)$ are bounded above. Thus, in Ω, system (1) is well posed. Hence, it is sufficient to study the dynamics of the system in Ω.

3.2. Existence of Equilibrium Points.

In the absence of influenza ($I_w = I_R = 0$), system (1) has a disease-free equilibrium, which is given by

$$E_0 = \left(S^0,\ V^0,\ 0,\ 0,\ 0\right) = \left(\frac{\Pi}{\phi + \mu},\ \frac{\phi\Pi}{\mu(\phi + \mu)},\ 0,\ 0,\ 0\right). \tag{15}$$

3.2.1. The Control Reproduction Number.

The control reproduction number, R_c, is a key threshold that determines the behaviour of the system in the presence of vaccination. In order to analyze the stability of system (1), we obtain the threshold condition for the establishment of the disease. Thus, we employ next-generation matrix operator method as explained in [60]. The matrices of new infections and transition terms evaluated at the disease-free equilibrium are given by

$$\mathbf{F} = \begin{bmatrix} \dfrac{\Pi\beta_w(\phi(1-\varepsilon) + \mu)}{\mu(\mu + \phi)} & 0 \\[3ex] 0 & \dfrac{\Pi\overline{\beta}_r(\phi(1-\varepsilon) + \mu)}{\mu(\mu + \phi)} \end{bmatrix},$$

$$\mathbf{V} = \begin{bmatrix} b + \alpha + \mu + a_w & 0 \\ -b & \mu + a_r + \alpha_r \end{bmatrix}. \tag{16}$$

The dominant eigenvalue corresponding to the spectral radius $\rho(\mathbf{FV}^{-1})$ of the matrix $\mathbf{FV}^{-1}$ is the control reproduction number, which is given by

$$R_c = \max\{R_{cw},\ R_{cr}\}, \tag{17}$$

where

$$R_{cw} = \frac{\beta_w\pi(\mu + \phi(1-\varepsilon))}{\mu(\phi + \mu)(\alpha + b + a_w + \mu)},$$

$$R_{cr} = \frac{\overline{\beta}_r\pi(\mu + (1-\varepsilon)\phi)}{\mu(\phi + \mu)(\alpha_r + a_r + \mu)}. \tag{18}$$

R_{cw} is a measure of the average number of secondary wild-type influenza infections caused by a single infected individual introduced into the model population. On the other hand, R_{cr} gives the average number of secondary resistant influenza infections caused by one infected individual introduced into the model population.

From Theorem 2 in [60], we have the following results.

Proposition 1. *The disease-free equilibrium is locally asymptotically stable whenever R_c is less than unity and unstable otherwise.*

Proof. The Jacobian matrix evaluated at E_0 is obtained as

$$J(E_0) = \begin{bmatrix} -\phi - \mu & 0 & -\beta_w S^0 & -\overline{\beta_r} S^0 & \vartheta \\ \phi & -\mu & -(1-\varepsilon)\beta_w V^0 & -(1-\varepsilon)\overline{\beta_r} V^0 & 0 \\ 0 & 0 & \beta_w S^0 + (1-\varepsilon)\beta_w V^0 - Q_1 & 0 & 0 \\ 0 & 0 & b & \overline{\beta_r} S^0 + (1-\varepsilon)\overline{\beta_r} V^0 - Q_2 & 0 \\ 0 & 0 & \alpha & \alpha_r & -\vartheta - \mu \end{bmatrix},$$

(19)

where $Q_1 = \alpha + b + a_w + \mu$ and $Q_2 = \alpha_r + a_r + \mu$.

For the DFE to be locally stable, the eigenvalues of $J(E_0)$ must have negative real parts.

The characteristic polynomial of $J(E_0)$ is given by

$$P(\lambda) = (\lambda + \mu)(\lambda + \mu + \vartheta)(\lambda + \mu + \phi)$$
$$\cdot \left(\mu(\mu + \phi)(a_r + \lambda + \mu + \alpha_r) - \Pi\overline{\beta_r}(\mu - \varepsilon\phi + \phi) \right)$$
$$\cdot \left(\mu(\mu + \phi)(a_w + \alpha + b + \lambda + \mu) - \Pi\beta_w(\mu - \varepsilon\phi + \phi) \right).$$

(20)

Clearly, the following eigenvalues with negative real parts can be obtained from the polynomial (20): $\lambda_1 = -\mu$, $\lambda_2 = -\mu - \vartheta$, and $\lambda_3 = -\mu - \phi$. Other roots can be obtained from the remaining part of the polynomial (20), which is given by

$$P_1(\lambda) = \left(\mu(\mu + \phi)(a_r + \lambda + \mu + \alpha_r) - \Pi\overline{\beta_r}(\mu - \varepsilon\phi + \phi) \right)$$
$$\cdot \left(\mu(\mu + \phi)(a_w + \alpha + b + \lambda + \mu) - \Pi\beta_w(\mu - \varepsilon\phi + \phi) \right).$$

(21)

Hence, we obtain

$$\lambda_4 = \frac{-\mu(\mu + \phi)(a_r + \mu + \alpha_r) + \pi\overline{\beta_r}(\mu + \phi(1 - \varepsilon))}{\mu(\mu + \phi)},$$

$$\therefore \lambda_4 = -Q_2(1 - R_{cr}),$$

$$\lambda_5 = \frac{-\mu(\mu + \phi)(b + \alpha + \mu + a_w) + \pi\beta_w(\mu + \phi(1 - \varepsilon))}{\mu(\mu + \phi)},$$

$$\therefore \lambda_5 = -Q_1(1 - R_{cw}).$$

(22)

From (22), if $R_{cr} < 1$, then $\lambda_4 < 0$, and if $R_{cw} < 1$, then $\lambda_5 < 0$.

We therefore conclude that the disease-free equilibrium E_0 is locally asymptotically stable whenever $R_c < 1$. The biological implication of Proposition 1 is that if $R_c < 1$, influenza will be eliminated from the model population provided that the initial sizes of the subpopulations in various compartments of model (1) are in the basin of attraction of the influenza-free equilibrium.

3.2.2. Effective Reproduction Number. The effective reproduction number $(R_e(t))$ is the actual average number of secondary cases per primary case at calendar time t (for $t > 0$) [61]. $R_e(t)$ shows time-dependent variation due to decline in susceptible individuals and the implementation of control measures. The effective reproduction number is therefore used to characterize transmissibility in a population that is not entirely susceptible. It is the basic reproduction number times the fraction of the population that is susceptible to infection at time t.

The basic reproduction number (R_0) is the average number of secondary infections generated by a single infective individual in a totally susceptible population [60]. From model (1), the basic reproduction number is obtained as

$$R_0 = \max\left\{ \frac{\beta_w \pi \mu}{\mu^2(\alpha + b + a_w + \mu)}, \frac{\overline{\beta_r} \pi \mu}{\mu^2(\alpha_r + a_r + \mu)} \right\}.$$

(23)

Thus, the effective reproduction number $R_e(t) = f R_0$, where f is the fraction of population susceptible to infection at a time t.

3.3. Endemic Equilibria. The endemic equilibria of model (1) are the steady states where influenza may persist in the population. This happens when at least one of the infected classes of the model is nonempty. The rate of change in populations in each compartment is zero at equilibrium; hence, the right-hand side of (1) is set to zero as follows:

$$0 = \pi + \vartheta R^* - (\phi + \mu + \lambda_1 + \lambda_2)S^*,$$
$$0 = \phi S^* - ((1 - \varepsilon)\lambda_1 + (1 - \varepsilon)\lambda_2 + \mu)V^*,$$
$$0 = \lambda_1 S^* + (1 - \varepsilon)\lambda_1 V^* - (b + \mu + a_w + \alpha)I_w^*,$$
$$0 = \lambda_2 S^* + (1 - \varepsilon)\lambda_2 V^* + bI_w^* - (\mu + \alpha_r + a_r)I_R^*,$$
$$0 = \alpha I_w^* + \alpha_r I_R^* - (\vartheta + \mu)R^*.$$

(24)

Next, S^*, V^*, I_w^*, I_R^*, and R^* are solved from (24) in terms of the two forces of infection, λ_1 and λ_2 to obtain

$$S^* = \frac{\pi + \vartheta R^*}{\mu + \phi + \lambda_1 + \lambda_2},$$

$$V^* = \frac{(\phi(\pi + \vartheta R^*))}{((\mu + \phi + \lambda_1 + \lambda_2)(\mu - (-1 + \varepsilon)\lambda_1 - (-1 + \varepsilon)\lambda_2))},$$

$$I_w^* = \frac{((\pi + \vartheta R^*)\lambda_1(\mu + \phi - \varepsilon\phi - (-1 + \varepsilon)\lambda_1 - (-1 + \varepsilon))\lambda_2))}{(Q_1(\mu + \phi + \lambda_1 + \lambda_2)(\mu - (-1 + \varepsilon)\lambda_1 - (-1 + \varepsilon)\lambda_2))},$$

$$I_R^* = \frac{((\pi + \vartheta R^*)(\mu + \phi - \varepsilon\phi - (-1 + \varepsilon)\lambda_1 - (-1 + \varepsilon)\lambda_2)(b\lambda_1 + Q_1\lambda_2))}{(Q_1 Q_2(\mu + \phi + \lambda_1 + \lambda_2)(\mu - (-1 + \varepsilon)\lambda_1 - (-1 + \varepsilon)\lambda_2))},$$

$$R^* = \frac{(\pi(\mu + \phi - \varepsilon\phi - (-1 + \varepsilon)\lambda_1 - (-1 + \varepsilon)\lambda_2(\alpha Q_2\lambda_1 + \alpha_r(b\lambda_1 + Q_1\lambda_2))))}{(-\vartheta(\alpha Q_2 + b\alpha_r)\lambda_1(\mu + \phi - \varepsilon\phi - (-1 + \varepsilon)\lambda_1 + \lambda_2 - \varepsilon\lambda_2) + Q_4)}.$$

(25)

where

$$Q_1 = \alpha + b + a_w + \mu,$$
$$Q_2 = \alpha_r + a_r + \mu,$$
$$Q_3 = \vartheta + \mu,$$
$$Q_4 = Q_1(\vartheta\alpha_r\lambda_2(-\mu + (-1 + \varepsilon)\phi + (-1 + \varepsilon)\lambda_1$$
$$+ (-1 + \varepsilon)\lambda_2 + Q_2 Q_3)(\mu + \phi + \lambda_1 + \lambda_2)$$
$$\cdot (\mu - (-1 + \varepsilon)\lambda_1 + \lambda_2 - \varepsilon\lambda_2).$$

(26)

Upon dividing and simplifying the two expressions for λ_1 and λ_2, we obtain the following polynomial:

$$p(\lambda_1, \lambda_2) = \pi Q_3 \lambda_1 \Big(\big(\mu + \phi - \varepsilon\phi - (-1+\varepsilon)\lambda_1 - (-1+\varepsilon)\lambda_2 \big)$$
$$\cdot \big(-Q_2 \beta_w \lambda_2 + \overline{\beta_r}(b\lambda_1 + Q_1\lambda_2) \big) \Big). \tag{27}$$

Note that if $\lambda_1 = 0$ in the equation obtained when polynomial (27) is set to zero, then clearly $\lambda_2 = 0$. This gives the disease-free equilibrium previously obtained in (15). The solutions to the remaining part of the polynomial (27), described by (28), define the possible endemic states of system (1).

$$p(\lambda_1^*, \lambda_2^*) = \big(\mu + \phi - \varepsilon\phi - (-1+\varepsilon)\lambda_1 - (-1+\varepsilon)\lambda_2 \big)$$
$$\cdot \big(-Q_2 \beta_w \lambda_2 + \overline{\beta_r}(b\lambda_1 + Q_1\lambda_2) \big) = 0. \tag{28}$$

The existence of the endemic equilibrium points for system (1) depends on the solutions of (28), and the roots of the equation must be real and positive to guarantee existence of the endemic equilibrium point(s). Due to mathematical complexity, we are not able to express explicitly the endemic steady states of system (1). We shall however represent the polynomial in (28) graphically as shown in Figure 5.

From the surface plot in Figure 5, it can be observed that there exist endemic steady states for the two-strain influenza model. The steady states only exist for positive values of $p(\lambda_1, \lambda_2)$. The endemic equilibria exist in the case where only the wild-type strain is present, the case where only the resistant strain exists or both strains coexist.

3.3.1. Existence of an Endemic State with Wild-Type Strain Only.

There exists an endemic state when the wild-type strain persists and the resistant strain dies out. Solving (1) in terms of λ_1 yields

$$S^* = \frac{\pi + \vartheta R^*}{\mu + \phi + \lambda_1},$$

$$V^* = \frac{(\phi(\pi + \vartheta R^*))}{((\mu + \phi + \lambda_1)(\mu + \lambda_1 - \varepsilon\lambda_1))},$$

$$I_w^* = \frac{-((\pi + R^*)\lambda_1(-\mu - \phi + \varepsilon\phi - \lambda_1 + \varepsilon\lambda_1))}{(Q_1(\mu + \phi + \lambda_1)(\mu + \lambda_1 - \varepsilon\lambda_1))},$$

$$R^* = \frac{\alpha\pi\lambda_1(\mu + \phi - \varepsilon\phi - (-1+\varepsilon))}{(Q_1 Q_3(\mu + \phi + \lambda_1)(\mu - (-1+\varepsilon)\lambda_1) + \alpha\vartheta\lambda_1(-\mu + (-1+\varepsilon)\phi + (-1+\varepsilon\lambda_1)))}. \tag{29}$$

Substituting I_w^* obtained in (29) into λ_1^* yields polynomial (30) given by

$$\lambda_1 \big(Q_1 Q_3(\mu + \phi + \lambda_1)(\mu - (-1+\varepsilon)\lambda_1) \big)$$
$$- \big(\mu + \phi - \varepsilon\phi - (-1+\varepsilon)\lambda_1 \big)\big(\phi Q_3 \beta_w + \alpha\vartheta\lambda_1 \big). \tag{30}$$

It is important to note that when $\lambda_1 = 0$, a wild-type strain-free equilibrium is obtained which is given by

$$\big(S^0, V^0, 0, 0 \big) = \left(\frac{\Pi}{\phi + \mu}, \frac{\phi\Pi}{\mu(\phi + \mu)}, 0, 0 \right). \tag{31}$$

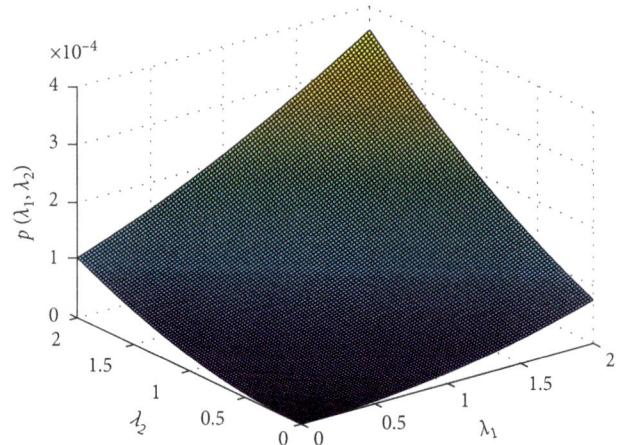

FIGURE 5: Endemic equilibrium points of the two-strain influenza model.

The remaining part of polynomial (30) can be expressed as

$$P(\lambda_1) = D_2\lambda_1^2 + D_1\lambda_1 + D_0. \tag{32}$$

where

$$D_2 = (1-\varepsilon)(Q_1 Q_3 - \alpha\vartheta),$$
$$D_1 = Q_3\big((-(-1+\varepsilon)\mu + \phi - \varepsilon\phi)Q_1 + (-1+\varepsilon)\pi\beta_w \big)$$
$$- \alpha(\mu + \phi - \varepsilon\phi)\vartheta, \tag{33}$$
$$D_0 = Q_3\big(\mu(\mu + \phi)Q_1(1 - R_{cw}) \big).$$

The roots of the quadratic equation obtained when the polynomial in (32) is set to zero can be obtained by the quadratic formula given by

$$\lambda_1 = \frac{-D_1 \pm \sqrt{D_1^2 - 4D_2 D_0}}{2D_2}. \tag{34}$$

Note that $D_0 > 0$ if $R_{cw} < 1$, $D_0 = 0$ if $R_{cw} = 1$, and $D_0 < 0$ if $R_{cw} > 1$. If $D_0 < 0$, the discriminant $\Delta = D_1^2 - 4D_2 D_0 > 0$ and (32) have a unique positive solution, and hence, the model system (1) has a unique wild-type influenza persistent equilibrium. If $R_{cw} < 1$, then $D_0 > 0$, and by adding the conditions $D_1 < 0$ and $\Delta > 0$, two positive real equilibria are obtained. If $R_{cw} = 1$, then $D_0 = 0$, and there is a unique nonzero solution of (32) which is positive if and only if $D_1 < 0$. The following theorem summarizes the existence of the wild-type influenza endemic equilibria.

Theorem 3. *The model system (1) has*

(i) *a unique endemic equilibrium if $R_{cw} > 1$*

(ii) *two endemic equilibria if $R_{cw} < 1$, $D_1 < 0$, and $\Delta > 0$*

(iii) *one positive equilibrium for $R_{cw} = 1$ and $D_1 < 0$*

(iv) *no wild-type influenza endemic equilibrium otherwise*

Epidemiologically, Theorem 3 item (ii) implies that bringing R_{cw} below unity does not suffice for the eradication of wild-type influenza since system (1) exhibits backward bifurcation when $R_{cw} < 1$. The existence of backward bifurcation indicates that in the neighbourhood of 1, for $R_{cw} < 1$, a stable wild-type influenza-free equilibrium coexists with a stable wild-type influenza persistent equilibrium. In order to eradicate the disease, the control reproduction R_{cw} should be decreased below the critical value R_{cw}^*. To obtain R_{cw}^*, the discriminant in (32) is set to zero and R_{cw} made the subject of the relation. This yields

$$R_{cw}^* = 1 - \frac{D_1^2}{4\mu(\mu + \phi)Q_1 Q_3 D_2}. \quad (35)$$

It follows that backward bifurcation occurs for values of R_{cw} such that $R_{cw}^* < R_{cw} < 1$. This is illustrated by Figure 6.

3.3.2. Existence of Resistant Influenza Strain Only Endemic State. There exists an endemic state when the resistant strain persists and the wild-type strain dies out. Solving (1) in terms of λ_2 and substituting I_R^* into λ_2^* yields the following equation:

$$\lambda_2\left(-Q_2 Q_3\left(\mu + \phi + \lambda_2\right)\left(\mu - (-1 + \varepsilon)\lambda_2\right)\right.$$
$$\left. + \left(\mu + \phi - \varepsilon\phi - (-1 + \varepsilon)\lambda_2\right)\left(\phi Q_3\overline{\beta_r} + \alpha_r \vartheta \lambda_2\right)\right) = 0. \quad (36)$$

When $\lambda_2 = 0$, resistant influenza-free equilibrium is obtained. The remaining part of polynomial (36) can be expressed as

$$P(\lambda_2) = A_2\lambda_2^2 + A_1\lambda_2 + A_0, \quad (37)$$

where

$$A_2 = (-1 + \varepsilon)\left(Q_2 Q_3 - \alpha_r \vartheta\right),$$
$$A_1 = \alpha_r \phi \vartheta(\varepsilon - 1) + Q_2 Q_3 \mu(1 - \varepsilon) + Q_2 Q_3 \phi(1 - \varepsilon)$$
$$\quad + Q_3\overline{\beta_r}\pi(\varepsilon - 1) - \alpha_r \mu \vartheta, \quad (38)$$
$$A_0 = Q_3\left(\mu(\mu + \phi)Q_2\left(1 - R_{cr}\right)\right).$$

Using the procedure as in Section 3.3.1, it can be shown that the system exhibits a backward bifurcation when $R_{cr} < 1$. This is illustrated by Figure 7.

4. Sensitivity Analysis

In order to curb the spread of influenza in a given population, it is essential to know the relative importance of the different parameters responsible for its transmission and prevalence. Influenza transmission and endemicity are directly related to R_c. As in [62, 63], the normalized forward sensitivity analysis is used for this model. The normalized sensitivity index which measures the relative change in a parameter k, with respect to the reproduction number R_c is given by $P_q = (k/R_c)(\partial R_c/\partial k)$,[64]. The sign of P_q determines the direction of changes, increasing (for positive P_q) and decreasing (for negative P_q) [65]. The sensitivity indices of the model reproduction number to the parameters in the model at the parameter values described in Table 2 are calculated. These indices reveal how crucial each parameter is to disease transmission and spread making it possible to

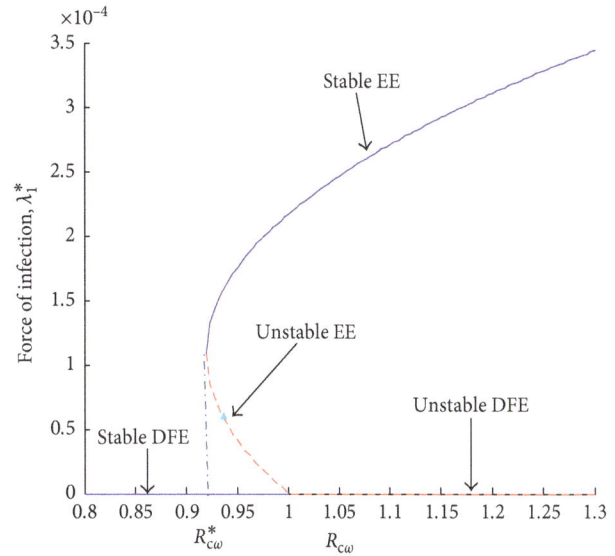

FIGURE 6: Force of infection, λ_1, versus control reproduction number, R_{cw}.

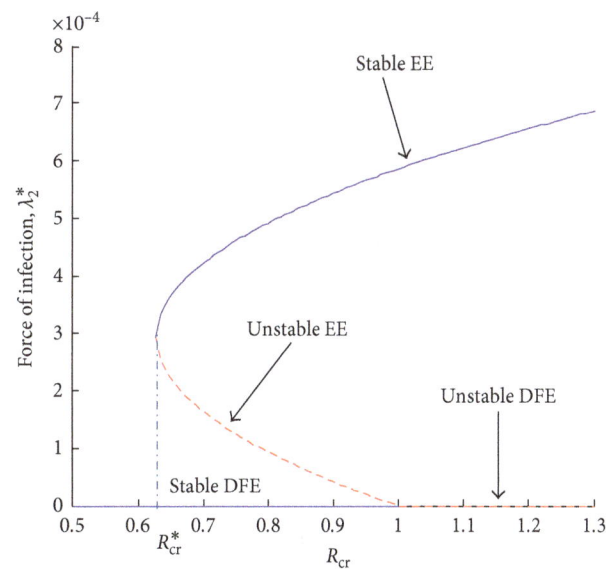

FIGURE 7: Force of infection, λ_2, versus control reproduction number, R_{cr}.

discover parameters that have a high impact on R_c and should be targeted by intervention strategies. The calculated sensitivity indices of R_c are given in Table 3.

Small variations in a highly sensitive parameter lead to large quantitative changes; hence, caution should be taken when handling such a parameter. A positive sensitivity index indicates that R_c is an increasing function of the corresponding parameter, and hence, an increase in the parameter while other factors are held constant leads to an increase in the reproduction number and could lead to disease spread [65]. On the other hand, a negative sensitivity index shows that an increase in the parameter while other factors are held constant leads to a decrease in the reproduction number, which could then lead to disease

TABLE 3: Sensitivity indices of R_{cw} and R_{cr}.

Parameter	Sensitivity index
Sensitivity indices of R_{cw}	
β_w	0.99999
π	1
ϕ	−0.2582418982
ε	−2.064509968
α	−0.6094452335
a_w	−0.0305027644
b	−0.3599326204
μ	−0.7418774828
Sensitivity indices of R_{cr}	
β_r	0.99999
π	1
b	0.02746556942
ϕ	−0.2582418983
ε	−2.064509968
α_r	−0.7724001063
a_r	−0.2271765018
μ	−0.7421814939

control. For instance, if the vaccination rate, ϕ, is increased by 10%, R_c would decrease by about 2.5%. Increasing the recruitment rate by 10% increases the R_c by 10%.

5. Numerical Simulation

5.1. Effects of Drug Resistance. For the parameter values in Table 2, as the drug resistance increases, the changes in the reproduction numbers can be observed as shown in Figure 8.

In conformity with the expectation, increased drug resistance leads to an increase in R_{cr}. It can also be observed that R_{cw} decreases with increased drug resistance. The implication of increased drug resistance on infected population is discussed in the next section.

5.1.1. Effects of Drug Resistance on Infected Population. The rate of drug resistance is varied holding all the other parameter values constant. Figures 9 and 10 are obtained.

It can be observed from Figure 9 that when there is no development of drug resistance ($b = 0$), the number of individuals infected with resistant strain decreases to zero. An increase in the rate of drug resistance leads to an increase in the number of individuals infected with resistant strain.

Next, the effect of drug resistance on individuals infected with wild-type strain is investigated.

From Figure 10, it can be observed that an increase in the rate of drug resistance leads to a decrease in the number of individuals infected with wild-type strain. For instance, when $b = 1$, the number of individuals infected with wild-type strain decrease to zero. This could be attributed to the mutation of the wild-type strain to resistant strain.

5.2. Effect of Vaccination on Reproduction Number and on Influenza Prevalence in the Model Population. Figures 11 and 12 show the population dynamics of the infected individuals in a case where there is no vaccination. The reproduction

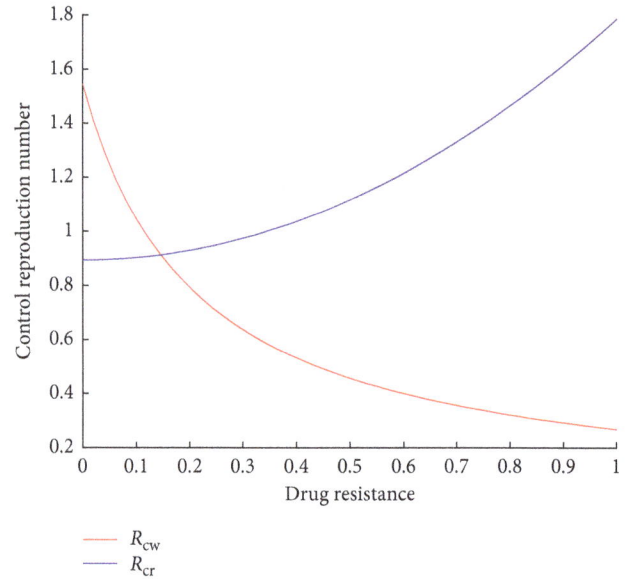

FIGURE 8: Relationship between reproduction numbers and drug resistance.

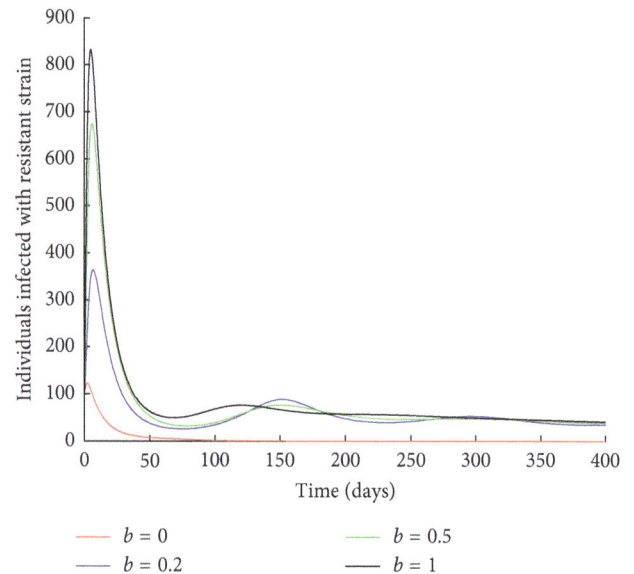

FIGURE 9: Effect of drug resistance on I_R class.

number of the resistant strain is obtained as 2.7762, while that of the wild-type strain is obtained as 3.0288.

Note that the reproduction number for the two cases is greater than one. It can be observed from Figures 11 and 12 that the resistant strain and the wild-type strain persist in the population.

Next, numerical simulation is done in the case where there is vaccination. Using the parameter values in Table 2, Figures 13 and 14 are obtained. The control reproduction number (17), R_{cr}, is obtained as 0.9059, and R_{cw} is obtained as 0.9883.

Note that the reproduction number in this case is less than one. Vaccination reduces the reproduction number. However, from Figures 13 and 14, it can be observed that

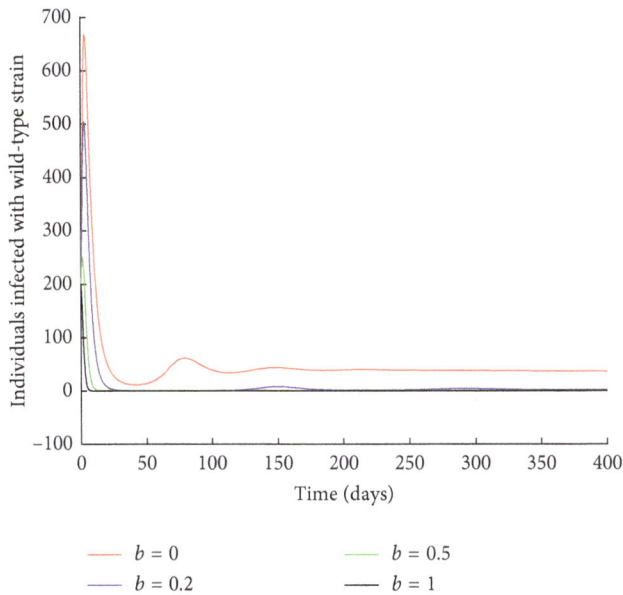

FIGURE 10: Effect of drug resistance on I_w class.

- $b = 0$
- $b = 0.2$
- $b = 0.5$
- $b = 1$

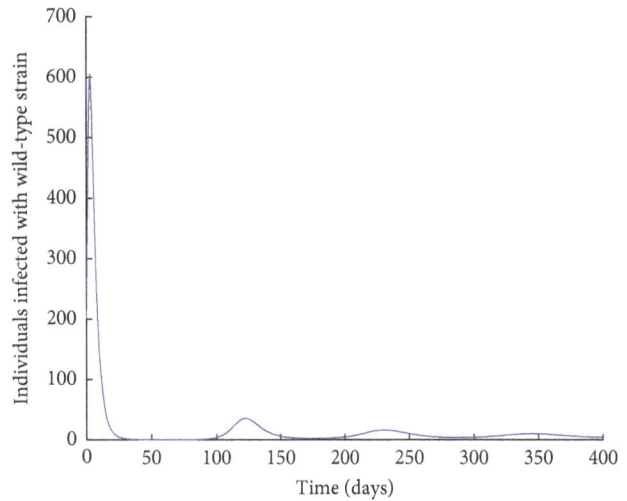

FIGURE 12: I_w individuals with no vaccination.

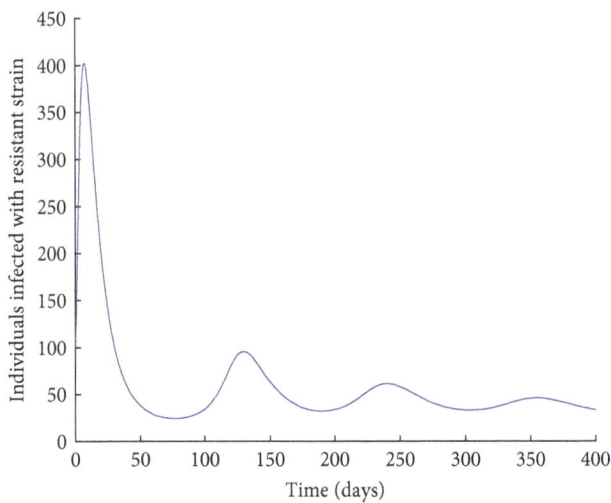

FIGURE 11: I_R individuals with no vaccination.

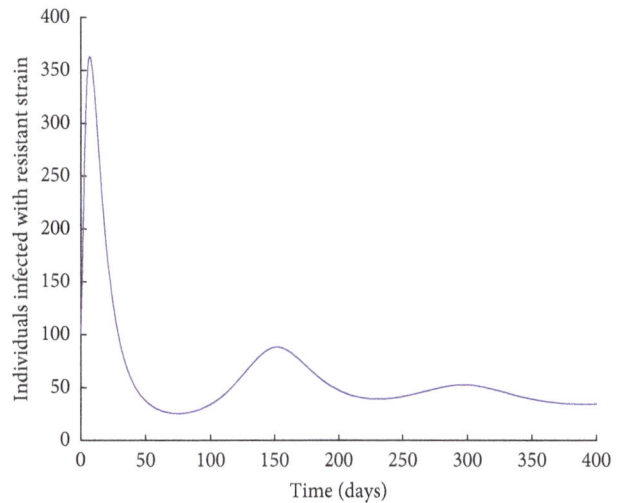

FIGURE 13: I_R individuals with vaccination.

both the resistant strain and the wild-type strain do not completely die out from the population despite the reproduction number being less than one. These findings are consistent with Figures 6 and 7 obtained in Sections 3.3.1 and 3.3.2, respectively. This shows that bringing the reproduction number below unity does not describe the necessary effort to curb the spread of influenza. Therefore, the intervention strategies should be carefully implemented to bring the reproduction number below the critical value. It can also be observed from Figures 11–14 that the level of persistence of the resistant strain is higher than that of the wild-type strain.

5.3. Effect of Transmission Rates β_w and β_r on Infected Population

5.3.1. Case 1: Effect of β_w on I_w Individuals. From Figure 15, it can be observed that the higher the transmission rate, the

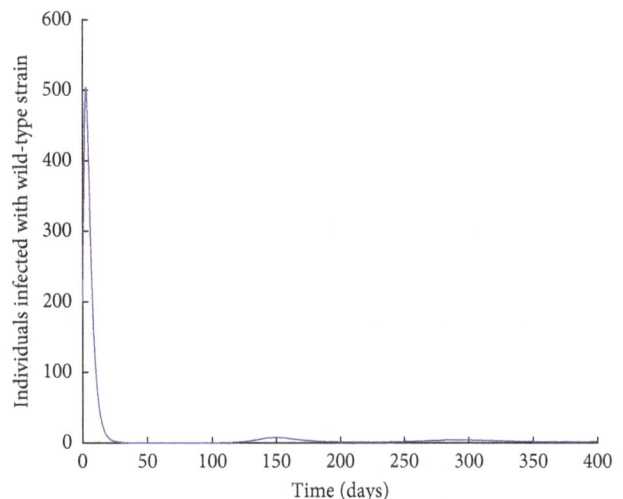

FIGURE 14: I_w individuals with vaccination.

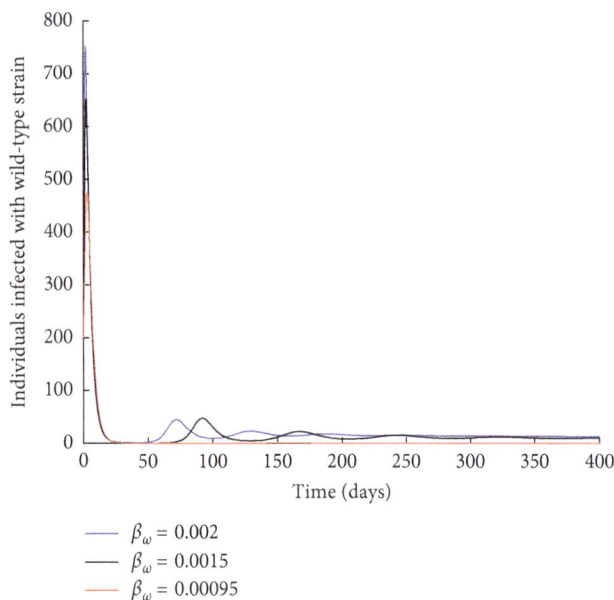

FIGURE 15: Effect of β_w on individuals infected with wild-type strain.

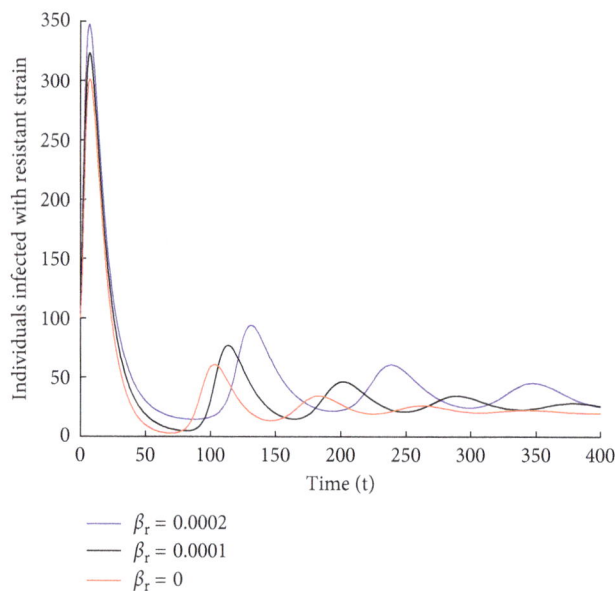

FIGURE 16: Effect of β_r on individuals infected with resistant strain.

higher the number of infected individuals. The number of infected individuals drastically decreases to zero within a short period of time but then starts to increase again shortly after and the disease does not completely die out after that (this is when $\beta_w = 0.002$ and 0.0015). When $\beta_w = 0.00095$, it can be observed that the number of infected individuals declines to zero and the disease completely dies out. It should be noted that for this case, the $R_{cw} = 0.9205$ which is below the critical value $R_{cw}^* = 0.9351$.

5.3.2. Case 2: Effect of β_r on I_R Individuals. It is observed from Figure 16 that the higher the transmission rate, the higher the number of infected individuals. It is also interesting to note that when $\beta_r = 0$, there still exist individuals infected with the resistant strain and the strain persists in the population. This shows that curbing the spread of the resistant strain is quite difficult. This could be due to the fact that the spread of the resistant strain is fuelled by two processes: transmission and mutation of the wild-type strain to resistant strain.

6. Conclusion

To completely wipe out influenza from a population continues to prove difficult. This is because the virus evolves very rapidly and is able to change from one season to the other. This is extensively explained in [3, 7, 9]. Results from our model show that vaccination reduces the reproduction number, and hence, it could be used as a control strategy. However, caution should be taken because influenza can still persist in case there is backward bifurcation. Results also show that it is easier to curtail the spread of the wild-type strain especially in a given season than the resistant strain. This could be through social distancing and issuing travel

bans to areas affected with the virus. For the resistant strain, social distancing could also be used as a control strategy in addition to reducing the mutation of the wild-type strain.

Conflicts of Interest

The authors declare that there are no conflicts of interest regarding the publication of this article.

References

[1] M. C. White and A. C. Lowen, "Implications of segment mismatch for influenza a virus evolution," *Journal of General Virology*, vol. 99, no. 1, pp. 3–16, 2017.

[2] J. K. Taubenberger and D. M. Morens, "Influenza viruses: breaking all the rules," *mBio*, vol. 4, no. 4, article e00365-13, 2013.

[3] CDC, *How the Flu Virus Can Change: Drift and Shift*, CDC, Atlanta, GA, USA, 2017, https://www.cdc.gov/flu/about/viruses/change.htm.

[4] G. J. Smith, D. Vijaykrishna, J. Bahl et al., "Origins and evolutionary genomics of the 2009 swine-origin H1N1 influenza a epidemic," *Nature*, vol. 459, no. 7250, p. 1122, 2009.

[5] WHO, *WHO/Europe—Influenza-Data and Statistics*, WHO, Geneva, Switzerland, 2017, http://www.euro.who.int/en/health-topics/communicable-diseases/influenza/data-and-statistics.

[6] CDC, *Clinical Signs and Symptoms of Influenza: Health Professionals–CDC*, CDC, Atlanta, GA, USA, 2017, https://www.cdc.gov/flu/professionals/acip/clinical.htm.

[7] A. Moscona, "Neuraminidase inhibitors for influenza," *New England Journal of Medicine*, vol. 353, no. 13, pp. 1363–1373, 2005.

[8] CDC, *Preventing the Flu: Good Health Habits Can Help Stop Germs–CDC*, CDC, Atlanta, GA, USA, 2017, https://www.cdc.gov/flu/protect/habits.htm.

[9] D. M. Matheka, J. Mokaya, and M. Maritim, "Overview of influenza virus infections in Kenya: past, present and future," *Pan African medical journal*, vol. 14, 2013.

[10] K. Cheng and P. Leung, "What happened in china during the 1918 influenza pandemic?," *International Journal of Infectious Diseases*, vol. 11, no. 4, pp. 360–364, 2007.

[11] N. Goeyvaerts, L. Willem, K. Van Kerckhove et al., "Estimating dynamic transmission model parameters for seasonal influenza by fitting to age and season-specific influenza-like illness incidence," *Epidemics*, vol. 13, pp. 1–9, 2015.

[12] P. R. Saunders-Hastings and D. Krewski, "Reviewing the history of pandemic influenza: understanding patterns of emergence and transmission," *Pathogens*, vol. 5, no. 4, p. 66, 2016.

[13] CDC, *Past Pandemics*, CDC, Atlanta, GA, USA, 2017, https://www.cdc.gov/flu/pandemic-resources/basics/past-pandemics.html.

[14] WHO, *WHO—Influenza*, WHO, Geneva, Switzerland, 2017, http://www.who.int/mediacentre/factsheets/2003/fs211/en/.

[15] CDC, *Seasonal Flu Death Estimate Increases Worldwide*, CDC, Atlanta, GA, USA, 2017, https://www.cdc.gov/media/releases/2017/p1213-flu-death-estimate.html.

[16] R. Hope-Simpson, "The role of season in the epidemiology of influenza," *Epidemiology & Infection*, vol. 86, no. 1, pp. 35–47, 1981.

[17] B. S. Finkelman, C. Viboud, K. Koelle, M. J. Ferrari, N. Bharti, and B. T. Grenfell, "Global patterns in seasonal activity of influenza A/H3N2, A/H1N1, and B from 1997 to 2005: viral coexistence and latitudinal gradients," *PLoS One*, vol. 2, no. 12, Article ID e1296, 2007.

[18] L. P.-C. Shek and B.-W. Lee, "Epidemiology and seasonality of respiratory tract virus infections in the tropics," *Paediatric Respiratory Reviews*, vol. 4, no. 2, pp. 105–111, 2003.

[19] M. A. Katz, B. D. Schoub, J. M. Heraud, R. F. Breiman, M. K. Njenga, and M.-A. Widdowson, "Influenza in Africa: uncovering the epidemiology of a long-overlooked disease," *Journal of Infectious Diseases*, vol. 206, no. 1, pp. S1–S4, 2012.

[20] WHO, *Influenza*, WHO, Geneva, Switzerland, 2017, http://www.who.int/influenza/gisrs_laboratory/updates/summaryreport_20171002/en/.

[21] WHO, *Influenza*, WHO, Geneva, Switzerland, 2018, http://www.who.int/influenza/gisrs_laboratory/updates/summaryreport/en/.

[22] RGA, *Seasonal Influenza and Mortality*, RGA, St. Louis, MO, USA, 2018, https://www.rgare.com/knowledge-center/articles/seasonal-influenza-and-mortality.

[23] A. Ku and L. Chan, "The first case of H5N1 avian influenza infection in a human with complications of adult respiratory distress syndrome and Reye's syndrome," *Journal of Paediatrics and Child Health*, vol. 35, no. 2, pp. 207–209, 1999.

[24] T. T. Hien, N. T. Liem, N. T. Dung et al., "Avian influenza a (H5N1) in 10 patients in Vietnam," *New England Journal of Medicine*, vol. 350, no. 12, pp. 1179–1188, 2004.

[25] R. Gao, B. Cao, Y. Hu et al., "Human infection with a novel avian-origin influenza a (H7N9) virus," *New England Journal of Medicine*, vol. 368, no. 20, pp. 1888–1897, 2013.

[26] B. Mazel-Sanchez, I. Boal-Carvalho, F. Silva, R. Dijkman, and M. Schmolke, "H5N1 influenza a virus PB1-F2 relieves HAX-1-mediated restriction of avian virus polymerase pa in human lung cells," *Journal of Virology*, vol. 92, no. 11, p. e00425–18, 2018.

[27] T. R. Hurtado, "Human influenza a (H5N1): a brief review and recommendations for travelers," *Wilderness & Environmental Medicine*, vol. 17, no. 4, pp. 276–281, 2006.

[28] F. Li, B. Choi, T. Sly, and A. Pak, "Finding the real case-fatality rate of H5N1 avian influenza," *Journal of Epidemiology & Community Health*, vol. 62, no. 6, pp. 555–559, 2008.

[29] WHO, *Influenza at the Human-Animal Interface*, WHO, Geneva, Switzerland, 2018, http://www.who.int/influenza/human_animal_interface/Influenza_Summary_IRA_HA_interface_25_01_2018_FINAL.pdf.

[30] H. Chen, H. Yuan, R. Gao et al., "Clinical and epidemiological characteristics of a fatal case of avian influenza a h10n8 virus infection: a descriptive study," *The Lancet*, vol. 383, no. 9918, pp. 714–721, 2014.

[31] Z. Zhang, R. Li, L. Jiang et al., "The complexity of human infected AIV H5N6 isolated from china," *BMC Infectious Diseases*, vol. 16, no. 1, p. 600, 2016.

[32] Y. Huang, X. Li, H. Zhang et al., "Human infection with an avian influenza a (H9N2) virus in the middle region of china," *Journal of Medical Virology*, vol. 87, no. 10, pp. 1641–1648, 2015.

[33] J. Yuan, L. Zhang, X. Kan et al., "Origin and molecular characteristics of a novel 2013 avian influenza a (H6N1) virus causing human infection in Taiwan," *Clinical Infectious Diseases*, vol. 57, no. 9, pp. 1367–1368, 2013.

[34] M. E. Alexander, C. Bowman, S. M. Moghadas, R. Summers, A. B. Gumel, and B. M. Sahai, "A vaccination model for transmission dynamics of influenza," *SIAM Journal on Applied Dynamical Systems*, vol. 3, no. 4, pp. 503–524, 2004.

[35] D. Guo, K. C. Li, T. R. Peters, B. M. Snively, K. A. Poehling, and X. Zhou, "Multi-scale modeling for the transmission of influenza and the evaluation of interventions toward it," *Scientific Reports*, vol. 5, no. 1, 2015.

[36] A. K. Srivastav and M. Ghosh, "Analysis of a simple influenza a (H1N1) model with optimal control," *World Journal of Modelling and Simulation*, vol. 12, no. 4, pp. 307–319, 2016.

[37] R. Mikolajczyk, R. Krumkamp, R. Bornemann, A. Ahmad, M. Schwehm, and H. Duerr, "Influenza–insights from mathematical modelling," *Deutsches Arzteblatt International*, vol. 106, no. 47, pp. 777–782, 2009.

[38] E. W. Larson, J. W. Dominik, A. H. Rowberg, and G. A. Higbee, "Influenza virus population dynamics in the respiratory tract of experimentally infected mice," *Infection and Immunity*, vol. 13, no. 2, pp. 438–447, 1976.

[39] M. Imran, T. Malik, A. R. Ansari, and A. Khan, "Mathematical analysis of swine influenza epidemic model with optimal control," *Japan Journal of Industrial and Applied Mathematics*, vol. 33, no. 1, pp. 269–296, 2016.

[40] S. Lee, G. Chowell, and C. Castillo-Chávez, "Optimal control for pandemic influenza: the role of limited antiviral treatment and isolation," *Journal of Theoretical Biology*, vol. 265, no. 2, pp. 136–150, 2010.

[41] O. Prosper, O. Saucedo, D. Thompson, G. Torres-Garcia, X. Wang, and C. Castillo-Chavez, "Modeling control strategies for concurrent epidemics of seasonal and pandemic H1N1 influenza," *Mathematical Biosciences and Engineering*, vol. 8, no. 1, pp. 141–170, 2011.

[42] M. Woolhouse and J. Farrar, "Policy: an intergovernmental panel on antimicrobial resistance," *Nature*, vol. 509, no. 7502, pp. 555–557, 2014.

[43] E. van der Vries, M. Schutten, P. Fraaij, C. Boucher, and A. Osterhaus, "Influenza virus resistance to antiviral therapy," *Advances in Pharmacology*, vol. 67, pp. 217–246, 2013.

[44] T. Li, M. C. Chan, and N. Lee, "Clinical implications of antiviral resistance in influenza," *Viruses*, vol. 7, no. 9, pp. 4929–4944, 2015.

[45] CDC, *About Antimicrobial Resistance—Antibiotic/ Antimicrobial Resistance*, CDC, Atlanta, GA, USA, 2017, https://www.cdc.gov/drugresistance/about.html.

[46] J. D. Hayes and C. R. Wolf, "Molecular mechanisms of drug resistance," *Biochemical Journal*, vol. 272, no. 2, p. 281, 1990.

[47] S. Blower, A. Aschenbach, H. Gershengorn, and J. Kahn, "Predicting the unpredictable: transmission of drug-resistant HIV," *Nature Medicine*, vol. 7, no. 9, pp. 1016–1020, 2001.

[48] S. Blower and P. Volberding, "What can modeling tell us about the threat of antiviral drug resistance?," *Current Opinion in Infectious Diseases*, vol. 15, no. 6, pp. 609–614, 2002.

[49] M. G. Ison, L. V. Gubareva, R. L. Atmar, J. Treanor, and F. G. Hayden, "Recovery of drug-resistant influenza virus from immunocompromised patients: a case series," *Journal of Infectious Diseases*, vol. 193, no. 6, pp. 760–764, 2006.

[50] A. Kamali and M. Holodniy, "Influenza treatment and prophylaxis with neuraminidase inhibitors: a review," *Infection and Drug Resistance*, vol. 6, p. 187, 2013.

[51] CDC, *Influenza Antiviral Drug Resistance*, CDC, Atlanta, GA, USA, 2017, https://www.cdc.gov/flu/about/qa/antiviralresistance.htm.

[52] F. G. Hayden and M. D. de Jong, "Emerging influenza antiviral resistance threats," *Journal of Infectious Diseases*, vol. 203, no. 1, pp. 6–10, 2011.

[53] M. Lipsitch, T. Cohen, M. Murray, and B. R. Levin, "Antiviral resistance and the control of pandemic influenza," *PLoS Medicine*, vol. 4, no. 1, p. e15, 2007.

[54] K. Jnawali, B. Morsky, K. Poore, and C. T. Bauch, "Emergence and spread of drug resistant influenza: a two-population game theoretical model," *Infectious Disease Modelling*, vol. 1, no. 1, pp. 40–51, 2016.

[55] J. M. McCaw, J. G. Wood, C. T. McCaw, and J. McVernon, "Impact of emerging antiviral drug resistance on influenza containment and spread: influence of subclinical infection and strategic use of a stockpile containing one or two drugs," *PLoS One*, vol. 3, no. 6, Article ID e2362, 2008.

[56] N. M. Ferguson, S. Mallett, H. Jackson, N. Roberts, and P. Ward, "A population-dynamic model for evaluating the potential spread of drug-resistant influenza virus infections during community-based use of antivirals," *Journal of Antimicrobial Chemotherapy*, vol. 51, no. 4, pp. 977–990, 2003.

[57] N. I. Stilianakis, A. S. Perelson, and F. G. Hayden, "Emergence of drug resistance during an influenza epidemic: insights from a mathematical model," *Journal of Infectious Diseases*, vol. 177, no. 4, pp. 863–873, 1998.

[58] ISG, *Vaccine Efficacy and Effectiveness*, Influenza Specialist Group, Melbourne, VIC, Australia, 2017, http://www.isg.org.au/index.php/vaccination/vaccine-efficacy-and-effectiveness/.

[59] CDC, *Flu Vaccine Coverage Remains Low This Year*, Centers for Disease Control and Prevention, Atlanta, GA, USA, 2017, https://www.cdc.gov/media/releases/2016/p1207-flu-vaccine-coverage.html.

[60] P. Van den Driessche and J. Watmough, "Reproduction numbers and sub-threshold endemic equilibria for compartmental models of disease transmission," *Mathematical Biosciences*, vol. 180, no. 1, pp. 29–48, 2002.

[61] H. Nishiura and G. Chowell, "The effective reproduction number as a prelude to statistical estimation of time-dependent epidemic trends," in *Mathematical and Statistical Estimation Approaches in Epidemiology*, pp. 103–121, Springer, Berlin, Germany, 2009.

[62] H. S. Rodrigues, M. T. T. Monteiro, and D. F. M. Torres, "Sensitivity analysis in a dengue epidemiological model," *Conference Papers in Science*, vol. 2013, Article ID 721406, 7 pages, 2013.

[63] N. Chitnis, J. M. Hyman, and C. A. Manore, "Modelling vertical transmission in vector-borne diseases with applications to rift valley fever," *Journal of Biological Dynamics*, vol. 7, no. 1, pp. 11–40, 2013.

[64] F. Hategekimana, S. Saha, and A. Chaturvedi, "Dynamics of amoebiasis transmission: stability and sensitivity analysis," *Mathematics*, vol. 5, no. 4, p. 58, 2017.

[65] G. Chowell and J. M. Hyman, *Mathematical and Statistical Modeling for Emerging and Re-emerging Infectious Diseases*, Springer, Berlin, Germany, 2016.

17

Detecting Depression using an Ensemble Logistic Regression Model based on Multiple Speech Features

Haihua Jiang,[1] Bin Hu [iD],[1] Zhenyu Liu,[2] Gang Wang,[3] Lan Zhang,[4] Xiaoyu Li,[2] and Huanyu Kang[2]

[1]Faculty of Information Technology, Beijing University of Technology, Beijing 100124, China
[2]Gansu Provincial Key Laboratory of Wearable Computing, School of Information Science and Engineering, Lanzhou University, Lanzhou 730000, China
[3]Beijing Anding Hospital of Capital Medical University, Beijing 100088, China
[4]Lanzhou University Second Hospital, Lanzhou 730030, China

Correspondence should be addressed to Bin Hu; bh@bjut.edu.cn

Academic Editor: Raul Alcaraz

Early intervention for depression is very important to ease the disease burden, but current diagnostic methods are still limited. This study investigated automatic depressed speech classification in a sample of 170 native Chinese subjects (85 healthy controls and 85 depressed patients). The classification performances of prosodic, spectral, and glottal speech features were analyzed in recognition of depression. We proposed an ensemble logistic regression model for detecting depression (ELRDD) in speech. The logistic regression, which was superior in recognition of depression, was selected as the base classifier. This ensemble model extracted many speech features from different aspects and ensured diversity of the base classifier. ELRDD provided better classification results than the other compared classifiers. A technique for identifying depression based on ELRDD, ELRDD-E, was here suggested and tested. It offered encouraging outcomes, revealing a high accuracy level of 75.00% for females and 81.82% for males, as well as an advantageous sensitivity/specificity ratio of 79.25%/70.59% for females and 78.13%/85.29% for males.

1. Introduction

Worldwide, over 300 million people of different ages have clinical depression [1]. The rise in the prevalence of this disease has been connected to a group of important outcomes [2]. At the most extreme, patients with depression may commit suicide [3]. To halt the onset of clinical depression, advance intervention can offer a pivotal action to ease the burden of the disease. However, current depression diagnosis methods rely on self-report of patient and clinical opinion [4], which risk several subjective biases. Therefore, a convenient and objective method for detecting depression is of primary importance.

Depressed speech is distinguished invariably by clinicians as monotone, uninteresting, and spiritless [5]. The acoustic qualities of speech can be affected by the emotional state of a person with depression [6]. Therefore, depression can be detected by analyzing changes in the acoustical characteristics of speech. Several approaches have been proposed to reveal correlations between depression and acoustic features for depressed speech classification. To improve the effect of classification, many features were extracted in early studies. However, it is still unclear which acoustic features are most effective for detecting depression especially in Mandarin speech. Furthermore, an objective method based on speech is still in need.

This study investigates the classification performance of multiple speech features which were extracted from subjects to identify depression in those who spoke Mandarin language. To develop an effective objective method and improve the classification result, we propose an ensemble logistic regression model for detecting depression (ELRDD), which contributes to depression recognition based on speech in several ways. First, to make the best use of speech features, it extracts many speech features from different aspects and ensures diversity of the feature spaces and the base classifiers. Second, to overcome the problem of dimensionality curse, the feature subspace dimensionality of each base classifier is lower than the all features space, while a feature reduction method is also used to avoid the curse of dimensionality. Third, a logistic regression model as the base classifier offers probabilities for every class, so the ensemble classifier could make the greatest use of the uncertain information to acquire the best classification outcomes.

The rest of the paper is structured as follows: Section 2 reviews the related work. Section 3 describes the speech database used for this study. Section 4 provides a detailed description of our methodology. Section 5 describes the experiments and results, and Section 6 presents the conclusions.

2. Related Work

Darby and Hollien [7] performed an introductory evaluation of patients with major depression, and they discovered that listeners could discern various distinct characteristics in depressed speech. A variety of speech features have been explored for detecting depression. Mundt et al. [4], Stassen et al. [8], and Hönig et al. [9] reported correlations between F_0 variables and depression. However, Alpert et al. [10], Cannizzaro et al. [11], and Yang et al. [12] reported no significant correlation between F_0 variables and depression. Low et al. [13], Moore et al. [14], and Ooi et al. [15, 16] evaluated classification systems with prosodic, glottal, and spectral features. Low et al. [17], Valstar et al. [18], Alghowinem et al. [19], and Jiang et al. [20] used low-level descriptors and statistical characteristics to identify depression. Cummins et al. [21, 22], Sturim et al. [23], Alghowinem et al. [24], and Joshi et al. [25] investigated mel-frequency cepstrum coefficients (MFCC) and found that the recognition performance was statistically significant for depression classification. An evaluation by Scherer et al. [26–28] revealed a tight connection between voice quality features and the degree of depression. Quatieri and Malyska [29] and Ozdas et al. [30] discovered that depressed subjects showed increased energy levels on the glottal spectrum.

The support vector machine (SVM) and the Gaussian mixture model (GMM) are the most popular classification technologies used for detecting depression in speech. Moore et al. [14] studied 15 depressed subjects and 18 healthy controls and used quadratic discriminant analysis to construct a classifier. They reported accuracies of 91% (with sensitivity to specificity 89%/93%) for males and 96% (with sensitivity to specificity 98%/94%) for females. Their analysis showed that glottal features were more discriminating than prosodic features. Cohn et al. [31] recruited 57 depressed patients and used fundamental frequency and speak-switch duration as inputs to a logistic regression (LR) classifier. They reported an accuracy of 79% (with sensitivity to specificity 88%/64%) when classifying subjects who either responded or did not respond to treatment for depression. Low et al. [13] examined 139 adolescents (71 healthy and 68 depressed) who spoke English, and they used a gender-independent GMM classifier that incorporated glottal, prosodic, and spectral features. They reported classification results of 67–69% for males and 70–75% for females. Ooi

et al. [16] studied 30 participants (15 were at risk of depression and 15 were not at risk) who spoke English and presented an ensemble method using GMM classifiers that used prosodic and glottal features. They reported a classification result of 74% (with sensitivity to specificity 77%/70%). Alghowinem et al. [32] recruited 30 controls and 30 depressed patients who spoke English. They summarized low-level descriptors and statistical features and compared the following classifiers: SVM, GMM, Multilayer Perceptron Neural Network (MLP), and Hierarchical Fuzzy Signature (HFS). They concluded that SVM and GMM had better classification performance. Helfer et al. [33] studied 35 subjects whose Hamilton Depression Scale (HAMD) scores were below 7 or above 17, respectively. They used associated dynamic and the first three formant trajectories as features and reported that SVM performed better than GMM when classifying depression severity. Jiang et al. [20] studied 170 subjects and proposed a computational methodology based on SVM (STEDD). They documented accuracies of 75.96% (with sensitivity to specificity of 77.36%/74.51%) for females and 80.30% (with sensitivity to specificity of 75.00%/85.29%) for males. It should be noted that most of these previous studies were usually limited to small depressed samples and focused on participants who spoke Western languages.

To the best of our knowledge, there has been little research exploring the ensemble classifier for detecting depression based on speech. However, ensemble logistic regression has been used effectively in other research fields [34–39]. In these previous studies, two methods were used to deal with the feature spaces. In one method, all feature spaces were used in each base classifier [34–36]. In the other method, the feature spaces were randomly partitioned into several subspaces [37–39]. It should be mentioned that the feature subspace dimensionality of the previous remained higher, and the variety of the feature subspaces of the last-mentioned could not be guaranteed and the classification outcome was unsteady.

3. Speech Database

In our research, all the subjects were native Chinese speakers between the ages of 18 and 55 and had at least an elementary school education [40]. First, every participant was required to fill in a preassessment booklet that contained general information and demographic information, including health history, age, gender, educational status, and employment. Second, every participant was chosen by psychiatrists based on the *Diagnostic and Statistical Manual Of Mental Disorders* (DSM-IV) [41] rules. Finally, all the subjects were interviewed by psychiatrists to complete the patient health questionnaire-9 (PHQ-9) [42]. These subjects were then divided into two groups depending upon the PHQ-9 scores: depressed patients (PHQ-9 $\geq$ 5) and healthy controls (PHQ-9 < 5). Depressed patients were diagnosed as having pure depression, and they did not experience any other mental illnesses. The controls had no previous or ongoing mental disorder and were matched to the depressed patients based on demographics.

Following the completion of the clinical evaluations, our recording experiment began and it consisted of three parts:

an interview assignment, a reading assignment, and a picture detailing assignment. The interview assignment was made up of 18 questions, and the topics were taken from the Self-Rating Depression Scale (SDS), HAMD, and DSM-IV. The following are sample questions: How do you evaluate yourself? What is the most important present you have ever been given, and how did it make you feel? What do you enjoy doing when you are not able to fall asleep? Please detail any plans you may have for an upcoming vacation. Please tell us about a friend, including their age, type of employment, personality, and pastimes. What situations could make you become desperate? The reading assignment consisted of a short story named "*The North Wind and the Sun*" [43] and three sets of words with neutral (e.g., center, since), positive (e.g., outstanding, happy), and negative (e.g., depression, wail) emotions. The picture detailing assignment involved four dissimilar pictures. Three of them, which had neutral, positive, and negative faces, were obtained from the Chinese Facial Affective Picture System (CFAPS). The last picture titled "*Crying Woman*" was chosen from the Thematic Apperception Test (TAT) [9]. In this assignment, participants were requested to openly detail the four pictures.

We collected speech recordings in a quiet, soundproof, clean laboratory. The ambient noise level in the laboratory was kept below 60 dB. The speech signals were documented with a 24-bit sampling depth and 44.1 kHz sampling rate. We segmented and labeled all these recordings manually and retained only subject voice signals. These recordings were stored in an uncompressed WAV format. The database utilized in this evaluation contained speech recordings from 85 controls (34 males and 51 females) and 85 depressed individuals (32 males and 53 females). The speech of each subject was split into 29 recordings depending on different subtasks. In all, this study utilized 4,930 speech recordings. The overall lengths of speech during the interview, picture detailing, and reading were 52,427 s, 16,203 s, and 21,425 s, respectively. The average duration of speech recording was 18.3 s.

4. Methods

In light of gender variations in depressive indications [44], there are two classification methods: gender-independent modeling (GIM) and gender-dependent modeling (GDM). Low et al. [13] discovered that GDM outperformed GIM. In our study, we used GDM, in which females and males were modeled independently. The proposed framework for the ELRDD is detailed in Figure 1. In the next sections of our paper, features extraction, features reduction, and modeling techniques are recounted.

4.1. Features Extraction and Reduction. The acoustic speech features explored in the literature can be divided into three main categories: prosodic features, spectral features, and glottal features. Each of the three categories comprises several subcategories. MFCC was one of the most frequent spectral features utilized in speech parameters, and the classification outcomes were statistically significant in identifying depression [22–25]. Therefore, MFCC was

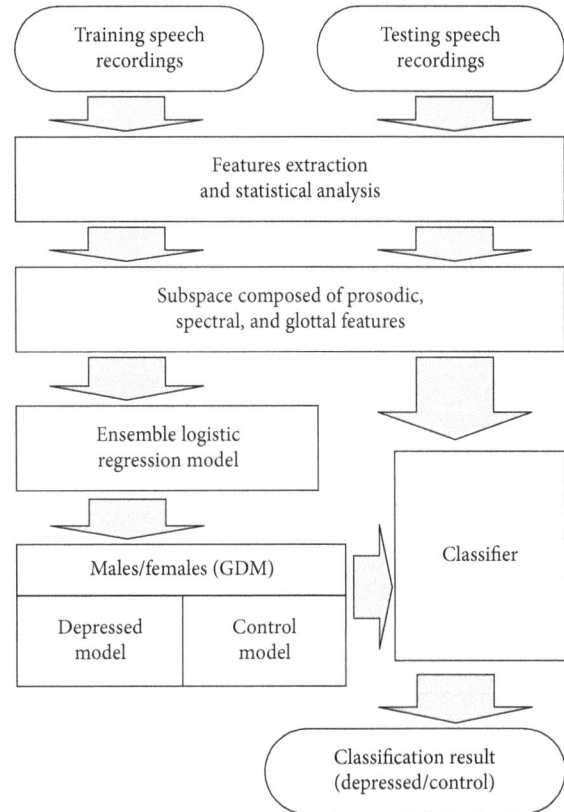

FIGURE 1: Block diagram of the ensemble logistic regression model for detecting depression (ELRDD).

separated from spectral features as a main category. For convenience, the prosodic features are abbreviated PROS, the spectral features are abbreviated SPEC, and the glottal features are abbreviated GLOT. Table 1 presents a summary of the main speech feature categories, subcategories, the number of features, and the statistical functions. Since PROS, SPEC, MFCC, and GLOT were extracted using very different feature extraction methods, they can describe speech from diverse aspects. Thus, feature vectors were complementary to one another. Then, if the feature subspaces of the ensemble classifier were made up of a few of these feature vectors, these subspaces will have a larger diversity. We combined one or more of these four features to form 15 different feature spaces. Table 2 displays these subspaces made up of various feature vectors, in which PROS + SPEC suggests that the subspace is made up of the feature vectors of PROS and SPEC, and MFCC + PROS + SPEC + GLOT suggests that the space is made up of every one of the features. The glottal features were calculated using the TTK Aparat toolbox [45], and the prosodic and spectral features were calculated using the open-source software openSMILE [46].

Compared with the dimensionality of the whole feature space, the dimensionalities of feature subspaces had been reduced considerably, but some dimensionalities of the subspaces were still very high. We applied and compared principal component analysis (PCA), kernel PCA, Laplacian, Isomap, Landmark Isomap, and locally linear embedding (LLE) to reduce feature space dimensionality. We employed

TABLE 1: Summary of speech features.

Main category	Subcategory	Number of features	Functions
MFCC	MFCC (0–14)	630	Corresponding delta coefficients appended
SPEC	Flux	42	21 functions utilized
	Centroid	42	maxPos, minPos
	Entropy	42	Mean, std dev
	Roll-off	168	Skewness, kurtosis
	Band energies	84	Quartile 1/2/3
PROS	PCM loudness	42	Quartile range (2–1)/(3–2)/(3–1)
	Log mel-frequency band (0–7)	336	Linear regression error Q/A
	LSP frequency (0–7)	336	Linear regression coeff. 1/2
	F_0 envelope	42	Percentile 1/99
	Voicing probability	42	Percentile range (99–1)
	F0final, ShimmerLocal	76	19 functions by eliminating the minimum value and the
	JitterLocal, JitterDDP	76	Range functions from the 21 abovementioned functions
	Pitch onsets, duration	2	No functions
GLOT	GLT	27	Mean, max, min
	GLF	5	Mean, max, min
Total		1992	

TABLE 2: Subspaces composed of several different feature vectors.

No.	Subspace	No.	Subspace	No.	Subspace
1	MFCC	2	PROS	3	SPEC
4	GLOT	5	MFCC + PROS	6	MFCC + SPEC
7	MFCC + GLOT	8	PROS + SPEC	9	PROS + GLOT
10	SPEC + GLOT	11	MFCC + PROS + SPEC	12	MFCC + PROS + GLOT
13	MFCC + SPEC + GLOT	14	PROS + SPEC + GLOT	15	MFCC + PROS + SPEC + GLOT

LLE, because it outperformed other methods and preserved the local geometry of high dimensional data [47].

4.2. Ensemble Classification. Given that training data $X = \{X^{(1)}, X^{(2)}, \ldots, X^{(K)}\}$ and its label $Y = \{Y^{(1)}, Y^{(2)}, \ldots, Y^{(K)}\}$, where $X^{(k)} = \{x_1^{(k)}, x_2^{(k)}, \ldots, x_N^{(k)}\}$ is one of the feature subspaces of training points, the value of each label in $Y^{(k)} = \{y_1^{(k)}, y_2^{(k)}, \ldots, y_N^{(k)}\}$ was set to 1 for the depressed patients and 0 for the controls. Given test input data $x = \{x^{(1)}, x^{(2)}, \ldots, x^{(K)}\}$, where $x^{(k)}$ included in Table 2 is a feature subspaces of x, the outputs $P(L = 1|x)$ and $P(L = 0|x)$ providing the 1 and 0 estimated probabilities are given by

$$P(L = 1|x) = \sum_{k=1}^{K} P\left(L = 1|x^{(k)}; w^{(k)}\right)$$
$$= \sum_{k=1}^{K} \frac{\exp\left(w^{(k)} \cdot x^{(k)}\right)}{1 + \exp\left(w^{(k)} \cdot x^{(k)}\right)},$$
(1)

$$P(L = 0|x) = \sum_{k=1}^{K} P\left(L = 0|x^{(k)}; w^{(k)}\right)$$
$$= \sum_{k=1}^{K} \frac{1}{1 + \exp\left(w^{(k)} \cdot x^{(k)}\right)},$$
(2)

where $w = \{w^{(1)}, w^{(2)}, \ldots, w^{(K)}\}$ are the parameters of the ensemble logistic regression model. The log-likelihood function under this model is as follows:

$$l(w) = \sum_{k=1}^{K} l\left(w^{(k)}\right)$$
$$= \sum_{k=1}^{K} \sum_{i=1}^{N} \left[y_i^{(k)}\left(w^{(k)} \cdot x_i^{(k)}\right) - \log\left(1 + \exp\left(w^{(k)} \cdot x_i^{(k)}\right)\right)\right],$$
(3)

where maximizing $l(w)$ produces a maximum likelihood estimator for w.

According to Section 4.1, the complete algorithm of ELRDD is outlined in Algorithm 1.

To validate ELRDD, SVM, GMM, and LR were compared as classifiers for detecting depression. SVM and GMM were usually employed for recognition of depression, while LR was taken as the base classifier for ELRDD. We utilized the expectation-maximization (EM) algorithm to approximate the GMM parameters of every Gaussian component and a radial basis function (RBF) as SVM's kernel function. Then, we looked for the most adequate parameters with a grid search utilizing five-fold cross validation on our training dataset with the LIBSVM toolbox [48].

To demonstrate that ELRDD outperforms other ensemble classifiers, three classic classifiers were compared: adaboost decision tree, bagging decision tree, and random forest. They depicted the speech recordings by the feature spaces made up of MFCC, PROS, SPEC, and GLOT. Because males and females were modeled separately, the number of base classifiers for each classifier depended on gender. These numbers were chosen from 15, 50, 100, 200,

---

Input: training speech recordings $\{s_1, s_2, \ldots, s_n\}$ and its label $\{y_1, y_2, \ldots, y_n\}$ and testing speech recordings $\{r_1, r_2, \ldots, r_m\}$.

Output: depressed patient or healthy control labels of $\{r_1, r_2, \ldots, r_m\}$.

//Training process

Step 1: extract MFCC, PROS, SPEC, and GLOT features for each speech recording from $\{s_1, s_2, \ldots, s_n\}$, and compute the feature statistics as listed in Table 1.

Step 2: in terms of Table 2, 15 feature subspaces are constructed $\{X^{(1)}, X^{(2)}, \ldots, X^{(15)}\}$, where $\{X(k) = x_1^{(k)}, x_2^{(k)}, \ldots, x_n^{(k)}\}$.

For $k = 1$ to 15

Step 3: feature reduction for $X(k)$ is achieved using LLE.

End

Step 4: maximize Equation (3) to achieve the trained classifier model.

//Testing process

Step 5: extract MFCC, PROS, SPEC, and GLOT features for each speech recording from $\{r_1, r_2, \ldots, r_m\}$, and compute the feature statistics as listed in Table 1.

Step 6: in terms of Table 2, 15 feature subspaces are constructed $\{D^{(1)}, D^{(2)}, \ldots, D^{(15)}\}$, where $\{D(k) = d_1^{(k)}, d_2^{(k)}, \ldots, d_n^{(k)}\}$.

For $k = 1$ to 15

Step 7: feature reduction for $D(k)$ is achieved using LLE.

End

Step 8: based on the trained classifier model, apply Equations (1) and (2) to compute the probabilities that the testing samples belong to depressed patients $\{p_1, p_2, \ldots, p_m\}$ or healthy controls $\{q_1, q_2, \ldots, q_m\}$, and then output the category label whose probability is greater.

ALGORITHM 1: ELRDD.

300, 400, and 500, which yielded the best classification outcomes.

ELRDD computed the probabilities that each speech recording belonged to depressed and healthy subjects. To improve recognition performance, classifying a subject as depressed patient or healthy control could use the classification results of more than one speech recording. In our study, each participant had 29 speech recordings, and the final classification result could depend on all these speech recordings. Therefore, we proposed ELRDD-E, which can be summarized as Algorithm 2.

We examined the precise classifications of the controls and the depressed patients in sensitivity, specificity, and accuracy. The controls were distinguished as the negative cases, and the depressed patients were distinguished as the positive cases. When examining performance, each of the three parameters of a well-performing method would have high values, but if a compromise was required, it was sensible to acquire the greatest accuracy while obtaining an optimum sensitivity/specificity ratio (ideally > 1). We employed a speaker-independent split of test and train data and used a ten-fold cross validation. The one-way analysis of variance (ANOVA) and the least significant difference (LSD) tests were conducted to establish if variations in the classification outcomes were statistically significant. The level of significance was set as $p < 0.05$.

5. Experiments and Results

5.1. Experiment Using Individual and Ensemble Classifiers for Males. Table 3 reveals the classification outcomes of every individual classifier for males. It can be noted that the chosen speech features impacted the recognition performance of classifiers. For example, SVM had the best specificity and accuracy with SPEC + GLOT. In contrast, LR achieved the best specificity and accuracy with PROS + SPEC, and GMM achieved the best accuracy with MFCC + PROS + SPEC. In addition, ANOVA and LSD tests were carried out on the four speech feature subspaces (MFCC, PROS, SPEC, and GLOT) over the ten-fold cross validation outcomes utilizing SVM, GMM, and LR classifiers. The accuracy, sensitivity, and specificity significantly varied between the four feature subspaces ($p < 0.05$). The accuracy and sensitivity of GLOT were worse in comparison to MFCC, PROS, and SPEC ($p < 0.05$), and the accuracy and specificity of SPEC and PROS were greater than MFCC ($p < 0.05$). ANOVA and LSD tests were also carried out on paired classifiers over the ten-fold cross validation outcomes. The specificity and accuracy of SVM, GMM, and LR were alike ($p > 0.05$), and the sensitivity of LR and GMM was greater than SVM ($p < 0.05$).

Table 4 shows the recognition performance of ELRDD and existing ensemble classifiers for males. The number of base classifiers for adaboost decision tree, bagging decision tree, and random forest was set to 300, 500, and 400, respectively, which yielded the best classification results. From Tables 3 and 4, it was discovered that ELRDD outperformed the greatest outcome of individual classifiers in accuracy and sensitivity in the identification of depression. Following ANOVA and LSD tests being conducted on paired ensemble classifiers over the ten-fold cross validation outcomes, we discovered that ELRDD also outperformed the contrasted current ensemble classifiers for males in sensitivity and accuracy ($p < 0.05$), and specificity was alike ($p > 0.05$).

5.2. Experiment Using Individual and Ensemble Classifiers for Females. Table 5 reveals the classification outcomes of every individual classifier for females. Following ANOVA and LSD tests being carried out on paired classifiers over the

Input: training speech recordings $\{s_1, s_2, \ldots, s_{n*29}\}$ of subject $\{b_1, b_2, \ldots, b_n\}$ and its label $\{y_1, y_2, \ldots, y_{n*29}\}$ and testing speech recordings $\{r_1, r_2, \ldots, r_{29}\}$ of subject g.
Output: depressed patient or healthy control label of subject g.
    Step 1: call the training process of ELRDD; the inputs are $\{s_1, s_2, \ldots, s_n\}$ and $\{y_1, y_2, \ldots, y_{n*29}\}$.
    For $k = 1$ to 29
    Step 2: call the testing process of ELRDD; the input is r_k of subject g and the outputs are probability pk for depressed patients and probability q_k for healthy controls.
    End
    Step 3: $p = p_1 + p_2 + \cdots + p_{29}, q = q_1 + q_2 + \cdots + q_{29}$, if the value of p is larger than q, subject g is classified as depressed; otherwise, g is classified as a control.

ALGORITHM 2: ELRDD-E.

TABLE 3: Classification outcomes of each individual classifier for males.

Features	SVM			GMM			LR		
	Sen. (%)	Spe. (%)	Acc. (%)	Sen. (%)	Spe. (%)	Acc. (%)	Sen. (%)	Spe. (%)	Acc. (%)
MFCC	56.14	64.91	60.66	62.72	58.22	60.40	62.50	60.75	61.60
PROS	61.96	70.39	66.30	61.75	74.14	68.13	63.15	71.10	67.24
SPEC	**63.36**	73.94	68.81	65.84	71.60	68.81	**67.35**	70.69	69.07
GLOT	36.32	60.95	49.01	47.95	54.26	51.20	44.07	54.56	49.48
MFCC + PROS	60.67	69.78	65.36	63.69	70.49	67.19	65.41	68.36	66.93
MFCC + SPEC	59.05	72.72	66.09	64.55	69.17	66.93	63.58	69.07	66.41
MFCC + GLOT	53.56	66.53	60.24	61.96	60.65	61.29	61.10	60.75	60.92
PROS + SPEC	63.25	73.83	68.70	62.72	74.14	68.60	67.13	**72.21**	**69.85**
PROS + GLOT	60.99	71.60	66.46	61.96	72.92	67.61	62.82	71.20	67.14
SPEC + GLOT	62.61	**75.15**	**69.07**	65.19	70.89	68.13	66.70	70.99	68.91
MFCC + PROS + SPEC	60.99	72.92	67.14	65.63	72.31	**69.07**	64.55	70.39	67.56
MFCC + PROS + GLOT	59.59	72.62	66.30	63.36	69.27	66.41	62.82	67.24	65.10
MFCC + SPEC + GLOT	60.24	72.82	66.72	65.84	69.98	67.97	64.66	68.66	66.72
PROS + SPEC + GLOT	60.02	73.83	67.14	62.82	**74.24**	68.70	64.12	71.91	68.13
MFCC + PROS + SPEC + GLOT	61.85	73.12	67.66	**66.27**	71.30	68.86	64.33	**72.21**	68.39

Maximum of sensitivity (sen.), specificity (spe.), and accuracy (acc.) is shown in bold.

TABLE 4: Recognition performance of each classifier for males.

Classifier	Number of base classifiers	Sensitivity (%)	Specificity (%)	Accuracy (%)
Adaboost decision tree	300	58.94	67.14	63.17
Bagging decision tree	500	59.48	70.28	65.05
Random forest	400	59.05	70.99	65.20
ELRDD	15	67.35	73.94	70.64

ten-fold cross validation outcomes, it can be noted that LR functioned as well as SVM and GMM ($p > 0.05$), and the greatest experimental outcome of LR outperformed SVM and GMM, which was in agreement with the outcomes for males. In addition, ANOVA and LSD tests were also conducted on the four speech feature subspaces (MFCC, PROS, SPEC, and GLOT) over the ten-fold cross validation outcomes utilizing SVM, GMM, and LR classifiers for females. The accuracy and specificity significantly varied between the four feature subspaces ($p < 0.05$). The accuracy and specificity of GLOT were worse than that of MFCC, PROS, and SPEC ($p < 0.05$), and the sensitivity of PROS was better than that of GLOT ($p < 0.05$).

Table 6 shows the recognition performances of ensemble classifiers for females. The number of base classifiers for adaboost decision tree, bagging decision tree, and random forest was set to 200, 300, and 300, respectively, which yielded the best classification results. After the LSD test, ELRDD still outperformed the other ensemble classifiers for females in terms of sensitivity ($p < 0.05$), and specificity and accuracy were similar ($p > 0.05$).

5.3. Experiment Using ELRDD-E. The classification outcomes of ELRDD-E are presented in Table 7. The outcomes of utilizing STEDD [20], which is an efficient technique according to speech types and emotions to identify depression in the identical database, are also included for comparison. From this table, it was found that ELRDD-E outperformed the results of Adaboost Decision Tree, Bagging Decision Tree, and Random Forest in terms of accuracy and sensitivity ($p < 0.05$). It also can be noted that ELRDD-E performed greater than STEDD in classification sensitivity and accuracy for males, while they had the same specificity. Further, ELRDD-E provided better sensitivity than STEDD for females, while STEDD performed minutely better in specificity and accuracy. It can be concluded that ELRDD-E provided very promising results and was effective for detecting depression.

TABLE 5: Classification outcomes of each individual classifier for females.

Features	SVM			GMM			LR		
	Sen. (%)	Spe. (%)	Acc. (%)	Sen. (%)	Spe. (%)	Acc. (%)	Sen. (%)	Spe. (%)	Acc. (%)
MFCC	63.24	57.27	60.31	56.47	66.06	61.17	62.79	61.80	62.30
PROS	67.21	60.65	63.99	51.72	73.29	62.30	64.35	66.73	65.52
SPEC	60.64	63.35	61.97	52.44	73.70	62.87	63.05	64.91	63.96
GLOT	56.60	42.53	49.70	51.33	50.44	50.90	52.70	46.11	49.47
MFCC + PROS	**67.53**	61.06	64.36	56.86	71.54	64.06	**64.93**	66.06	65.48
MFCC + SPEC	66.10	61.60	63.89	**57.78**	69.78	63.66	63.24	65.99	64.59
MFCC + GLOT	63.05	57.20	60.18	55.63	64.84	60.15	62.66	60.24	61.47
PROS + SPEC	64.09	**64.50**	64.29	51.01	**73.83**	62.20	63.63	**67.61**	65.58
PROS + GLOT	67.47	59.16	63.40	52.31	72.08	62.00	63.37	66.73	65.02
SPEC + GLOT	61.09	60.31	60.71	51.79	70.99	61.21	61.87	62.75	62.30
MFCC + PROS + SPEC	64.74	62.41	63.59	56.47	73.09	**64.62**	64.41	67.41	65.88
MFCC + PROS + GLOT	67.08	62.27	**64.72**	55.50	72.62	63.89	64.74	67.14	**65.92**
MFCC + SPEC + GLOT	63.37	62.68	63.03	57.71	69.37	63.43	62.39	63.42	62.90
PROS + SPEC + GLOT	64.15	63.42	63.79	51.53	73.43	62.27	63.11	67.07	65.05
MFCC + PROS + SPEC + GLOT	65.00	63.22	64.13	56.02	72.96	64.32	63.44	**67.61**	65.48

Maximum of sensitivity (sen.), specificity (spe.), and accuracy (acc.) are shown in bold.

TABLE 6: Recognition performance of each classifier for females.

Classifier	Number of base classifiers	Sensitivity (%)	Specificity (%)	Accuracy (%)
Adaboost decision tree	200	59.34	69.91	64.52
Bagging decision tree	300	58.75	68.56	63.56
Random forest	300	59.66	68.56	64.03
ELRDD	15	65.71	67.68	66.68

TABLE 7: Classification outcomes of ELRDD-E.

Gender	Classifier	Sensitivity (%)	Specificity (%)	Accuracy (%)
Male	ELRDD-E	78.13	85.29	81.82
	Adaboost decision tree	65.63	82.35	74.24
	Bagging decision tree	65.63	79.41	72.73
	Random forest	62.50	79.41	71.21
	STEDD	75.00	85.29	80.30
Female	ELRDD-E	79.25	70.59	75.00
	Adaboost decision tree	64.15	76.47	70.19
	Bagging decision tree	62.26	74.51	68.27
	Random forest	66.04	76.47	71.15
	STEDD	77.36	74.51	75.96

6. Discussion

Table 3 shows the classification outcomes of each individual classifier for males. It can be noted that the optimal features for every classifier varied. These results indicate that each feature vector could provide complementary information for the different classifiers. Moreover, it was impossible for each classifier to utilize the same feature subspace that worked best for other classifiers. This indirectly indicates that it is necessary to develop classifiers from multiple feature subsets. Results showed that SPEC and PROS features performed better than MFCC and GLOT features for males.

Table 5 reveals the classification outcomes of every individual classifier for females. It can be observed that each classifier yielded the best classification result using different feature subspaces. These outcomes suggest that every feature was complementary and offered various classifiers with different information, which was also in agreement with the discoveries for males. It was noted that utilizing SPEC, PROS, and MFCC features offered significantly better classification outcomes for females compared to utilizing GLOT features.

From Tables 3 and 5, it can be concluded that using GLOT features provided worst classification outcomes among these four feature vectors. This result is contrary to the findings of two earlier studies. Low et al. [13] and Ooi et al. [15] observed that glottal features performed better than prosodic and spectral features. The disparity may be due to the fact that previous researchers focused on participants who spoke Western languages, while all the participants in this work spoke Mandarin. The assignments used in the previous studies were also different from ours. It also can be observed that the performance of LR was no worse than that of SVM and GMM with most feature subspaces. Furthermore, the best experimental result of LR outperformed SVM and GMM. This was one of the reasons that LR was chosen as the base classifier.

Tables 4 and 6 show the recognition performances of classifiers. It can be observed that ELRDD had a better recognition effect than other classifiers. This result could be due to the fact that ELRDD could ensure the diversity of the feature subspaces and utilize more information provided by features. Moreover, compared with the other three existing ensemble classifiers, the number of base classifiers in ELRDD was much smaller.

7. Conclusion

In this evaluation, we initially contrasted the outcomes of three varying individual classifiers utilizing 15 feature

subspaces to determine the connection between speech features and the performance of classifiers. It was observed that classifier performance was sensitive to the features used for both males and females. Since each feature subspace contained different information of the speech recordings, it was reasonable to integrate suitable speech features. It was noted that utilizing SPEC and PROS features offered significantly better classification outcomes for males than utilizing MFCC and GLOT features ($p < 0.05$). It was discovered that utilizing GLOT features offered significantly worse classification outcomes for females than utilizing SPEC, PROS, and MFCC features ($p < 0.05$). It was also discovered that LR performed minutely better than SVM base classifier.
and GMM, which was a reason for LR being selected as the

Second, we revealed an ensemble methodology for the classification of depression, ELRDD. It was noted that ELRDD, which was developed from multiple feature subsets, outperformed both the individual classifiers and the other ensemble classifiers including SVM, GMM, LR, adaboost decision tree, bagging decision tree, and random forest. ELRDD revealed an accuracy level of 70.64% for males and 66.68% for females, as well as a sensitivity/specificity ratio of 67.35%/73.94% for males and 65.71%/67.68% for females.

Finally, based on ELRDD, we proposed ELRDD-E, which utilized the classification results of all 29 speech recordings of each subject in our dataset. This methodology offered extremely encouraging outcomes, revealing an increased accuracy level of 81.82% for males and 75.00% for females, as well as an advantageous sensitivity/specificity females.
ratio of 78.13%/85.29% for males and 79.25%/70.59% for

While the experimental outcomes are promising, a possible limitation of this research is that speech may have additional features that pertain to depression. A future direction of this study is to investigate improvements in feature extraction and selection strategy.

Conflicts of Interest

The authors declare that there are no conflicts of interest regarding the publication of this paper.

Acknowledgments

This work was supported by the National Basic Research Program of China (973 Program) (no. 2014CB744600).

References

[1] World Health Organization, *Depression Fact Sheet*, WHO, Geneva, Switzerland, 2018, http://www.who.int/en/news-room/fact-sheets/detail/depression.

[2] R. C. Kessler, P. Berglund, O. Demler et al., "The epidemiology of major depressive disorder: results from the national comorbidity survey replication (NCS-R)," *JAMA*, vol. 289, no. 23, pp. 3095–3105, 2003.

[3] K. Hawton, C. Casanas i Comabella, C. Haw, and K. Saunders, "Risk factors for suicide in individuals with depression: a systematic review," *Journal of Affective Disorders*, vol. 147, no. 1–3, pp. 17–28, 2013.

[4] J. C. Mundt, P. J. Snyder, M. S. Cannizzaro, K. Chappie, and D. S. Geralts, "Voice acoustic measures of depression severity and treatment response collected via interactive voice response (IVR) technology," *Journal of Neurolinguistics*, vol. 20, no. 1, pp. 50–64, 2007.

[5] C. Sobin and H. A. Sackeim, "Psychomotor symptoms of depression," *American Journal of Psychiatry*, vol. 154, pp. 4–17, 1997.

[6] N. Cummins, S. Scherer, J. Krajewski, S. Schnieder, J. Epps, and T. F. Quatieri, "A review of depression and suicide risk assessment using speech analysis," *Speech Communication*, vol. 71, pp. 10–49, 2015.

[7] J. K. Darby and H. Hollien, "Vocal and speech patterns of depressive patients," *Folia Phoniatrica et Logopaedica*, vol. 29, pp. 279–291, 1977.

[8] H. H. Stassen, S. Kuny, and D. Hell, "The speech analysis approach to determining onset of improvement under antidepressants," *European Neuropsychopharmacology*, vol. 8, no. 4, pp. 303–310, 1998.

[9] F. Hönig, A. Batliner, E. Nöth, S. Schnieder, and J. Krajewski, "Automatic modelling of depressed speech: relevant features and relevance of gender," in *Proceedings of Fifteenth Annual Conference of the International Speech Communication Association*, pp. 1248–1252, ISCA, Singapore, September 2014.

[10] M. Alpert, E. R. Pouget, and R. R. Silva, "Reflections of depression in acoustic measures of the patient's speech," *Journal of Affective Disorders*, vol. 66, no. 1, pp. 59–69, 2001.

[11] M. Cannizzaro, B. Harel, N. Reilly, P. Chappell, and P. J. Snyder, "Voice acoustical measurement of the severity of major depression," *Brain and Cognition*, vol. 56, no. 1, pp. 30–35, 2004.

[12] Y. Yang, C. Fairbairn, and J. Cohn, "Detecting depression severity from vocal prosody," *IEEE Transactions on Affective Computing*, vol. 4, pp. 142–150, 2012.

[13] L. A. Low, N. C. Maddage, M. Lech, L. B. Sheeber, and N. B. Allen, "Detection of clinical depression in adolescents speech during family interactions," *IEEE Transactions on Biomedical Engineering*, vol. 58, no. 3, pp. 574–586, 2011.

[14] E. Moore, M. Clements, J. W. Peifer, and L. Weisser, "Critical analysis of the impact of glottal features in the classification of clinical depression in speech," *IEEE Transactions on Biomedical Engineering*, vol. 55, no. 1, pp. 96–107, 2008.

[15] K. E. B. Ooi, M. Lech, and N. B. Allen, "Multichannel weighted speech classification system for prediction of major depression in adolescents," *IEEE Transactions on Biomedical Engineering*, vol. 60, no. 2, pp. 497–506, 2013.

[16] K. E. B. Ooi, M. Lech, and N. B. Allen, "Prediction of major depression in adolescents using an optimized multi-channel weighted speech classification system," *Biomedical Signal Processing and Control*, vol. 14, pp. 228–239, 2014.

[17] L. A. Low, N. C. Maddage, M. Lech, L. B. Sheeber, and N. B. Allen, "Influence of acoustic low-level descriptors in the detection of clinical depression in adolescents," in *Proceedings of IEEE International Conference on Acoustics, Speech and Signal Processing (ICASSP)*, pp. 5154–5157, IEEE, Dallas, TX, USA, March 2010.

[18] M. Valstar, B. Schuller, K. Smith et al., "3D dimensional affect and depression recognition challenge," in *Proceedings of 4th*

ACM International Workshop on Audio/Visual Emotion Challenge (AVEC'14), pp. 3–10, ACM, Orlando, FL, USA, November 2014.

[19] S. Alghowinem, R. Goecke, M. Wagner, J. Epps, M. Breakspear, and G. Parker, "Detecting depression: a comparison between spontaneous and read speech," in *Proceedings of IEEE International Conference on Acoustics, Speech and Signal Processing (ICASSP)*, pp. 7547–7551, IEEE, Vancouver, Canada, 2013.

[20] H. H. Jiang, B. Hu, Z. Y. Liu et al., "Investigation of different speech types and emotions for detecting depression using different classifiers," *Speech Communication*, vol. 90, pp. 39–46, 2017.

[21] N. Cummins, J. Epps, M. Breakspear, and R. Goecke, "An investigation of depressed speech detection: features and normalization," in *Proceedings of Interspeech*, pp. 2997–3000, ISCA, Florence, Italy, August 2011.

[22] N. Cummins, J. Epps, V. Sethu, and J. Krajewski, "Variability compensation in small data: oversampled extraction of i-vectors for the classification of depressed speech," in *Proceedings of IEEE International Conference on Acoustics, Speech and Signal Processing (ICASSP) 2014*, pp. 970–974, IEEE, Florence, Italy, May 2014.

[23] D. Sturim, P. A. Torres-Carrasquillo, T. F. Quatieri, N. Malyska, and A. McCree, "Automatic detection of depression in speech using Gaussian mixture modeling with factor analysis," in *Proceedings of Interspeech*, pp. 2983–2986, ISCA, Florence, Italy, August 2011.

[24] S. Alghowinem, R. Goecke, M. Wagner, J. Epps, M. Breakspear, and G. Parker, "From joyous to clinically depressed: mood detection using spontaneous speech," in *Proceedings of FLAIRS Conference*, pp. 141–146, AAAI Press, Marco Island, FL, USA, May 2012.

[25] J. Joshi, R. Goecke, S. Alghowinem et al., "Multimodal assistive technologies for depression diagnosis and monitoring," *Journal on Multimodal User Interfaces*, vol. 7, no. 3, pp. 217–228, 2013.

[26] S. Scherer, G. Stratou, J. Gratch, and L. Morency, "Investigating voice quality as a speaker-independent indicator of depression and PTSD," in *Proceedings of Interspeech*, pp. 847–851, ISCA, Lyon, France, August 2013.

[27] S. Scherer, G. Stratou, M. Mahmoud, J. Boberg, and J. Gratch, "Automatic behavior descriptors for psychological disorder analysis," in *Proceedings of 10th IEEE International Conference and Workshops on Automatic Face and Gesture Recognition (FG)*, pp. 1–8, IEEE, Shanghai, China, April 2013.

[28] S. Scherer, G. Stratou, and L. P. Morency, "Audiovisual behavior descriptors for depression assessment," in *Proceedings of 15th ACM on International Conference on Multimodal Interaction (ICMI)*, pp. 135–140, ACM, New York, NY, USA, 2013.

[29] T. F. Quatieri and N. Malyska, "Vocal-source biomarkers for depression: a link to psychomotor activity," in *Proceedings of Interspeech*, pp. 1059–1062, ICSA, Portland, OR, USA, September 2012.

[30] A. Ozdas, R. G. Shiavi, S. E. Silverman, M. K. Silverman, and D. M. Wilkes, "Investigation of vocal jitter and glottal flow spectrum as possible cues for depression and near-term suicidal risk," *IEEE Transactions on Biomedical Engineering*, vol. 51, no. 9, pp. 1530–1540, 2004.

[31] J. F. Cohn, T. S. Kruez, I. Matthews et al., "Detecting depression from facial actions and vocal prosody," in *Proceedings of 3rd International Conference on Affective Computing and Intelligent Interaction and Workshops*, pp. 1–7, IEEE, Amsterdam, Netherlands, September 2009.

[32] S. Alghowinem, R. Goecke, M. Wagner, J. Epps, T. Gedeon, and M. Breakspear, "A comparative study of different classifiers for detecting depression from spontaneous speech," in *Proceedings of IEEE International Conference on Acoustics, Speech and Signal Processing (ICASSP) 2013*, pp. 8022–8026, IEEE, Vancouver, Canada, May 2013.

[33] B. S. Helfer, T. F. Quatieri, J. R. Williamson, D. D. Mehta, R. Horwitz, and B. Yu, "Classification of depression state based on articulatory precision," in *Proceedings of Interspeech*, pp. 2172–2176, ISCA, Lyon, France, August 2013.

[34] A. Sebti and H. Hassanpour, "Body orientation estimation with the ensemble of logistic regression classifiers," *Multimedia Tools and Applications*, vol. 76, no. 22, pp. 23589–23605, 2017.

[35] H. Wang, Q. S. Xu, and L. F. Zhou, "Large unbalanced credit scoring using lasso-logistic regression ensemble," *Plos One*, vol. 10, no. 2, Article ID e0117844, 2015.

[36] P. D. Prasad, H. N. Halahalli, J. P. John, and K. K. Majumdar, "Single-trial EEG classification using logistic regression based on ensemble synchronization," *IEEE J. Biomed. Health*, vol. 18, no. 3, pp. 1074–1080, 2014.

[37] N. Lim, H. Ahn, H. Moon, and J. J. Chen, "Classification of high-dimensional data with ensemble of logistic regression models," *Journal of Biopharmaceutical Statistics*, vol. 20, no. 1, pp. 160–171, 2010.

[38] H. Kuswanto, A. Asfihani, Y. Sarumaha, and H. Ohwada, "Logistic regression ensemble for predicting customer defection with very large sample size," in *Proceedings of Third Information Systems International Conference*, pp. 86–93, Elsevier, Amsterdam, Netherlands, December 2015.

[39] K. Lee, H. Ahn, H. Moon, R. L. Kodell, and J. J. Chen, "Multinomial logistic regression ensembles," *Journal of Biopharmaceutical Statistics*, vol. 23, no. 3, pp. 681–694, 2013.

[40] Z. Y. Liu, B. Hu, L. H. Yan et al., "Detection of depression in speech," in *Proceedings of International Conference on Affective Computing and Intelligent Interaction (ACII)*, pp. 743–747, IEEE, Xi'an, China, September 2015.

[41] American Psychiatric Association, *Diagnostic and Statistical Manual of Mental Disorders*, American Psychiatric Association, Washington, DC, USA, 4th edition, 1994.

[42] K. Kroencke, R. Spitzer, and J. Williams, "The phq-9: validity of a brief depression severity measure," *Journal of General Internal Medicine*, vol. 16, pp. 606–613, 2001.

[43] D. J. France, R. G. Shiavi, S. Silverman, M. Silverman, and M. Wilkes, "Acoustical properties of speech as indicators of depression and suicidal risk," *IEEE Transactions on Biomedical Engineering*, vol. 47, no. 7, pp. 829–837, 2000.

[44] S. Nolenhoeksema and J. S. Girgus, "The emergence of gender differences in depression during adolescence," *Psychological Bulletin*, vol. 115, no. 3, pp. 424–443, 1994.

[45] M. Airas, "TKK Aparat: an environment for voice inverse filtering and parameterization," *Logopedics Phoniatrics Vocology*, vol. 33, no. 1, pp. 49–64, 2008.

[46] F. Eyben, M. Wöllmer, and B. Schuller, "Opensmile-the Munich versatile and fast open-source audio feature extractor," in *Proceedings of 18th ACM International Conference on Multimedia*, pp. 1459–1462, ACM, Firenze, Italy, October 2010.

[47] J. Chen and Y. Liu, "Locally linear embedding: a survey," *Artificial Intelligence Review*, vol. 36, no. 1, pp. 29–48, 2011.

[48] C. C. Chang and C. J. Lin, "LIBSVM: a library for support vector machines," *ACM Transactions on Intelligent Systems and Technology*, vol. 2, no. 3, pp. 1–27, 2011.

18

Structure Optimization for Large Gene Networks based on Greedy Strategy

Francisco Gómez-Vela (ID),[1] **Domingo S. Rodriguez-Baena,**[1] and **José Luis Vázquez-Noguera**[2]

[1]*Division of Computer Science, Pablo de Olavide University, 41013 Seville, Spain*
[2]*Carrera de Ingeniería Informática, Universidad Americana, Asunción, Paraguay*

Correspondence should be addressed to Francisco Gómez-Vela; fgomez@upo.es

Academic Editor: Ting Hu

In the last few years, gene networks have become one of most important tools to model biological processes. Among other utilities, these networks visually show biological relationships between genes. However, due to the large amount of the currently generated genetic data, their size has grown to the point of being unmanageable. To solve this problem, it is possible to use computational approaches, such as heuristics-based methods, to analyze and optimize gene network's structure by pruning irrelevant relationships. In this paper we present a new method, called GeSOp, to optimize large gene network structures. The method is able to perform a considerably prune of the irrelevant relationships comprising the input network. To do so, the method is based on a greedy heuristic to obtain the most relevant subnetwork. The performance of our method was tested by means of two experiments on gene networks obtained from different organisms. The first experiment shows how GeSOp is able not only to carry out a significant reduction in the size of the network, but also to maintain the biological information ratio. In the second experiment, the ability to improve the biological indicators of the network is checked. Hence, the results presented show that GeSOp is a reliable method to optimize and improve the structure of large gene networks.

1. Background

One of the most important challenges in systems biology is to understand how individual biological components behave and interact in the context of large and complex systems [1]. This knowledge provides the opportunity of controlling and/or optimizing different parts of biological processes to generate a specific effect in the whole system. Therefore, this system-wide view may lead to new applications in areas such as biotechnology and medicine [2]. In particular, the high amount of data generated in the last years allows the inference of relationships between DNA, RNA, proteins, and other cellular components. The sum of these interactions leads to various types of interaction networks (including protein-protein interaction, metabolic, signalling, and transcription-regulatory networks) called gene networks for the sake of simplicity.

Gene networks are usually inferred from gene expression data and have been widely used to model gene relationships in a biological process [3]. In the last decade, many computational approaches have been proposed for the reverse engineering of gene networks [4]. However, the continuous advances in high-throughput technologies enable carrying out large-scale analyses on the DNA and RNA levels the same as on the protein and metabolite level. As a result, the sources of data from which the gene networks are inferred have increased in size, complexity, and diversity [2]. Due to this, new computational challenges have arisen. For example, some methods have been redesigned to improve their performance during large-scale dataset processing [5]. Other research works have focused their efforts on integrating different sources of data for a more accurate gene network reconstruction, such as the work of [6], in which time data sets from different perturbation experiments are simultaneously considered, or that in [7], where the proposed model integrates big data of diverse types to increase both the power and accuracy of networks inference. Different inference algorithms are combined for reconstructing genome-scale and high-quality gene network from massive-scale RNA-seq samples in [8]. Even other works, like [9], adapt known gene network construction methods to highly parallel execution using distributed high-throughput computing resources.

As a result of these new researches, inferred gene networks are more complex and larger. This fact makes it difficult to visually detect interesting connections between nodes, even though analysis tools have been created recently to apply both advanced statistics and innovative visualization strategies to support efficient knowledge extraction from gene networks [10]. Regarding the gene network structure, some pieces of evidence, like those from the analysis of metabolism and genetic regulatory networks, have proven most biological networks to be sparse, following a scale-free topology. That is, the nodal degree distribution of the network is a power law distribution [11]. Scale-free networks are highly nonuniform; that is, most of the nodes have only a few links while a few nodes have a very large number of links, which are called Hubs. Hubs in a network play a crucial role in how the information is processed in the network since they connect different highly interconnected group of nodes (modules) that could represent different biological functions [12]. Nowadays, the generation of gene networks with a scale-free topology is harder due to the great size and complexity of the networks obtained from the high quantity of data available, so the optimization of gene network structures is currently an important challenge.

In this paper, a new method for automatic optimization of the topology of a large gene network is presented. The method, called Gene Network Structure Optimization (GeSOp), is a backward elimination procedure based on a greedy heuristic method to perform a prune of the irrelevant relationships of the input network. Through this novel method, large genetic networks can improve their topological characteristics without losing their biological information.

1.1. Related Works. Explicit structure optimization methods examine networks models and apply a scoring function to assess the degree to which the resulting structure explains the data, while penalizing the complexity of the model. For this aim, interactions are added and/or removed until the best score is reached. Therefore, heuristic search algorithms are one of the most used techniques since exploring all possible combinations of interactions is an NP-hard problem, specially with very big and complex networks [2, 13]. Several optimization techniques have been developed. However, they are usually limited by the high dimensionality of the problem, as well as computational power required for large networks [14].

Some research works use evolutionary techniques. To reduce the large search spaces, elitist selection method is often used in genetic algorithms, ensuring that the algorithm does not waste time in the rediscovery of previously discarded partial solutions. For example, in [15], a random Boolean network is evolved to look for an accurate model based only on experimental data, without taking into account prior biological knowledge. Other research works use other methods to improve the algorithm's performance, like [16] that proposes a multiagent genetic algorithm to reconstruct large-scale gene regulatory networks. This algorithm is based on fuzzy cognitive maps and includes efficient search operators to reduce the search space.

The optimization algorithms that are based on one objective function, for example, error minimization, can lead to over-fitting and many false positive connections in large networks inference. For example, in [17], the inference problem of N genes is decomposed into $N \times (N - 1)$ different regression problems, in which the expression level of a target gene is predicted from the expression level of a potential regulation gene by using the sum of squared residuals and the Pearson correlation coefficient. To reduce the over-fitting phenomena, some works use multiple objective functions and/or add prior biological knowledge to infer an accurate network model. For example, authors in [18] import some a priori regulatory information about extracted gene networks from existing publications or biological web sites with the aim of enhancing veracity of the network. The proposal presented in [19] was the first one to incorporate functional association databases. They create undirected, confidence-weighted likelihood matrix by means of pairwise confidence scores from those databases and use it to infer gene networks, improving their accuracy.

Other works focus their efforts on looking for scale-free properties. For example, in [20], a new proposal is presented which takes the scale-free topology into account as prior information to prune the search space during the inference process. This way, the search space traversed by the method integrates the exploration of all predictors sets combinations, like when having a small number of combinations, when performing a floating search, or when the number of combinations becomes excessive.

This process is guided by scale-free prior information. In [21], informative prior based on scale-free property is also used to improve inference accuracy. In particular, during a Bayesian-based inference process, prior knowledge about scale-free properties is used to evaluate the relative importance of nodes from the linkage characteristics of the entire network.

As can be observed, most research works in literature integrate different network structure optimization strategies within the inference process. Therefore, these optimization efforts depend on concrete input data and the network generation tasks. In this sense, to the best of our knowledge, the new method proposed in this paper is the first one that is independent of the network inference process. As a result, this method is able to optimize any input gene network.

2. Materials and Methods

In this section, the methods and the different materials used in this paper are presented. Firstly, the GeSOp method to optimize large gene network structures is exhaustively described. Secondly, the gene network generation method applied in the experimentation will be presented, along with the input datasets and biological databases used.

2.1. Gene Network Structure Optimization. GeSOp is a novel method for large gene networks topology optimization.

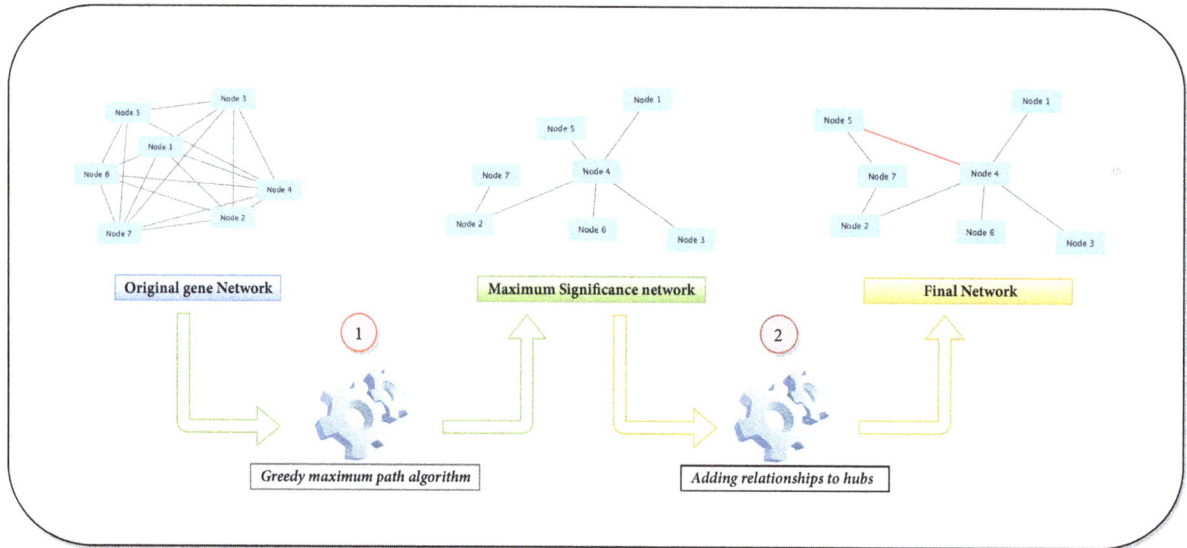

FIGURE 1: GeSOp method is composed of two different steps: 1. application of a greedy algorithm to prune the original network and 2. detection of Hubs in the resulting network and their enrichment by adding new interactions.

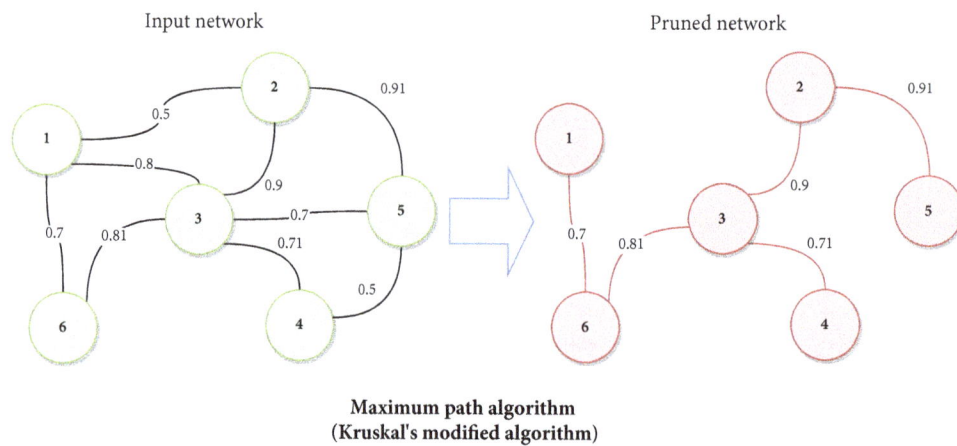

FIGURE 2: Representation of step 1, in which an input network is pruned using the maximum path algorithm.

The method uses undirected influence networks since they represent the highest level of abstraction in the gene networks as was discussed in [3]. Due to this, our method can be applied for a larger number of networks since almost any gene network can be transformed into a nondirected influence network.

The main goal of the GeSOp is to transform the input gene network into a simpler and more efficient network in terms of information transfer, keeping the biological meaningfulness [2]. For this aim, a new backward removal procedure composed of two different steps has been developed. Initially, GeSOp uses a greedy-based heuristic strategy to prune the original network and select the most biologically relevant interactions. Then, the method looks for the most connected nodes (Hubs) in the resultant network and proceeds by adding relevant interactions which were pruned on the previous step. A description of the general schema of the method, along with a toy example, is shown in Figure 1.

A complete description of the two steps and a pseudocode of the method are detailed below.

Step1: Greedy Maximum Relevance Path. The first step of GeSOp uses a greedy-based heuristic algorithm to perform a prune of the input network, taking into account most relevant interactions from a biological point of view (see Figure 2). To do so, a modification of Kruskal's algorithm for the shortest path problem in graphs has been developed [22].

In particular, our method does not select the shortest path between nodes. On the contrary, it selects the longest path according to the weight of edges. Therefore, the relationships with the highest level of significance are selected with respect to the weight of the edges for later network reconstruction.

As a result, the pruned network generated contains the same number of genes (nodes) as the original network but it keeps only most relevant relationships. Hence, it implies a large reduction in terms of the number of edges, while

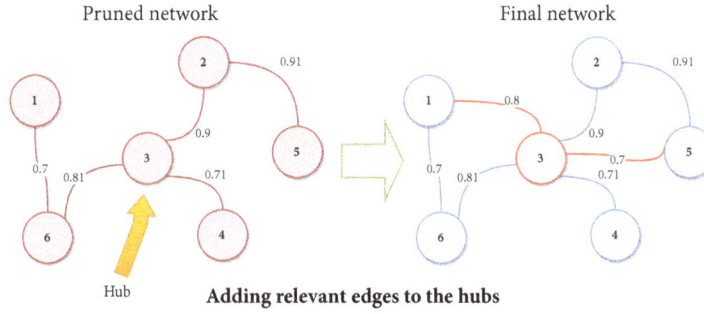

FIGURE 3: An example of the second step of our method, in which the Hubs of the pruned network are identified and relevant edges are added to them. Note that the relationships are added if their weight exceeds the Th_β; in this example, $Th_\beta \geq 0.7$.

still depending on the degree of connectivity of the original network, as is shown in Figure 2.

Step2: Addition of Missing Relationships. As is mentioned in Section 1, Hubs have been reported to have special properties regarding their neighbouring nodes in a gene network. Due to this, in this second step, a topological analysis of the pruned network is performed in order to identify network's Hubs. For this aim, Hubs are selected as those nodes whose connection degree exceeds average network connectivity [12]. A toy example is depicted in Figure 3, where the node "3" is identified as a Hub on the left network.

After the Hubs identification, a threshold (Th_β) is set to determine which relationships of those removed in step 1 should be added to the Hubs. The threshold Th_β is an input parameter of GeSOp algorithm (see Algorithm 1) and it is determined by the user. In this sense, the user may select the threshold which better fits the problem studied. Thus, a new relationship is added to the final network if exceeding Th_β. The process is represented in Figure 3, where two pruned relationships are added to the Hub node in the network on the right.

The final network is generated after each Hub of the pruned networks is processed.

A general pseudocode of the complete method described in this paper is presented in Algorithm 1.

Finally, the complexity of GeSOp combines the complexity of the Step1 ($\Theta(E\log(V))$) and the Step2 ($\Theta(V(E^2))$) resulting in and average case complexity of

$$\Theta\left(E\log\left(V\right)\right) + \Theta\left(V\left(E^2\right)\right), \tag{1}$$

where V and E represent the number of genes and relationships of the input network, respectively.

2.2. Input Datasets.
In this section, experimental datasets used for the generation of input gene network used to test GeSOp implementation are shown. In particular, we have selected two different datasets from two different organisms with different features.

Saccharomyces cerevisiae Cell Cycle Dataset. The first dataset used was the one presented by Spellman et al. [23], in relation to the well-known Yeast Cell Cycle. This microarray describes

```
input: Input Network, G := ⟨V, E⟩
       V: genes, E: relationships
input: Relevant Threshold, Th_β
output: Final network, G_β := ⟨V, E_ε⟩
, where E_ε ∈ E
/*Step1: maximum path graph*/
G_β ← maximumPathAlgorithm(G);
/*Step2: adding missing edges to Hubs nodes*/
i ← 0;
for v_i ∈ V do
    if isHub(v_i) then
        j ← 0;
        for e_j ∈ E do
            if contains(e_j, v_i) ∧ e_j.weight ≥ Th_β then
                G_β ← addEdge(e_j);
            end
            j ← j + 1
        end
    end
    i ← i + 1
end
Return G_β;
```

ALGORITHM 1: A general pseudocode of the proposed method. The algorithm is divided into two different steps.

the expression level of 5521 genes in samples from yeast cultures, which were synchronized by three independent methods: α factor arrest, elutriation, and arrest of a cdc15 temperature-sensitive mutant. Particularly, we focus on data generated by cdc15 experiments.

Homo sapiens Single Nucleotide Polymorphism (SNP) Dataset. In order to prove the usefulness of our proposed method, the *Homo sapiens* SNP, presented in the work of Hodo et al. [24], has been also selected. This dataset was obtained to study associations of interleukin 28B with carcinoma recurrence in patients with chronic hepatitis C, and it contains information about 54616 genes of *Homo sapiens*.

2.3. Gene Networks Generation Methods.
In the following, the methods used to extract gene networks from the two datasets

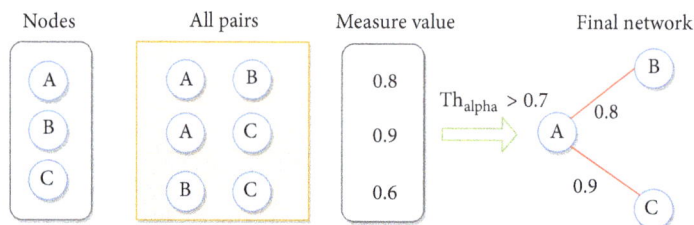

FIGURE 4: An example of the generation of the input networks. Note that the relationships are added if their weight exceeds the Th_α.

presented above are described. In total, three networks were generated for each dataset. Gene networks based on information theory are one of the most widely used types in literature [2] since they are able to identify coexpression relationships among genes. In this sense, we have selected this kind of networks since they are computationally simple and allow the fitting of large datasets. In particular, three standard measures from information theory to generate coexpression gene networks have been used: **Spearman's** correlation algorithm, **Kendall's** Rank correlation algorithm [1, 25], and **Symmetric Uncertainty** measure (SU) [26, 27].

Gene networks were constructed by calculation of the presented measures (Kendall, Spearman, and SU) from the expression levels in each pair of genes from the input datasets. If the result of the measure exceeds a determinate threshold (here after Th_α) selected by the user, a new edge is added to the network between the nodes as is represented by Figure 4.

For our study, we have selected a low threshold, $Th_\alpha = 0.5$, in order to obtain over-connected networks as was discussed in [3].

2.4. Biological Databases. The aim of this section is to present the biological databases used as reference in the experiment section.

In particular, we have selected three different databases: (a) the GeneMANIA database for evaluating yeast and human networks, (b) YeastNet database for yeast, and (c) HumanNet for human.

GeneMANIA [28] contains information presented in the form of web application for generating hypotheses about gene functions. A prediction server uses a large set of functional association data, including protein and genetic interactions, pathways, coexpression, colocalization, and protein domain similarities. The information stored in GeneMANIA is freely available online. This information is stored in a structure categorized by organisms, where genes (nodes) are related (gene-gene relationship) if at least one piece of evidence of this relation exists in the literature.

YeastNet, which was presented in [29], is a probabilistic functional gene network obtained from 5794 protein-coding genes of the yeast extracted from *Saccharomyces cerevisiae* Genome Database [30]. This network combines protein-protein interactions, protein-DNA interactions, coexpression, phylogenetic conservation, and also literature information, in total covering 102803 linkages among 5483 yeast proteins.

Finally **HumanNet**, which was presented in [31], is a probabilistic functional gene network of 18714 validated protein-coding genes of *Homo sapiens*. It is constructed by modified Bayesian integration of 21 types of "omics" data from multiple organisms. Each data type is weighted according to how well it associates known genes to a biological function in *Homo sapiens*. Each interaction in HumanNet has an associated log-likelihood score that rates the probability of a relationship representing a true functional linkage between two genes.

3. Results and Discussion

The performance of the proposed method was tested by means of two different experiments. The aim of the first experiment is proving that the networks processed by our method do not lose rate of biological information. To this end, we have used different networks, generated using standard methods of literature, and different databases (see Sections 2.3 and 2.4). In the second experiment, a topological analysis of different networks is carried out to check how biological structure indicators are improved.

3.1. Biological Information Analysis. The aim of this experiment is to show how the networks processed by our method reduce the size of the network, keeping their biological information ratio. To do so, for each dataset used, we present a comparison, in terms of size and performance, between the original inferred network and those optimized by GeSOp.

3.1.1. Performance Evaluation. The quality of the optimized networks was assessed by a direct comparison with a gold standard, that is, the biological databases presented in Section 2.2. To compute the quality measures, the following indices were defined as they were presented in [32]:

(i) **True positives (TP):** both networks contain the gene-gene relationship evaluated.

(ii) **False positives (FP):** the input network contains a relationship which is not present in the biological database.

(iii) **True negatives (TN):** the relationships are not present neither in the input network nor in the biological database.

(iv) **False negatives (FN):** the relationship exists in the biological database but it does not in the input network.

TABLE 1: Results of yeast cell cycle networks processed with GeSOp. As it is shown, networks are significantly reduced in size.

	Yeast								
	Kendall			Spearman			SU		
	Input	GeSOp	diff. %	Input	GeSOp	diff. %	Input	GeSOp	diff. %
Nodes	5466	5466	-	5521	5521	-	4802	4802	-
Edges	619552	10801	-98.25 %	2555009	446704	-82.51%	145329	26421	-81.81%

Once these indices are obtained, other measures used in the literature have been selected to rate the quality of gene networks [2, 3], *Precision* and *Recall* [2, 33], which are defined below.

$$Precision = \frac{TP}{TP + FP} \qquad (2)$$

$$Recall = \frac{TP}{TP + FN} \qquad (3)$$

3.1.2. Yeast Experiment. As was stated before, in this subsection, the results obtained by the networks generated by the Yeast Cell Cycle dataset are presented. The input networks were generated using a $Th_\alpha = 0.5$ as cut-off to generate over-connected networks as was introduced in [3]. On the other hand, GeSOp uses a threshold $Th_\beta = 0.7$ for adding relationships. We have selected this threshold as relevant correlation value as was also discussed in [3].

The first analysis is presented in Table 1, in which the number of nodes and edges of the original networks and the optimized ones are exposed.

The table presents the different results obtained by the networks generated by the following methods: Kendall, Spearman, and SU. The first column of each method represents the original input network (network obtained by method on the dataset with $T_h = 0.5$) and the second one ("GeSOp") the final network obtained by our method. On the other hand, the rows of the table represent the number of nodes presented in the network ("Nodes") and the number of relationships comprising the network ("edges"), respectively. Finally, the column "diff. %" represents the difference between the number of edges of the input and final network.

Firstly, it is worth mentioning that the network generation methods present different results for the same dataset. Spearman's method is the one that obtains larger networks since the method is able to find less strictness coexpression levels. On the other hand, SU's method is the most restrictive, as this technique is based on detecting not only the lineal dependencies, but also the nonlinear ones. Finally, Kendall's method is more restrictive than the Spearman method but more relaxed than the SU's.

Regarding the size of the networks, results show that the networks optimized by GeSOp have reduced their size from 81, 81% to 98.25%, in terms of number of edges. Note that GeSOp preserves the nodes, as was described previously. These results represent a significant size reduction, which implies that the final networks are simpler and more user-friendly for researchers in terms of size and visualization.

Once it has been shown that GeSOp is capable of carrying out a reduction in the size of gene networks, it is also important to check if these optimized networks keep the ratio of biological information that they originally contained. For this aim, Tables 2 and 3 are presented. In them, for each method of generation (i.e., Kendall, Spearman, and SU), three columns are displayed. The columns "Input" represent the results for the input network, columns "GeSOp" represent the optimized networks generated by GeSOp. In addition, the results obtained by the networks computed only in step 1 of our method are presented in the "Pruned" columns. The rows "Precision" and "Recall" indicates the ratio of biological information of the networks according to the biological databases used.

Results show that the networks do not suffer any loss of information. On the contrary, the value of the Precision measure for these networks is increased. For example, in the case of the Kendall's network compared to YeastNet, Precision value goes from 0.01 to 0.09, which is a significant improvement. This behaviour is also presented in the Spearman's and SU's networks, where Precision's values increase from 0.01 to 0.02.

Regarding the Recall, it has been reduced in all the networks optimized by our method. This fact makes sense, since Recall value is inversely proportional to the number of FN, which are the relationships that are present in the biological databases. Therefore, our method for reducing the size of the network is inherently increasing the number of FN. Thus, the greater the database used to rate the network, the lower the value of its Recall because there will be more FN.

3.1.3. Homo sapiens Experiment. In this subsection, the experiments carried out by means of the human SNP dataset are described. The obtained networks were generated using the same parameters as in the previous section ($Th_\alpha = 0.5$ and $Th_\beta = 0.7$).

The analysis carried out on the size of the different human networks is shown in Table 4. The results follow the same pattern as of the yeast networks. Spearman is the method which presents the larger network while SU presents the smaller.

GeSOp is able to reduce considerably the size of the networks (e.g., −85.68% for Kendall's network and −89.46% for Spearman's), but the case of SU's network is remarkable. In this case, the reduction is about −40.08%, which is significantly lower than the rest of the cases. This result is consistent with the fact that the SU's network is significantly smaller than the rest of the studied networks, so it is difficult to reduce the size of this network without losing biologically

TABLE 2: Yeast's network results against YeastNet.

	Kendall			Spearman			SU		
	Input	Pruned	GeSOp	Input	Pruned	GeSOp	Input	Pruned	GeSOp
TP	8331	94	909	19706	64	6589	1744	94	436
FP	444362	4035	9449	1864316	4374	328473	102890	3496	20850
Precision	0.01	0.02	0.094	0.01	0.01	0.02	0.01	0.026	0.02
Recall	0.08	$9.18 \cdot 10^{-4}$	0.009	0.2	$6.25 \cdot 10^{-4}$	0.006	0.01	$9.18 \cdot 10^{-4}$	0.004

TABLE 3: Yeast's network results against GeneMANIA.

	Kendall			Spearman			SU		
	Input	Pruned	GeSOp	Input	Pruned	GeSOp	Input	Pruned	GeSOp
TP	194918	1942	7863	692753	1909	147360	43991	1722	10281
FP	400383	3273	8423	1770378	3326	293279	95244	2824	18206
Precision	0.32	0.37	0.48	0.28	0.36	0.33	0.31	0.37	0.36
Recall	0.04	$4.01 \cdot 10^{-4}$	0.016	0.08	$3.94 \cdot 10^{-4}$	0.003	0.009	$3.56 \cdot 10^{-4}$	0.002

TABLE 4: Results of human SNP networks processed with GeSOp. The size of the networks is also significantly reduced.

	Human								
	Kendall			Spearman			SU		
	Input	GeSOp	diff. %	Input	GeSOp	diff. %	Input	GeSOp	diff. %
Nodes	8068	8068	-	31061	31061	-	1431	1431	-
Edges	68329	9783	-85.68%	5387473	567590	-89.46%	1871	1121	-40.08%

TABLE 5: Human's network results against GeneMANIA.

	Kendall			Spearman			SU		
	Input	Pruned	GeSOp	Input	Pruned	GeSOp	Input	Pruned	GeSOp
TP	17144	1282	2085	351686	1305	52563	525	299	303
FP	26416	2759	3116	2512234	11646	248969	745	545	553
Precision	0.39	0.31	0.4	0.12	0.10	0.18	0.40	0.35	0.36
Recall	0.0024	$1.83 \cdot 10^{-4}$	$2.98 \cdot 10^{-4}$	0.04	$1.86 \cdot 10^{-4}$	0.0075	$0.7 \cdot 10^{-4}$	$0.4 \cdot 10^{-4}$	$0.43 \cdot 10^{-4}$

TABLE 6: Human's network results against HumanNet.

	Kendall			Spearman			SU		
	Input	Pruned	GeSOp	Input	Pruned	GeSOp	Input	Pruned	GeSOp
TP	4216	276	586	46850	141	8202	125	77	77
FP	35931	3291	4084	2465035	10540	258413	1045	699	711
Precision	0.10	0.07	0.12	0.01	0.01	0.03	0.10	0.09	0.09
Recall	0.008	$5.79 \cdot 10^{-4}$	0.001	0.09	$2.95 \cdot 10^{-4}$	0.017	$2.4 \cdot 10^{-4}$	$1.61 \cdot 10^{-4}$	$1.66 \cdot 10^{-4}$

relevant relationships. Due to this result, it is possible to argue that GeSOp performs better with larger gene networks which contain spurious relationships.

The biological validation of the different networks using GeneMANIA and HumanNet databases (see Section 2.2 for more details) is presented in Tables 5 and 6, respectively.

The validation results follow the same pattern as for the yeast networks. The accuracy value increases for all cases except for SU's networks. As was discussed above, it is difficult to prune small networks without losing relevant relationships. Even so, the loss of Precision value is very small (0.04 with GeneMANIA and 0.01 on HumanNet).

In conclusion, the results obtained by both experiments show how GeSOp is able to perform a pruning process on large networks, by reducing their size while keeping their ratio of biological information. The relevance of our method became more evident since, as was discussed in literature [14], the optimization usually implies loss of information in the majority of the cases. However, for almost all analyzed cases, Precision of the network is improved by GeSOp.

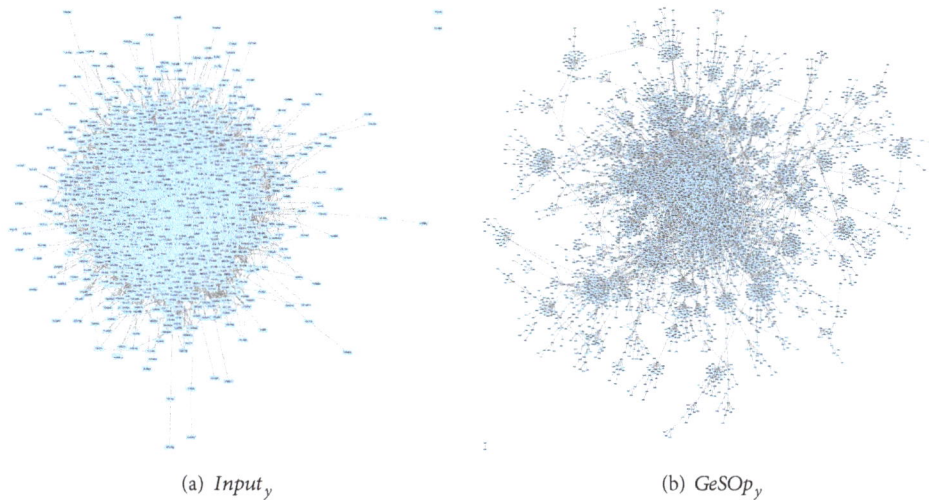

(a) $Input_y$ (b) $GeSOp_y$

FIGURE 5: Visual comparison of yeast network. The original Kendall's network is shown on (a). On (b), the final network obtained with GeSOp is depicted. As can be observed, the optimized network presents a scale-free topology.

3.2. Topological Analysis. In this section, the ability of GeSOp to improve the topology of gene networks is analyzed.

As was stated in Section 1, biological networks usually follow topological patterns, in particular the scale-free topology. The topology of a network is crucial to understand the biological network's architecture and performance [34]. Therefore, gene networks inferred by computational methods should present this type of topology [3]. Based on this assumption, we present a topological analysis of some of the networks optimized by GeSOp in the previous section. The objective is to identify if their topology indicators have been improved in terms of scale-free topology.

Scale-free networks have a structure containing only a few Hubs, among some other features. The most important and commonly used topological features of scale-free networks are presented [35, 36] as follows:

(i) **Characteristic path length (CPL):** The CPL of a network indicates the shortest path length between two nodes, averaged over all pairs of nodes comprising the network. A high path length indicates that the network is in a linear chain. A lower value means that is more compact. Scale-free networks usually have a great CPL.

(ii) **Diameter:** The diameter of a network indicates the maximal distance between two nodes. As in the case of CPL, a greater diameter of the network indicates that it follows a biological pattern.

(iii) **Clustering coefficient:** For one node, this coefficient can be calculated as the number of links among the nodes within its neighbourhood divided by the number of links that are possible among them. A high clustering coefficient for a network is another indicator of the existence of biological relationships.

(iv) **Graph density:** The density of a network defines the ratio of the number of edges to the number of possible edges. Gene networks are generally sparsely connected. Therefore, a low density should indicate biological meaning in the network.

(v) **The node degree distribution:** It indicates the ratio of nodes in the network with degree k. Scale-free networks usually follow a power law: $P(k) \sim k^{\gamma}$, where γ is a constant (≥ 0). A high γ is an indicator of a scale-free topology.

For this experiment, the networks obtained by Kendall's method on Yeast and Human datasets have been used as reference, for the sake of simplicity. Thus, we present a topological study for four networks, the originals (named "$Input_{organism}$") and the processed ones (hereafter "$GeSOP_{organism}$"). Visual representation of the networks is depicted in Figures 5 and 6, where it is possible to check the topological differences of the networks.

As can be seen in the figures, the optimized networks ("$GeSOp_x$") present a more linear and less compact topology than the input ones, so they fit better with the scale-free topology. In addition, an exhaustive topological analysis of the four networks has been carried out based on the indicators presented above. The topological analysis of the network has been performed using the tool Network Analyzer [37] and the results obtained are depicted in Table 7.

The results presented in Table 7 show that the networks improve their topological indicators once they are processed by GeSOp. Moreover, it is possible to argue that these networks follow a biological pattern according to [36]. That is, after the optimization process, networks show, on the one hand, a lower mean clustering coefficient and density. On the other hand, they present higher characteristic path length, diameter, and γ constant. These results mean that networks have improved in terms of the biological relevance of their relationships.

Moreover, the optimized networks present characteristics closer to a scale-free topology as their node degree distribution follows a power law with $\gamma \geq 0$[34] (see Figure 7).

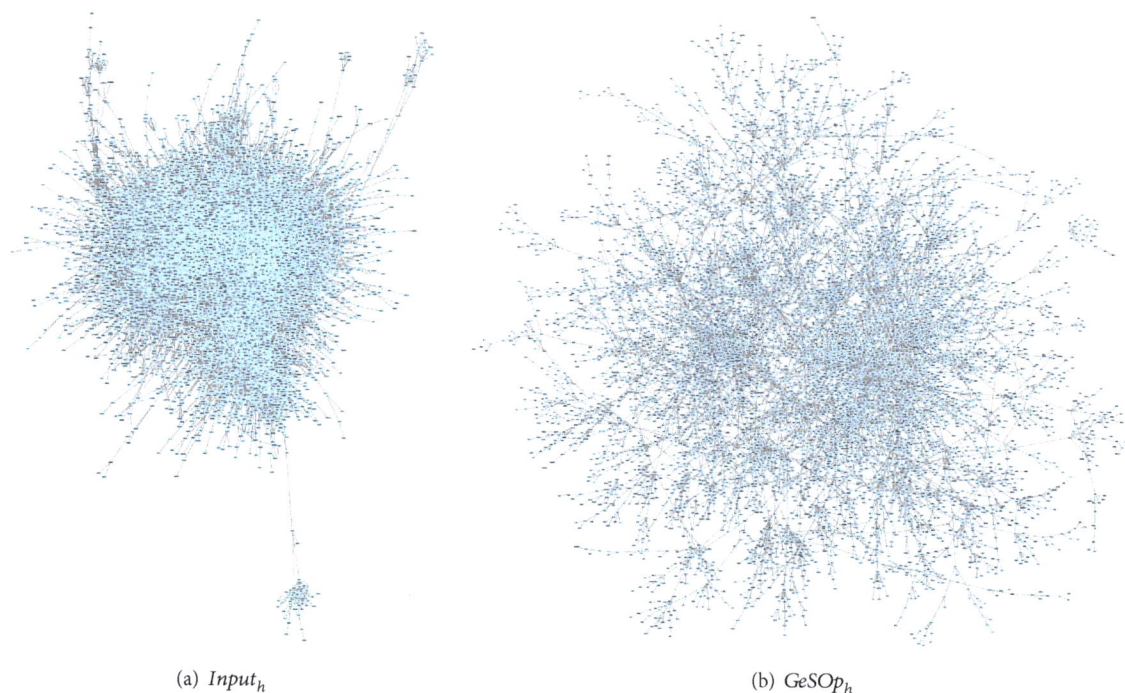

(a) $Input_h$

(b) $GeSOp_h$

FIGURE 6: Visual comparison of human networks used in this experiment. The original Kendall's network is shown on (a). On (b), the optimized network obtained with GeSOp is depicted.

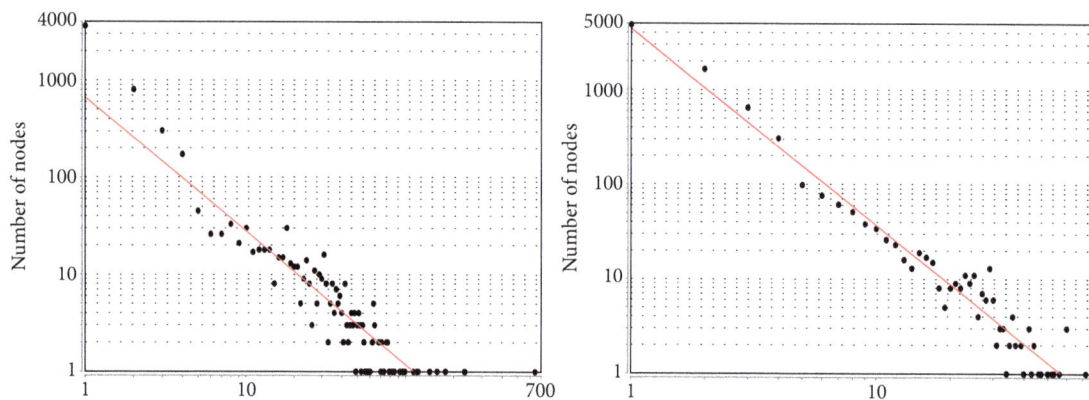

FIGURE 7: Node degree for the optimized networks obtained with GeSOp. The fitted power law indicates that the networks follow a scale-free topology.

TABLE 7: Topological indicator of four selected networks. The results presented show how the optimized networks obtained by GeSOp improve their indicators.

	Network	Clust. coef.	CPL	Diameter	Density	Gamma (γ)
Yeast	$Input_y$	0.411	2.697	9	0.041	0.845
	$GeSOp_y$	0.085	6.156	20	0.001	1.375
Human	$Input_h$	0.21	4.954	19	0.003	1.394
	$GeSOp_h$	0.024	10.84	33	~ 0.000	2.079

This fact can be verified by the results presented in column "Gamma" of Table 7, in which the values of γ (from power law) are improved in the optimized networks.

The results generated by this second experiment probes that GeSOp is a reliable method to improve the topological features of the gene networks, in terms of biological structure.

4. Conclusions

In this work, a new backward elimination method for optimization of large gene networks structure, namely, GeSOp, has been presented. The method, which is based on a greedy strategy, is able to perform a drastic reduction of size of the input network in terms of the number of gene-gene relationships. The prune of the less biologically significant relationships produces simpler and more user-friendly networks for researchers in terms of size and visualization.

On one hand, the results presented show that the method is able not only to perform a prune of the input network, but also to keep the ratio of the biological information presented in the original network. Furthermore, for almost all studied cases, this ratio is improved. On the other hand, topological analyses carried out in the experiments show how networks optimized by GeSOp improve their biological indicators by acquiring a scale-free topology. Finally, regarding the generated results, it is possible to argue that the relevance of our method becomes evident for the processing and optimization of large gene networks.

As future works, we will work on the inclusion of previous biological knowledge, in form of gene networks as gold standard, in the second step of the methodology. Thus, the method will take into account not only the existing Hubs in the input network, but also the genes that have a great relevance in the networks used as gold standard. Another future work is based on the implementation; we are working in paralleling implementation of the algorithm to improve its performance.

Data Availability

In this section, we provide the links to the datasets and databases presented above. In particular, the links for the datasets are as follows:

(1) **Yeast dataset**: https://www.ncbi.nlm.nih.gov/geo/query/acc.cgi?acc=GSE23

(2) **Human dataset**: https://www.ncbi.nlm.nih.gov/geo/query/acc.cgi?acc=GPL570

and those for the databases are as follows:

(1) **GeneMANIA**: http://genemania.org/data/

(2) **YeastNet**: https://www.inetbio.org/yeastnet/

(3) **HumanNet**: http://www.functionalnet.org/humannet/

Conflicts of Interest

The authors declare that they have no conflicts of interest.

References

[1] Y. X. R. Wang and H. Huang, "Review on statistical methods for gene network reconstruction using expression data," *Journal of Theoretical Biology*, vol. 362, pp. 53–61, 2014.

[2] M. Hecker, S. Lambeck, S. Toepfer, E. van Someren, and R. Guthke, "Gene regulatory network inference: data integration in dynamic models—a review," *BioSystems*, vol. 96, no. 1, pp. 86–103, 2009.

[3] F. Gómez-Vela, C. D. Barranco, and N. Díaz-Díaz, "Incorporating biological knowledge for construction of fuzzy networks of gene associations," *Applied Soft Computing*, vol. 42, pp. 144–155, 2016.

[4] D. Marbach, R. J. Prill, T. Schaffter, C. Mattiussi, D. Floreano, and G. Stolovitzky, "Revealing strengths and weaknesses of methods for gene network inference," *Proceedings of the National Acadamy of Sciences of the United States of America*, vol. 107, no. 14, pp. 6286–6291, 2010.

[5] A. Lachmann, F. M. Giorgi, G. Lopez, and A. Califano, "ARACNe-AP: gene network reverse engineering through adaptive partitioning inference of mutual information," *Bioinformatics*, vol. 32, no. 14, pp. 2233–2235, 2016.

[6] N. Omranian, J. M. O. Eloundou-Mbebi, B. Mueller-Roeber, and Z. Nikoloski, "Gene regulatory network inference using fused LASSO on multiple data sets," *Scientific Reports*, vol. 6, Article ID 20533, 2016.

[7] F. Petralia, P. Wang, J. Yang, and Z. Tu, "Integrative random forest for gene regulatory network inference," *Bioinformatics*, vol. 31, no. 12, pp. i197–i205, 2015.

[8] H. Yu, B. Jiao, L. Lu et al., "NetMiner-an ensemble pipeline for building genome-wide and high-quality gene co-expression network using massive-scale RNA-seq samples," *PLoS ONE*, vol. 13, no. 2, p. e0192613, 2018.

[9] W. L. Poehlman, M. Rynge, D. Balamurugan, N. Mills, and F. A. Feltus, "OSG-KINC: high-throughput gene co-expression network construction using the open science grid," in *Proceedings of the 2017 IEEE International Conference on Bioinformatics and Biomedicine (BIBM)*, pp. 1827–1831, Kansas City, MO, November 2017.

[10] J. Xia, E. E. Gill, and R. E. W. Hancock, "NetworkAnalyst for statistical, visual and network-based meta-analysis of gene expression data," *Nature Protocols*, vol. 10, no. 6, pp. 823–844, 2015.

[11] A. Barabási and Z. N. Oltvai, "Network biology: understanding the cell's functional organization," *Nature Reviews Genetics*, vol. 5, no. 2, pp. 101–113, 2004.

[12] R. R. Vallabhajosyula, D. Chakravarti, S. Lutfeali, A. Ray, and A. Raval, "Identifying Hubs in protein interaction networks," *PLoS ONE*, vol. 4, no. 4, Article ID e5344, 2009.

[13] Y. Wang, X. Zhang, and L. Chen, "Optimization meets systems biology," *BMC Systems Biology*, vol. 4, no. Suppl 2, p. S1, 2010.

[14] S. A. Thomas and Y. Jin, "Reconstructing biological gene regulatory networks: where optimization meets big data," *Evolutionary Intelligence*, vol. 7, no. 1, pp. 29–47, 2014.

[15] M. R. Mendoza and A. L. Bazzan, "Evolving random boolean networks with genetic algorithms for regulatory networks reconstruction," in *Proceedings of the the 13th annual conference*, p. 291, Dublin, Ireland, July 2011.

[16] J. Liu, Y. Chi, and C. Zhu, "A dynamic multiagent genetic algorithm for gene regulatory network reconstruction based on fuzzy cognitive maps," *IEEE Transactions on Fuzzy Systems*, vol. 24, no. 2, pp. 419–431, 2016.

[17] J. Xiong and T. Zhou, "Gene regulatory network inference from multifactorial perturbation data using both regression and correlation analyses," *PLoS ONE*, vol. 7, no. 9, Article ID e43819, 2012.

[18] J. Li and X.-S. Zhang, "An optimization model for gene regulatory network reconstruction with known biological information," in *Proceedings of the First International Symposium on Optimization and Systems Biology*, pp. 35–44, 2007.

[19] M. E. Studham, A. Tjärnberg, T. E. M. Nordling, S. Nelander, and E. L. L. Sonnhammer, "Functional association networks as priors for gene regulatory network inference," *Bioinformatics*, vol. 30, no. 12, pp. I130–I138, 2014.

[20] F. M. Lopes, D. C. Martins Jr., J. Barrera, and R. M. Cesar Jr., "A feature selection technique for inference of graphs from their known topological properties: revealing scale-free gene regulatory networks," *Information Sciences*, vol. 272, pp. 1–15, 2014.

[21] B. Yang, J. Xu, B. Liu, and Z. Wu, "Inferring gene regulatory networks with a scale-free property based informative prior," in *Proceedings of the 8th International Conference on BioMedical Engineering and Informatics (BMEI '15)*, pp. 542–547, October 2015.

[22] D. B. West, *Introduction to Graph Theory*, Prentice-Hall of India Private Limited, New Delhi, India, 2000.

[23] P. T. Spellman, G. Sherlock, M. Q. Zhang et al., "Comprehensive identification of cell cycle-regulated genes of the yeast Saccharomyces cerevisiae by microarray hybridization," *Molecular Biology of the Cell (MBoC)*, vol. 9, no. 12, pp. 3273–3297, 1998.

[24] Y. Hodo, M. Honda, A. Tanaka et al., "Association of interleukin-28B genotype and hepatocellular carcinoma recurrence in patients with chronic hepatitis C," *Clinical Cancer Research*, vol. 19, no. 7, pp. 1827–1837, 2013.

[25] P. A. Jaskowiak, R. J. G. B. Campello, and I. G. Costa, "On the selection of appropriate distances for gene expression data clustering," *BMC Bioinformatics*, vol. 15, article no. S2, 2014.

[26] L. Song, P. Langfelder, and S. Horvath, "Comparison of co-expression measures: mutual information, correlation, and model based indices," *BMC Bioinformatics*, vol. 13, no. 1, article no. 328, 2012.

[27] H. Liu, L. Liu, and H. Zhang, "Ensemble gene selection for cancer classification," *Pattern Recognition*, vol. 43, no. 8, pp. 2763–2772, 2010.

[28] D. W. Farley, S. L. Donaldson, O. Comes et al., "The Gene-MANIA prediction server: biological network integration for gene prioritization and predicting gene function," *Nucleic Acids Research*, vol. 38, no. 2, pp. W214–W220, 2010.

[29] H. Kim, J. Shin, E. Kim et al., "YeastNet v3: a public database of data-specific and integrated functional gene networks for Saccharomyces cerevisiae," *Nucleic Acids Research*, vol. 42, no. 1, pp. D731–D736, 2014.

[30] J. M. Cherry, E. L. Hong, and C. Amundsen, "Saccharomyces genome database: the genomics resource of budding yeast," *Nucleic Acids Research*, pp. D700–D705, 2012.

[31] I. Lee, U. M. Blom, P. I. Wang, J. E. Shim, and E. M. Marcotte, "Prioritizing candidate disease genes by network-based boosting of genome-wide association data," *Genome Research*, vol. 21, no. 7, pp. 1109–1121, 2011.

[32] E. R. Dougherty, "Validation of inference procedures for gene regulatory networks," *Current Genomics*, vol. 8, no. 6, pp. 351–359, 2007.

[33] D. M. Powers, "Evaluation: from precision, recall and f-measure to roc, informedness, markedness and correlation," *International Journal of Machine Learning Technology*, vol. 2, no. 1, pp. 37–63, 2011.

[34] N. T. Doncheva, Y. Assenov, F. S. Domingues, and M. Albrecht, "Topological analysis and interactive visualization of biological networks and protein structures," *Nature Protocols*, vol. 7, no. 4, pp. 670–685, 2012.

[35] G. A. Pavlopoulos, M. Secrier, C. N. Moschopoulos et al., "Using graph theory to analyze biological networks," *BioData Mining*, vol. 4, no. 1, article 10, 2011.

[36] W. Winterbach, P. V. Mieghem, M. Reinders, H. Wang, and D. D. Ridder, "Topology of molecular interaction networks," *BMC Systems Biology*, vol. 7, article no. 90, 2013.

[37] Y. Assenov, F. Ramírez, S.-E. Schelhorn, T. Lengauer, and M. Albrecht, "Computing topological parameters of biological networks," *Bioinformatics*, vol. 24, no. 2, pp. 282–284, 2008.

19

A Patient-Independent Significance Test by Means of False-Positive Rates in Selected Correlation Analysis of Brain Multimodal Monitoring Data

Rupert Faltermeier [ID],[1] **Martin A. Proescholdt** [ID],[1] **Stefan Wolf**,[2] **Sylvia Bele** [ID],[1] and **Alexander Brawanski**[1]

[1]*Department of Neurosurgery, University Hospital Regensburg, Regensburg, Germany*
[2]*Department of Neurosurgery, University Hospital Charite, Berlin, Germany*

Correspondence should be addressed to Rupert Faltermeier; rupert.faltermeier@ukr.de

Academic Editor: Michele Migliore

Recently, we introduced a mathematical toolkit called selected correlation analysis (sca) that reliably detects negative and positive correlations between arterial blood pressure (ABP) and intracranial pressure (ICP) data, recorded during multimodal monitoring, in a time-resolved way. As has been shown with the aid of a mathematical model of cerebral perfusion, such correlations reflect impaired autoregulation and reduced intracranial compliance in patients with critical neurological diseases. Sca calculates a Fourier transform-based index called selected correlation (sc) that reflects the strength of correlation between the input data and simultaneously an index called mean Hilbert phase difference (mhpd) that reflects the phasing between the data. To reliably detect pathophysiological conditions during multimodal monitoring, some thresholds for the abovementioned indexes sc and mhpd have to be established that assign predefined significance levels to that thresholds. In this paper, we will present a method that determines the rate of false positives for fixed pairs of thresholds (lsc, lmhpd). We calculate these error rates as a function of the predefined thresholds for each individual out of a patient cohort of 52 patients in a retrospective way. Based on the deviation of the individual error rates, we subsequently determine a globally valid upper limit of the error rate by calculating the predictive interval. From this predictive interval, we deduce a globally valid significance level for appropriate pairs of thresholds that allows the application of sca to every future patient in a prospective, bedside fashion.

1. Introduction

In critical neurological pathologies such as subarachnoid hemorrhage (SAH) or traumatic brain injury (TBI), two major mechanisms of neuronal damage have been identified [1–3]. The primary injury consists of direct tissue damage due to contusion, laceration, or intracranial hemorrhage, which can only be influenced therapeutically to a limited degree. In contrast, secondary injury is caused by a self-propagating biochemical cascade leading to neuronal dysfunction and death over hours and weeks after the initial insult, which could be a potential treatment target. However, despite promising results of translational research in this field, the clinical studies applying neuroprotective compounds have been uniformly disappointing [4]. Due to the lack of causative treatment, the primary focus of neurointensive care therefore provides the optimal physiological environment in order to minimize secondary injury and foster early regenerative processes [5]. To achieve this goal, it is mandatory to detect pathophysiological conditions such as impaired cerebral autoregulation and reduced intracranial compliance prior to irreversible neuronal damage [6, 7]. Consequently, multimodal brain monitoring has been established to obtain a robust biophysical signature and to tailor an individualized therapy for each patient [8, 9].

In an earlier study, we could demonstrate with the aid of a mathematical model of cerebral perfusion and oxygen supply that severely reduced cerebral compliance in combination with a defective autoregulation leads to a positive correlation between ABP and ICP data, whereas a severely reduced cerebral compliance in combination with an intact cerebral autoregulation leads to a negative correlation between the abovementioned signals [10, 11]. Therefore, we have developed a mathematical toolkit called selected correlation analysis (sca) that reliably detects positive and negative correlations in ABP and ICP data recorded during multimodal monitoring at an intensive care unit.

This method calculates two indices, the selected correlation (sc) and the mean Hilbert phase difference (mhpd) of two isochronous data windows of ABP and ICP data, whereby the sc value serves as a measure for the strength of correlation between the data windows and mhpd reflects the phasing between the data windows. The medical relevance of positive correlations detected by calculation of sc and mhpd values was demonstrated in previous studies including a comparison with the well-established PRx calculations as an index for autoregulation failure [12]. The goal of this work is to assign significance levels to specified pairs of thresholds (lsc, lmhpd) to reliably detect the abovementioned pathophysiological conditions. Furthermore, to make this computerized analysis method available as a point of care tool to support goal-directed clinical decision making, we attempted to establish patient-independent significance levels for these pairs of thresholds which would allow to apply sca prospectively to every future patient in a prospective, bedside fashion.

2. Methods

2.1. Patient Population.
To determine the significance of different threshold settings (lsc, lmhpd) and test the resulting error rates for normal distribution, we analyzed continuous measurements of ABP and ICP data of a patient cohort of 52 patients (32 female; 20 male) with a mean age of 50.4 years. The patients received multimodal brain monitoring either for the treatment of subarachnoid hemorrhage ($n = 43$; 82.7%) or traumatic brain injury ($n = 9$; 17.3%). A detailed description of the baseline characteristics is provided in Table 1. The study was performed in accordance to the Declaration of Helsinki and was approved by the local ethics review boards. The patients were treated either at the University Regensburg Medical Center ($n = 25$; 48.1%) or at the University Hospital Charite, Berlin ($n = 27$; 51.9%). The baseline parameters between the two patient subcohorts were balanced except for the diagnosis, which showed significantly more patients with SAH in the Berlin subcohort ($p = 0.001$). Informed consent was obtained from the patients or their relatives; the data were stored and analyzed after anonymization according to the study protocol. Intracranial pressure (ICP) monitoring was carried out either via an external ventricular drain (EVD) or a parenchymal ICP probe (Raumedic, Helmbrechts, Germany). Follow-up was completed up to March 2017, the mean

follow-up time was 53.8 months, and no patient was lost for follow-up. The neurological outcome was measured by the Glasgow Outcome Scale at the last follow-up, and the median score was 3 (range: 1–5, Table 1).

2.2. Mathematical Framework of Selected Correlation Analysis.
Selected correlation analysis (sca) is a method to detect correlations between two data windows of fixed length. The different elements of this analysis method are illustrated in Figure 1. Thereby, information about correlation is gained by fast Fourier transform of the data and subsequent analysis in frequency space. This approach permits the detection of correlation in a specific frequency band, allowing a differentiation between the correlation of fast or slow components of the signals. Additionally, the whole spectral information about correlation is condensed to a simple value, called sc, which serves as a measure for the degree of correlation between two data windows in a specific frequency range [13, 14].

Let $X := \{x_1, \ldots, x_N\}$ be a time series of ABP or ICP data of length N. A fixed segment or window $X^{s,k}(t)$ of such a time series can be represented as a function in time. An individual window is defined by its starting point k and its length s:

$$X^{s,k}(t) := \left\{ x_{k+t-1} \in X \mid 1 \leq t \leq s; \; k + s - 1 \leq N; \; s \equiv 2^{u \in \mathbb{N}} \right\}. \tag{1}$$

In the following, we will use such windows of ABP and ICP data as input for multitaper power spectrum (mtms) analysis and multitaper coherence spectrum (mtmc) analysis [15]. This spectral analysis will transform the discrete time domain of the windows, indexed by t, into the discrete frequency domain of the spectra, indexed by f with range $1 \leq f \leq s/2$:

$$\begin{aligned} S^s(k, f) &:= \text{mtms of } X^{s,k}(t), \\ C^s(k, l, f) &:= \text{tmc of } X^{s,k}(t) \text{ and } Y^{s,l}(t). \end{aligned} \tag{2}$$

The multitaper method comes along with a built-in statistical test for the significance of each single frequency f. Using this significance test for each individual frequency, we define the so-called pointwise selected correlation (PSC):

$$\text{PSC}^s(k, l) := (\text{psc}_1, \ldots, \text{psc}_{s/2}) \text{ with}$$
$$\text{psc}_f := \begin{cases} 1, & \text{if } S^s(k, f) \wedge S^s(l, f) \wedge C^s(k, l, f) \text{ significant,} \\ 0, & \text{otherwise.} \end{cases} \tag{3}$$

The above-defined PSC tuple contains information whether a frequency is significant in all three spectra, or not. Being significant in both power spectra assures that the specific frequency contributes essentially to the original signals. If this frequency is additionally significant in the coherence spectrum, a strong correlation between the input signals for this frequency is implied.

Baseline characteristics of the retrospective patient cohort treated for subarachnoid hemorrhage (SAH) or traumatic brain injury (TBI).

Parameter	Number (%)
N	52
Gender (f/m)	32/20 (61.5/38.5)
Age (mean)	50.4 (range: 16.4–72.4)
Diagnosis (SAH/TBI)	43/9 (82.7/17.3)
GCS at admission (median)	7 (range: 3–14)
GOS at last follow-up (median)	3 (range: 1–5)

Note. The retrospective patient cohort was analyzed for false-positive readings of the sca method. To illustrate the initial clinical condition and patient outcome, the Glasgow Coma Scale (GCS) rates at admission and the Glasgow Outcome Score (GOS) value at last follow-up are reported.

Using N successive pairs of isochronous windows as input for the above-described PSC calculations produces a time-resolved sequence of PSC tuples. From this sequence, we can deduce a measure for the average activity of the frequencies by calculating the mean pointwise selected correlation (MPSC):

$$\text{MPSC}^s(f) := \left(\frac{1}{N}\right) * \sum_{j=1}^{j=N} \text{PSC}_f^s(j, j). \tag{4}$$

The MPSC tuple is used to potentially identify frequency intervals, which basically carry information about correlations between the input data. Having found such a frequency interval $U = (m, \ldots, n)$, the next step is to determine time sequences in the data sets, where strong correlations occur with respect to U. A simple measure for the strength of correlation of a pair of windows with respect to U is gained by summing up all elements of the appropriate PSC tuple belonging to U and dividing this sum by the length of U. This measure is called selected correlation (sc):

$$\text{sc}^{s,m,n}(k, l) := \frac{1}{n-m+1} \sum_{f=m}^{f=n} \text{PSC}_f^s(k, l), \tag{5}$$

$$\text{with } 1 \leq m < n \leq \frac{s}{2}.$$

Predefining a threshold lsc, a pair of windows will be called selected correlated if $\text{sc} > \text{lsc}$. Using isochronous windows as input while shifting the starting points $\widetilde{t}$ along the time axis produces time-resolved information about the degree of correlation:

$$\text{sc}^{s,m,n}(\widetilde{t}) := \frac{1}{n-m+1} \sum_{f=m}^{f=n} \text{PSC}_f^s(\widetilde{t}, \widetilde{t}). \tag{6}$$

2.2.1. Hilbert Phase Differences.

With the abovementioned sc index, we can identify windows exhibiting a strong correlation between the input data. In order to assign the model predicted pathophysiological conditions, identified by positive and negative correlations, we also have to determine the phasing of the input data. The phasing of the data can be determined by using the so-called Hilbert transform, a mathematical approach to transform a real-valued function $s(t)$ into the complex plain:

$$s_{\text{analytic}}(t) := s(t) + i * \widetilde{s}(t) = A(t) * e^{i*\varphi(t)},$$

$$\text{with } \widetilde{s}(t) := \pi^{-1} P \cdot V \cdot \int_{-\infty}^{\infty} \frac{s(\tau)}{t-\tau} d\tau. \tag{7}$$

By calculating the Hilbert transformation of two windows $X^{s,k}(t)$, $Y^{s,l}(t)$, we are able to determine the associated phases $\varphi_X(t)$, $\varphi_Y(t)$ of the data and the Hilbert phase difference hpd(t):

$$\text{hpd}(t) := \varphi_X(t) - \varphi_Y(t)$$

$$= \arctan\left(\frac{\widetilde{X}^{s,k}(t)Y^{s,l}(t) - X^{s,k}(t)\widetilde{Y}^{s,l}(t)}{X^{s,k}(t)Y^{s,l}(t) - \widetilde{X}^{s,k}(t)\widetilde{Y}^{s,l}(t)}\right). \tag{8}$$

As a simple measure for the phasing of two windows, we will use the mean value mhpd of hpd(t):

$$\text{mhpd}^s(k, l) := \frac{1}{s} * \sum_t \text{hpd}(t). \tag{9}$$

Analogous to the sc value, a pair of windows is called positively correlated (scp) if $\text{sc} > \text{lsc}$ and $\text{mhpd} < \text{lmhpd}_{\text{pos}}$. If $\text{sc} > \text{lsc}$ and $\text{mhpd} > \text{lmhpd}_{\text{neg}}$, the data windows will be called negatively correlated (scn).

2.3. Construction of Patient-Independent Significance Levels

2.3.1. Statistical Test.

With the aid of sc and mhpd values, we are able to identify positively and negatively correlated sections of the input data, but up to now, we do not know the specificity of such correlations. Therefore, we will establish a statistical test, which allows us to relate a significance to individual pairs of the thresholds (lsc, $\text{lmhpd}_{\text{pos}}$) and (lsc, $\text{lmhpd}_{\text{neg}}$) in a patient-independent fashion, so that the resulting threshold pairs can be used for prospective studies. This statistical test uses the fact that the mathematical model predicts isochronous correlations between ABP and ICP. Consequently, two segments of ABP and ICP with starting points far apart from each other should not correlate. If, for example, we use data windows containing one hour of data and a starting point of the ICP data, that is, five hours later than the starting point of the ABP data, then there should be no casual link between these data windows and therefore no correlation. But, due to measurement noise, a few of the frequencies included in the sc analysis may exhibit a significant correlation.

Using this observation, we can count how often such separated windows produce, for example, values (sc, mhpd_{pos}) higher than a predefined pair of threshold levels (lsc, $\text{lmhpd}_{\text{pos}}$). The resulting error rate for this fixed pair of thresholds then determines the significance for this specific pair of thresholds. Clearly, this only applies to cases where the offset between the input data windows is big enough to avoid autocorrelation effects. Such effects can be estimated using the so-called mean windowed autocorrelation (mwa):

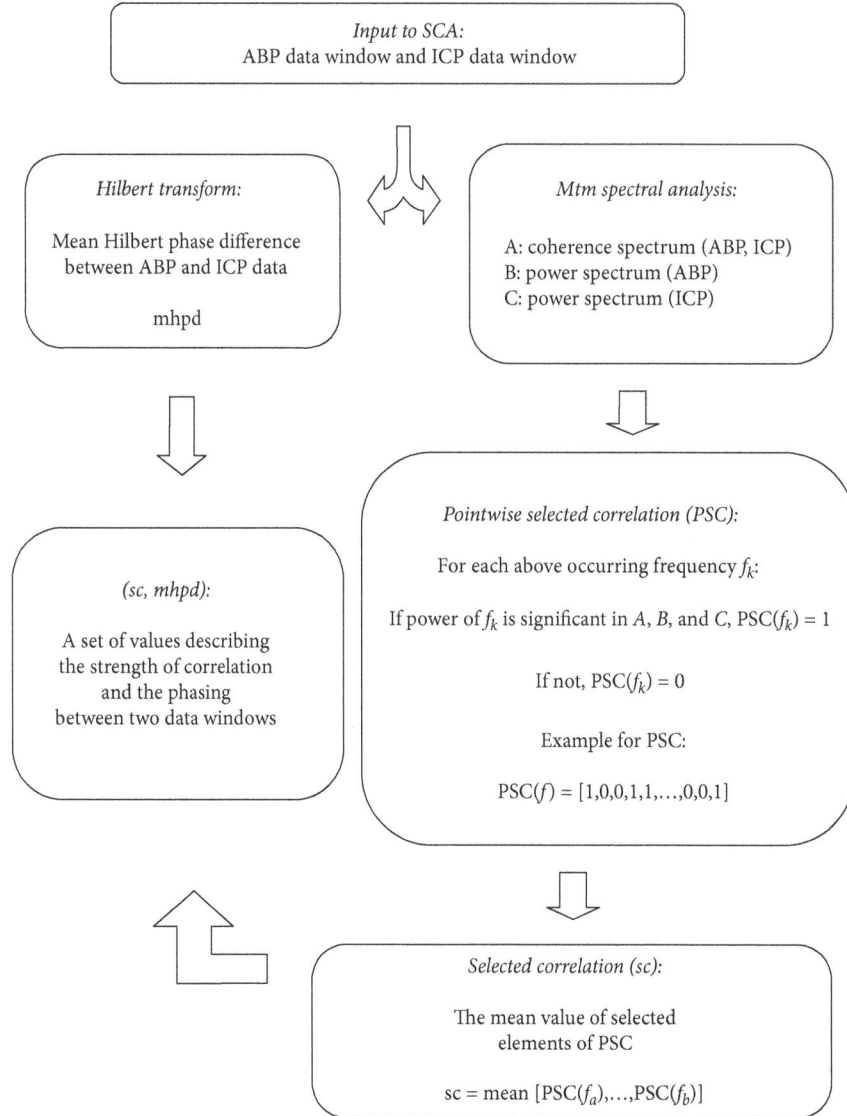

FIGURE 1: Selected correlation analysis (sca) illustrated as flowchart depicting the different elements of the method.

$$\text{mwa}^{s,R,m,n}(o) := \left(\frac{1}{R}\right) \sum_{i=1}^{i=R} \text{sc}^{s,m,n}(k_i, k_i + o),$$ (10)

with k_i random.

For offset o big enough to avoid autocorrelation, the values of mwa should become small and stable. With the knowledge of an appropriate offset o, we are able to calculate the error indices $ei^{s,m,n}(k, l, \text{lsc}, \text{lmhpd}_{\text{pos/neg}})$, for a predefined pair of thresholds (lsc, $\text{lmhpd}_{\text{pos/neg}}$) and a fixed pair of input windows with starting points k and l satisfying $l > k + o$:

$$ei^{s,m,n}\left(k,\, l,\, \text{lsc},\, \text{lmhpd}_{\text{pos}}\right)$$
$$:= \begin{cases} 1, & \text{if } \text{sc}^{s,m,n}(k,\, l) > \text{lsc} \wedge \text{mhpd}(k,\, l) < \text{lmhpd}_{\text{pos}}, \\ 0, & \text{otherwise}, \end{cases}$$
$$ei^{s,m,n}\left(k,\, l,\, \text{lsc},\, \text{lmhpd}_{\text{neg}}\right)$$
$$:= \begin{cases} 1, & \text{if } \text{sc}^{s,m,n}(k,\, l) > \text{lsc} \wedge \text{mhpd}(k,\, l) > \text{lmhpd}_{\text{neg}}, \\ 0, & \text{otherwise}. \end{cases}$$
(11)

Repeating this R times for different starting points leads to the error rate asc:

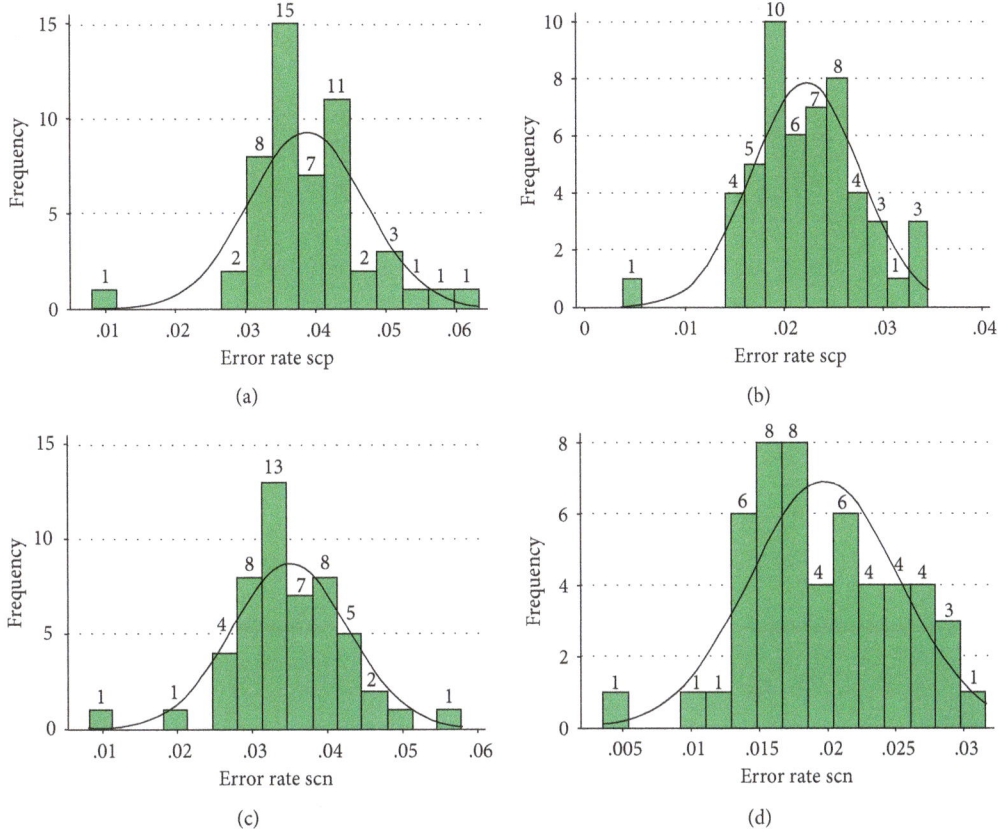

FIGURE 2: Frequency histograms illustrating the specific error rates for (a) scp lsc 0.056/lmhpd, (b) scp lsc 0.056/lmhpd 60, (c) scn lsc 0.056/lmhpd 110, and (d) scn lsc 0.056/lmhpd 120. The resulting error rates from all four parameter settings were defined to be normally distributed (modified Jarque–Bera test).

$$\mathrm{asc}^{s,R,m,n,o}\left(\mathrm{lsc},\ \mathrm{lmhpd}_{\mathrm{pos/neg}}\right)$$

$$:=\left(\frac{1}{R}\right)\sum_{i=1}^{i=R}ei^{s,m,n}\left(k_i,\ l_i,\ \mathrm{lsc},\ \mathrm{lmhpd}_{\mathrm{pos/neg}}\right), \qquad (12)$$

$$\text{with } k_i \text{ random: } l_i > k_i + o,$$

which indicates the percentage of obviously uncorrelated input windows that induce (sc, mhpd$_{\mathrm{pos/neg}}$) values higher than some predefined thresholds (lsc, lmhpd$_{\mathrm{pos/neg}}$). In other words, the error rate asc represents the percentage of false positives. Therefore, for a particular pair of thresholds (lsc, lmhpd$_{\mathrm{pos/neg}}$), we are now able to assign a significance to the detection of windows labeled scp or labeled scn:

$$\mathrm{sig}_{\mathrm{scp/scn}}\left(\mathrm{lsc},\ \mathrm{lmhpd}_{\mathrm{pos/neg}}\right)$$
$$=\left(1-\mathrm{asc}^{s,R,m,n,o}\left(\mathrm{lsc},\ \mathrm{lmhpd}_{\mathrm{pos/neg}}\right)\right)*100. \qquad (13)$$

2.3.2. Patient-Independent Statistics. Now, we can use the above-described method to calculate the significance for a specific pair of thresholds (lsc, lmhpd$_{\mathrm{pos/neg}}$) for a specific patient using the patient's ABP and ICP time series as input selecting an offset *o* big enough to avoid autocorrelation effects. However, if we apply the same approach to a different

patient, the result for the identical thresholds may slightly vary, due to the individual conditions of measurement setup and noise components. In order to determine a significance level for a specific pair of thresholds that is universally valid, we use the following approach.

For a fixed pair of thresholds (lsc, lmhpd$_{\mathrm{pos/neg}}$), we first calculate the appropriate error rates asc(lsc, lmhpd$_{\mathrm{pos/neg}}$) for each patient included in the study. Then, we check whether the distribution of the resulting error rate values is normal or not. In case of a normal distribution, we are able to deduce an upper limit lasc$^{\mathrm{up}}_{\mathrm{scp/scn}} = \mu + z \cdot \sigma$ from the one-sided prediction interval $[-\infty, \mu + z \cdot \sigma]$ for different probability levels $c(z) \in [0, 1]$ defined by the above-mentioned standard score z [16]. The upper limit of the one-sided prediction interval represents a value that assures that all future measurements will produce error rates lower than this value with a probability of $c(z)$. Thus, the patient-independent significance for this specific pair of thresholds could be defined as follows:

$$\mathrm{sig}^{\mathrm{indep}}_{\mathrm{scp/scn}} = c(z) * \left(1 - \mathrm{lasc}^{\mathrm{up}}_{\mathrm{scp/scn}}\right) * 100. \qquad (14)$$

2.3.3. Statistics of the Individual Error Rates. For each set of error rates asc(lsc, lmhpd$_{\mathrm{pos/neg}}$), we computed mean, median, maximal/minimal values, standard deviation and

TABLE 2: One-sided prediction intervals with upper limits of error rates for 90%, 95%, and 99% probability levels.

Analysis type	Prediction interval			Patient-independent significance
Scp	90%	95%	99%	
lsc 0.056/lsc 60	0.0294	0.0316	0.0357	95.41
lsc 0.056/lmhpd 70	0.0506	0.0541	0.0606	93.07
Scn				
lsc 0.056/lmhpd 120	0.0264	0.0285	0.0324	96.65
lsc 0.056/lmhpd 110	0.0459	0.0490	0.0550	93.57

Note. The resulting patient-independent significance values for scp and scn are listed in the last column.

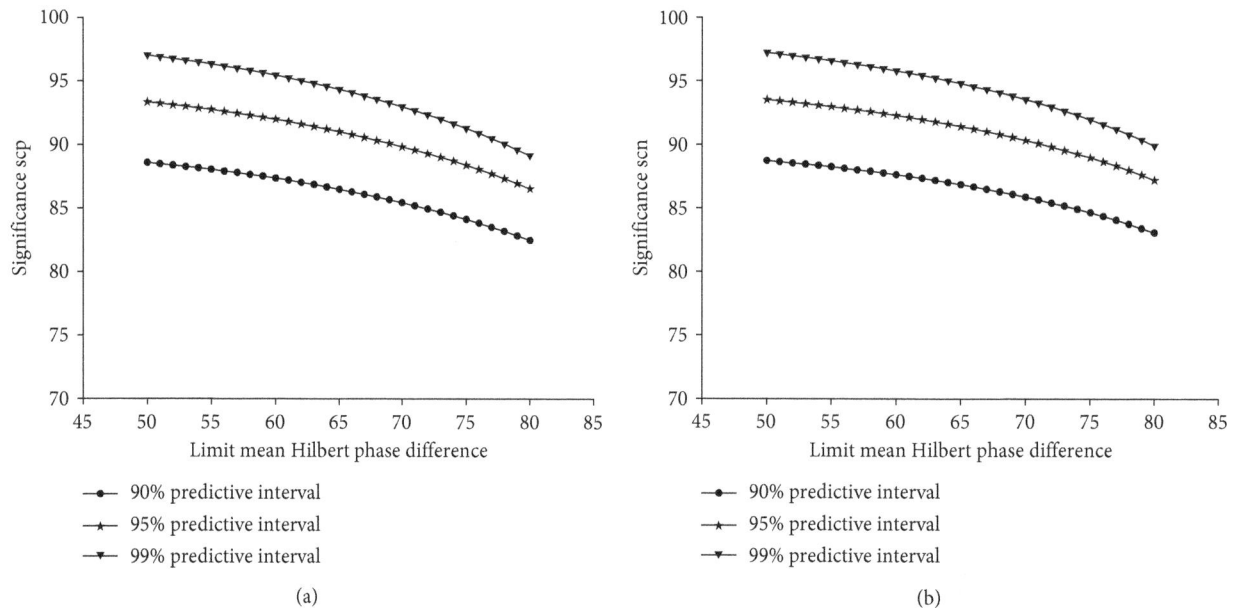

FIGURE 3: Relationship between patient-independent significance and mean Hilbert phase difference for scp (a) and scn (b).

error as well as variance, and 90–99% one-sided prediction intervals as population parameters. Subsequently, the error test results derived from different parameter settings of sca were analyzed for normal distribution using skewness–kurtosis testing (modified Jarque–Bera test). Differences in rates and proportions were analyzed by contingency tables and chi-square testing. Two-group comparisons were performed by computing Wilcoxon rank-sum tests.

3. Results

For the subsequent analysis, we used ABP and ICP data with sample frequency of 0.2 Hz and a window size s of 1024 points. The frequency band was set to $f \leq 0.00684$ Hz, an offset o of 5000 points was used, and R was set to one million [14]. With this, we calculated the error rates asc for different pairs of thresholds (lsc, $lmhpd_{pos/neg}$) consisting of the first 5 possible lsc values (0.000, 0.028, 0.056, 0.083, and 0.111) combined with lmhpd values from 50–80 degrees with a one-degree step size, for each patient separately.

The resulting error rate means for scp per parameter set ranged from 0.0033 to 0.205 and for scn from 0.0027 to 0.198. The scp-specific error rates were found to be normally distributed in a range of parameter settings from lsc

0.000/lmhpd 51 to lsc 0.111/lmhpd 50; in contrast, the scn-specific error rates were normally distributed from lsc 0.000/lmhpd 54 to lsc 0.083/lmhpd 66. Interestingly, the parameter settings, previously defined to be optimal for the clinical application of scp (lsc 0.056/lmhpd 70) [14], were found to be normally distributed for both scp- and scn-specific error test rates (Figure 2). To evaluate a threshold value, which would encompass any future patients for the error test result, we calculated the one-sided predictive intervals for 90–99% probability levels utilizing the error test results of our retrospective patient cohort [16]. The predictive intervals for both scp and scn analysis are listed in Table 2. Utilizing the upper limit of the 99% prediction interval would allow us to extrapolate that the error test result of any future patient will be within the determined interval with a probability of 99%. In addition, we calculated the resulting patient-independent significances according to the abovementioned formula. The results of this calculation are illustrated in Figure 3.

4. Discussion

The implementation of multimodal brain monitoring into neurointensive care management has two primary goals: (a) to detect reduced intracranial compliance due to brain edema, hydrocephalus, stroke, or intracranial hemorrhage [17] and (b) to uncover failure of the cerebral autoregulation [18, 19]. Since both aspects critically determine the therapeutic regimen, it would be ideal to have an integrative, computerized platform available, which unmasks these critical events in a timely fashion. Several indices focusing exclusively on autoregulation failure have been evaluated primarily to allow a more precise prognosis regarding mortality and functional outcome in patients with TBI and SAH [20]. Our approach, termed "selected correlation analysis" (sca) provides a mathematical tool set which allows the detection of both mechanisms, autoregulation failure and impaired intracranial compliance [13]. Regarding reduced intracranial compliance, we have validated our method utilizing a serial CT imaging approach [21]. In contrast, the sensitivity and specificity of autoregulation failure detection was substantiated by the comparison of our approach with the pressure reactivity index (PRx) as an established marker [12, 19]. One of the most significant drawbacks in time series analysis is type one error induced by autocorrelation effects, leading to potentially inadequate clinical treatment decisions [22, 23]. To ensure the exclusion of false-positive readings due to potential autocorrelation [24], we have implemented an error test into our method, which was hitherto calculated utilizing a retrospective patient cohort. However, for the bedside application of a sca monitor, it was mandatory to establish patient-independent significance levels for scp and scn. Statistically, this can be achieved by computing the prediction intervals of the 52 analyzed patients which would serve as a learning cohort. The upper patient-independent significance for the detection of scp deduced from the learning cohort does not profoundly differ from the values calculated for the sca parameter set optimization utilizing that cohort [14]. Additionally, the corresponding results for scn show very similar properties, and the applied statistical framework is capable of improving the resulting patient-independent significances with new patients added to the analysis and therefore enhancing the sample size. As a limitation of our study, the results of our error test calculation are based on a limited number of patients. It is conceivable that with increasing case numbers, the significances will be adjusted with the consequence of a higher sensitivity. In conclusion, our results provide a patient-independent pairs of threshold values for both scp and scn. Following the development of this patient-independent significance test for false-positive readings, we are now able to apply our method as a point of care system in a prospective fashion.

Conflicts of Interest

The authors declare that they have no conflicts of interest.

References

[1] J. Lok, W. Leung, S. Murphy et al., "Intracranial hemorrhage: mechanisms of secondary brain Injury," in *Intracerebral Hemorrhage Research*, J. H. Zhang and A. Colohan, Eds., pp. 63–68, Springer-Verlag Wien, Berlin, Germany, 2011.

[2] R. B. Borgens and P. Liu-Snyder, "Understanding secondary injury," *Quarterly Review of Biology*, vol. 87, no. 2, pp. 89–127, 2012.

[3] P. L. Reilly, "Brain injury: the pathophysiology of the first hours. 'Talk and Die revisited'," *Journal of Clinical Neuroscience*, vol. 8, no. 5, pp. 398–403, 2001.

[4] T. Zoerle, M. Carbonara, E. R. Zanier et al., "Rethinking neuroprotection in severe traumatic brain injury: toward bedside neuroprotection," *Frontiers in Neurology*, vol. 8, p. 354, 2017.

[5] A. H. Kramer and D. A. Zygun, "Neurocritical care: why does it make a difference?," *Current Opinion in Critical Care*, vol. 20, no. 2, pp. 174–181, 2014.

[6] J. Donnelly, M. Czosnyka, H. Adams et al., "Individualizing thresholds of cerebral perfusion pressure using estimated limits of autoregulation," *Critical Care Medicine*, vol. 45, no. 9, pp. 1464–1471, 2017.

[7] K. L. Kiening, W. N. Schoening, J. F. Stover, and A. W. Unterberg, "Continuous monitoring of intracranial compliance after severe head injury: relation to data quality, intracranial pressure and brain tissue PO_2," *British Journal of Neurosurgery*, vol. 17, no. 4, pp. 311–318, 2003.

[8] S. Jones, G. Schwartzbauer, and X. Jia, "Brain monitoring in critically neurologically impaired patients," *International Journal of Molecular Sciences*, vol. 18, no. 1, p. 43, 2016.

[9] G. Korbakis and P. M. Vespa, "Multimodal neurologic monitoring," in *Handbook of Clinical Neurology*, Vol. 140, pp. 91–105, Elsevier, New York, NY, USA, 2017.

[10] M. Böhm, R. Faltermeier, A. Brawanski, and E. W. Lang, "Mathematical modeling of human brain physiological data," *Physical Review E*, vol. 88, no. 6, p. 062711, 2013.

[11] A. Jung, R. Faltermeier, R. Rothoerl, and A. Brawanski, "A mathematical model of cerebral circulation and oxygen supply," *Journal of Mathematical Biology*, vol. 51, no. 5, pp. 491–507, 2005.

[12] M. A. Proescholdt, R. Faltermeier, S. Bele et al., "Detection of impaired cerebral autoregulation using selected correlation analysis: a validation study," *Computational and Mathematical Methods in Medicine*, vol. 2017, Article ID 8454527, 7 pages, 2017.

[13] R. Faltermeier, M. A. Proescholdt, S. Bele et al., "Windowed multitaper correlation analysis of multimodal brain monitoring parameters," *Computational and Mathematical Methods in Medicine*, vol. 2015, Article ID 124325, 8 pages, 2015.

[14] R. Faltermeier, M. A. Proescholdt, S. Bele et al., "Parameter optimization for selected correlation analysis of intracranial pathophysiology," *Computational and Mathematical Methods in Medicine*, vol. 2015, Article ID 652030, 7 pages, 2015.

[15] B. Babadi and E. N. Brown, "A review of multitaper spectral analysis," *IEEE Transactions on Biomedical Engineering*, vol. 61, no. 5, pp. 1555–1564, 2014.

[16] S. Geisser, "Non-Bayesian predictive approaches," in *Predictive Inference: An Introduction*, Chapman & Hall, New York, NY, USA, pp. 1–42, 1993.

[17] T. Howells, A. Lewen, M. K. Skold, E. Ronne-Engström, and P. Enblad, "An evaluation of three measures of intracranial compliance in traumatic brain injury patients," *Intensive Care Medicine*, vol. 38, no. 6, pp. 1061–1068, 2012.

[18] L. Rivera-Lara, A. Zorrilla-Vaca, R. G. Geocadin, R. J. Healy, W. Ziai, and M. A. Mirski, "Cerebral autoregulation-oriented therapy at the bedside: a comprehensive review," *Anesthesiology*, vol. 126, no. 6, pp. 1187–1199, 2017.

[19] M. Czosnyka and C. Miller, "Monitoring of cerebral autoregulation," *Neurocritical Care*, vol. 21, no. 2, pp. S95–S102, 2014.

[20] L. Rivera-Lara, A. Zorrilla-Vaca, R. Geocadin et al., "Predictors of outcome with cerebral autoregulation monitoring: a systematic review and meta-analysis," *Critical Care Medicine*, vol. 45, no. 4, pp. 695–704, 2017.

[21] R. Faltermeier, M. A. Proescholdt, and A. Brawanski, "Computerized data analysis of neuromonitoring parameters identifies patients with reduced cerebral compliance as seen on CT," in *Acta Neurochirurgica Supplementum*, vol. 114, pp. 35–38, Springer, Berlin, Germany, 2012.

[22] L. Glass and D. Kaplan, "Time series analysis of complex dynamics in physiology and medicine," *Medical Progress Through Technology*, vol. 19, no. 3, pp. 115–128, 1993.

[23] J. Arnau and R. Bono, "Autocorrelation problems in short time series," *Psychological Reports*, vol. 92, no. 2, pp. 355–364, 2003.

[24] A. Sivaganesan, G. T. Manley, and M. C. Huang, "Informatics for neurocritical care: challenges and opportunities," *Neurocritical Care*, vol. 20, no. 1, pp. 132–141, 2014.

20

Investigating the Relevance of Graph Cut Parameter on Interactive and Automatic Cell Segmentation

Kazeem Oyeyemi Oyebode [iD]**, Shengzhi Du** [iD]**, Barend Jacobus van Wyk,**
and Karim Djouani [iD]

Department of Electrical Engineering, Tshwane University of Technology, Pretoria, South Africa

Correspondence should be addressed to Shengzhi Du; dushengzhi@gmail.com

Academic Editor: Cristiana Corsi

Graph cut segmentation provides a platform to analyze images through a global segmentation strategy, and as a result of this, it has gained a wider acceptability in many interactive and automatic segmentation fields of application, such as the medical field. The graph cut energy function has a parameter that is tuned to ensure that the output is neither oversegmented (shrink bias) nor undersegmented. Models have been proposed in literature towards the improvement of graph cut segmentation, in the context of interactive and automatic cell segmentation. Along this line of research, the graph cut parameter has been leveraged, while in some instances, it has been ignored. Therefore, in this work, the relevance of graph cut parameter on both interactive and automatic cell segmentation is investigated. Statistical analysis, based on F1 score, of three publicly available datasets of cells, suggests that the graph cut parameter plays a significant role in improving the segmentation accuracy of the interactive graph cut than the automatic graph cut.

1. Introduction

Graph cut segmentation technique has become popular in recent times because of its ability in segmenting images into foreground and background using a global strategy. Therefore, it has become a useful tool in many segmentation application areas. One of such areas is the medical field, where the application of graph cut yields promising results in cell [1] and lung [2] segmentation. The automatic graph cut segmentation is useful as it speeds up cell segmentation, while the interactive segmentation provides the flexibility to select seed points when further investigation needs to be carried out in isolation. An example is the segmentation of an infected cell, in a particular region of an image.

The graph cut energy function is equipped with a parameter (λ) which can be tuned to ensure that objects are not oversegmented and undersegmented. The graph cut parameter has been explored and exploited in the area of interactive segmentation with good results [3–5]. Candemir and Akgul [3] proposed a model where object boundaries are extracted and are used to adapt the graph cut parameter around object boundaries, their approach is similar to the use of shape prior to adapt segmentation around object boundaries in order to mitigate the shrinkage of the object size after segmentation [4, 5]. The graph cut parameter can also be selected based on some predefined quality attributes of object [6]. In addition, Kirmizigul and Schlesinger [7] proposed an interactive segmentation approach where a range of λ is considered, and when there is a significant difference in segmentation output within a considered range of λ, a further division is carried out until segmentation outputs are almost the same within a given λ range. This may be considered as a trial and error approach where λ is initialized with a value and which is constantly increased until further increments does not yield any improvement. A similar approach to Candemir and Akgul [3] is investigated where a canny edge detector is used to obtain object boundaries, which is used to influence how weights are assigned to graph edges in the graph context [8].

Another method of interactive segmentation is proposed [9] where the parameter is learnt from the image. First, the user draws a line along the boundary of object to be segmented, then the object is then stripped and its pixel properties, such as cohesiveness, are learnt and used to inform the graph cut segmentation. The proposed interactive approach has the advantage of being able to segment a single object. However, when multiple objects are required to be segmented, the interaction with each object's boundaries may be a tedious task to undertake. The selection of λ based on experimental values, for cell segmentation, has also been researched [1]. A learning process for graph cut parameter is proposed [10] where segmentation is carried out iteratively. After each iteration, the segmentation result is compared with the ground truth, and then the graph cut parameters are adjusted in the next iteration to reflect an improved segmentation output over that obtained in the previous iteration. This is done until the recent segmentation output and the ground truth are almost similar. This approach to parameter learning may not be useful when ground truth of images is not available. Other related works [11–14] in respect of the selection of an appropriate parameter for image restoration have also been discussed. In addition, other approaches such as the Otsu thresholding, the k-means, and the template matching algorithms [15] have also been explored for cell segmentation. While some of the interactive segmentation methods proposed adapted λ in their graph cut methods, many automatic graph cut segmentation processes are carried out while ignoring the λ [16–18].

The focus of this paper is in three folds. Firstly, the relevance or the usefulness of graph cut parameter on graph cut segmentation is investigated. Admittedly, some existing researches have focused on investigating an optimal approach to graph cut parameter selection as discussed earlier. Secondly, the question of whether the graph cut parameter is useful to the investigation of both interactive and automatic segmentation is considered. This is a crucial consideration since most of the existing parameter selections focus on interactive segmentation only. Thirdly, the investigation of the effect of noise, on both interactive and automatic cell segmentation is carried out with respect to a constant λ. To the best of our knowledge, the investigation of the relevance of the graph cut parameter, in interactive and automatic cell segmentation, has not been carried out before.

2. Materials and Methods

2.1. A Graph.

A graph $G = (V, E)$, can be interpreted as having a set of nodes V and set of edges E. An example of this kind of graph is shown in Figure 1. In Figure 1, a, b, O, and B are nodes while O–a, a–B, b–B, a–b, and O–b are edges with corresponding weights 50, 20, 70, 18, and 22.

The idea behind the graph cut method is to discover, within a graphical network, the edge with the least flow capacity (edge with maximum flow, since the least capacity edge will have the maximum flow). A simple way to achieve this is to increase the flow (in this case liquid) from source node O to B (Figure 1). An edge capacity in the network may reach its saturation point, thereby be unable to accommodate further increase in the flow of liquid from O to B. At this point, the weakest link has been found in the network.

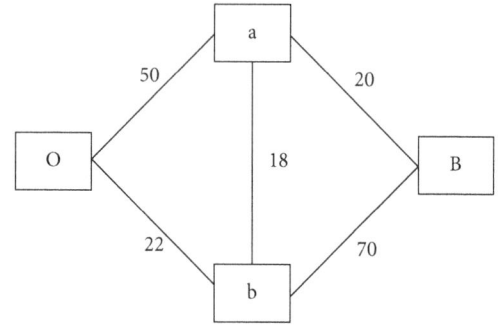

FIGURE 1: Weighted graph.

2.2. Graph Cut Segmentation.

The objective of graph cut segmentation is to assign a label $S \in \{0, 1\}$ to each pixel in a given image I where label "1" represents the foreground and "0" represents the background. Given I with observed grey-scale intensity level $M \in \{M_o, M_b\}$ (where M_o and M_b are observed foreground and background intensity levels), with x number of pixels, then the segmentation (S) of I into foreground and background, using the Bayesian model, is formulated in Equation (1), and I_a is the grey-scale intensity level of pixel a:

$$P(S \mid M) = \left(\prod_{a=1}^{x} P(I_a \mid S) * P(S) \right). \tag{1}$$

The maximum a posteriori (MAP) estimation for the segmentation of I is given in the following equation:

$$S_{\mathrm{MAP}} = \mathrm{argmax}_k \left(\prod_{a=1}^{x} P(I_a \mid S) * P(S) \right). \tag{2}$$

The negative logarithm of MAP in Equation (2) gives the following equation:

$$E(S) - \log \left(\prod_{a=1}^{x} P(I_a \mid S) \right) - \log P(S), \tag{3}$$

where $E(S)$ is the energy function that needs to be minimized in order to partition I into foreground and background. $E(S)$ can also be rewritten as seen in the following equation:

$$E(S) - \log \left(\prod_{a=1}^{x} -\log \left(P(I_a \mid S) \right) \right) - \log P(S). \tag{4}$$

In Equation (4), $-\log P(S)$ can be represented as a Markov Random Field (MRF) pairwise interaction between neighbouring pixels [19] a and b in Equation (5) where σ describes pixel similarity and N encapsulates neighbourhood pixels.

$$-\log P(S) = \sum_{(a,b) \in N} \exp \left(-\frac{I_a - I_b}{2\sigma^2} \right). \tag{5}$$

Therefore, the energy function can be rewritten as seen in the following equation:

$$E(S) = \lambda \left(\sum_{a=1}^{x} -\log\left(P\left(I_a \mid S\right)\right) \right) + \sum_{(a,b)\in N} \exp\left(-\frac{|I_a - I_b|^2}{2\sigma^2} \right). \tag{6}$$

In Equation (6), the first part of the equation is referred to as the data term while the second part is called the smoothness term. The parameter λ adjusts the relative importance of the data term to the smoothness term. There are several algorithms that can be used to minimize the energy function in Equation (6). One of such is the Ford Fulkerson algorithm [20]. Other algorithms [19, 21] are also proposed.

The Ford–Fulkerson [20] algorithm partitions a graph into two parts that are disjoint. In the image context, the image is partitioned into foreground (O) and background (B). The algorithm does this by finding the weakest link in a weighted graph network G of Figure 1. The weakest link(s) found globally (along the entire graph) invariably partition (s) the image into foreground and background. When this occurs, the algorithm has found the minimum cut (weakest link), where the maximum flow occurs. Assuming the data term in Equation (6) is used to assign weights to edges O–a, B–a, O–b, and B–b and the smoothness term is used to assign weight to the edge a–b in Figure (1), then Ford Fulkerson algorithm can be used to partition the graph into foreground (O) and background (B) as follows:

(1) Find the unsaturated path linking nodes O and B

(2) Saturate the discovered path with the minimum edge capacity in step 1

(3) Repeat steps 1 and 2 until all, path linking nodes O and B, are saturated

2.3. Investigating the Relevance of Graph Cut Parameter on Interactive and Automatic Cell Segmentation. The graph cut parameter within the context of the interactive and automatic segmentation on homogeneous, fairly homogeneous, and heterogeneous cell images is investigated. In both interactive and automatic cell segmentation strategies, the adaptation of the graph cut parameter is carried out at the cell boundaries in order to find out its relevance in mitigating the reduction in the size of objects (shrink bias). Shrink bias occurs when the boundary pixels of an object are absent after segmentation. It results in cells losing their actual size.

The approach of adapting the graph cut parameter, through object boundaries, is inspired by models discussed earlier [3, 4, 8], where the objective is to mitigate the shrink bias of graph cut. However, cell boundaries are extracted as discussed in [22]. Furthermore, the graph cut parameter value is varied to investigate its impact on the interactive and automatic graph cut segmentation. This approach is also similar to the model proposed in [7]. Equation (8) is used to adapt λ in Equation (7), while a_E is the set encapsulating boundary pixels (Equation (9)). Equation (9) shows how c is manipulated to adapt λ in Equation (8). In Equation (6), λ is set to 20, also in Equation (8), λ_1 is set to 20. An initial value

of 20 is selected to ensure the graph cut parameter is not too large nor not too small. In Equation (9), c_p is also set to 20.

$$E(S) = \lambda \left(\sum_{a=1}^{x} -\log\left(P\left(I_a \mid S\right)\right) \right) + \sum_{(a=1)\in N} \exp\left(-\frac{|I_a - I_b|}{2\sigma^2} \right), \tag{7}$$

$$\lambda = \lambda_1 * c, \tag{8}$$

$$c = \begin{cases} c_p, & a \in a_E \text{ at edge}(a - 0), \\ 0, & a \in a_E \text{ at edge}(a - B), \\ 1, & a \notin a_E. \end{cases} \tag{9}$$

The interactive segmentation provides a suitable platform to select foreground and background seed points on cell images. These seed points represent the observed intensity level M_O for foreground and M_B for background. Figure 2(b) shows how M_O and M_B are selected interactively. In addition, Figure 2(c) shows how M_O and M_B are selected automatically from the Otsu segmentation (white represents M_O and black represents M_B). M_O and M_B are used to build histograms of pixel intensity distribution for both foreground and background. These histograms are used to calculate the negative logarithm of the probability (data term in Equation (7)) of a given pixel intensity I_a being foreground (a–O) and background (a–B).

In the interactive approach, two types of interactive cell segmentation techniques are proposed. The first approach segments cell images with the static graph cut parameter (as observed in Algorithm 1), while the second segments with the adaptive graph cut parameter (Algorithm 2). As regards adapting λ on cell segmentation (Equation (7)), boundaries of cells are extracted as discussed in [22].

In the automatic cell segmentation, sample foreground and background pixels are selected automatically (Figure 2(c)). The selection is carried out on an Otsu segmented image to provide a coarse initial segmentation which serves as input for the selection of sample foreground and background pixels (seed points). This process is done automatically. The extraction of cell boundaries for the adaptation of graph cut parameter value is also undertaken as observed in [22]. This development gives rise to two kinds of automatic cell segmentation—the graph cut parameter when static λ (Algorithm 1) and the automatic cell segmentation (Algorithm 2) while adapting the graph cut parameter. In the evaluation section, the effect of noise on a given λ is also investigated.

3. Evaluation

The segmentation accuracies of the models are evaluated using the Accuracy Index (AI) metric (Equation (10)) and the F1scoremetric (Equation (11)). High values of AI and F1 score give good segmentation result. The F1 metric is also leveraged to investigate the statistical significance of a given model over another. The effect of noise is investigated on both interactive and automatic segmentation given a constant λ. The graph cut parameter is also varied to analyze its

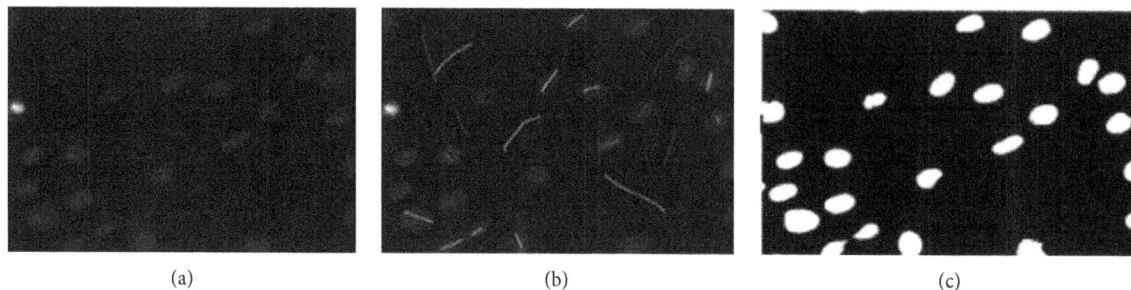

FIGURE 2: (a) Cell image. (b) Manual selection of sample foreground and background pixels. (c) Automatic selection of sample foreground and background pixels via Otsu thresholding.

impact on the interactive and automatic segmentation. Lastly, segmentation accuracies of models are also investigated under the Receiver Operating Characteristic (ROC) curves. The ROC curves give an account of the segmentation performance of a model using its false negative rate against its true positive rate. The Area Under the Curve (AUC) of a given ROC is then observed to determine its performance. An AUC close to 1 gives good segmentation output.

The AI metric evaluates segmentation accuracies based on the total number of correctly labeled pixels; it does not give an account of how a model performs based on its precision and recall, this is where the F1 metric becomes useful (Equation (11)), and it gives an account of how a model performs using the recall and precision. The ROC curves also investigate the performance of a model leveraging on its true positive and true negative rates.

Three publicly available datasets have been used for evaluation. The first is the U2OS [15] (1831 of fairly homogeneous cells of 49 images). The second is NIH3T3 [15] (2178 of heterogeneous cells of 49 images) while the third is the HT29 [23] (1291 of homogeneous cells of 24 images). These datasets are accompanied with their corresponding ground truths. Sample images of these datasets are shown in Figure 3. The graph cut algorithm proposed by Boykov and Jolly [21] is leveraged for the experiment, and its MATLAB implementation can be found in [24].

$$AI = \frac{TP + TN}{TP + TN + FP + FN}, \tag{10}$$

$$F1\ score = 2 \cdot \left(\frac{precision * recall}{precision + recall} \right), \tag{11}$$

$$precision = \left(\frac{TP}{TP + FP} \right), \tag{12}$$

$$recall = \left(\frac{TP}{TP + FN} \right). \tag{13}$$

True positive (TP) is the total number of foreground pixels found in the segmented image S (binary) that are found to be foreground pixels in the gold standard (ground truth) G. True negative (TN) is the total number of background pixels in the segmented image S that are found to be background pixels in G. False positive (FP) is the total number of foreground pixels in the segmented image S that are found to be background pixels in G. False negative (FN) is the total number of background pixels in the segmented image S that are found to be foreground pixels in G.

4. Results

4.1. Investigating the Relevance of Graph Cut Parameter on Interactive and Automatic Cell Segmentation. In Table 1 (where std is standard deviation), the segmentation results obtained by using the interactive graph cut segmentation is shown. It depicts that λ is both static and adaptive. On the U2OS dataset, it can be observed that the value of F1 (interactive segmentation) when λ is adaptive is high compared to when λ is static. This indicates that the shrink bias (reduction in the actual size) of graph cut is minimized when the graph cut parameter is adaptive. It can also be observed in Table 1, that is when λ is adaptive, a value for FN gives a score of 51947, whereas a score of 92152 is recorded when λ is static. This trend can also be observed in Tables 2 and 3. However, in Tables 4–6, one would notice that the F1 values are approximately the same when compared to the values of F1 in Tables 1–3.

In Tables 1–3, a reduction in the shrink bias of graph cut is observed (FN metric). There is a significant difference between the values of FN in the referenced tables. This is because the sample foreground pixels selected by the user (M_O) may not cover, sufficiently, the intensity levels of all foreground pixels in an image (including foreground boundary pixels). Hence, the introduction of adaptive λ helps to increase the edge weight (a–O) of pixels around cell boundaries and therefore reduces the graph cut shrink bias. The absence of this may result in cells losing their boundaries (after segmentation), culminating in the high FN value when λ is static (Tables 1–3). However, in Tables 4–6, the selection of foreground and background sample pixels are carried out automatically on an initial Otsu segmented image. This ensures that the variability of intensity levels of foreground pixels (M_O) is sufficiently captured. Thus, the assignment of edge weight reflects the true intensity level of pixels. As a result, adapting λ may have minimal effect on the shrink bias of graph cut as observed in F1 values in Tables 4–6. This analysis also applies to the AI index in all the six tables.

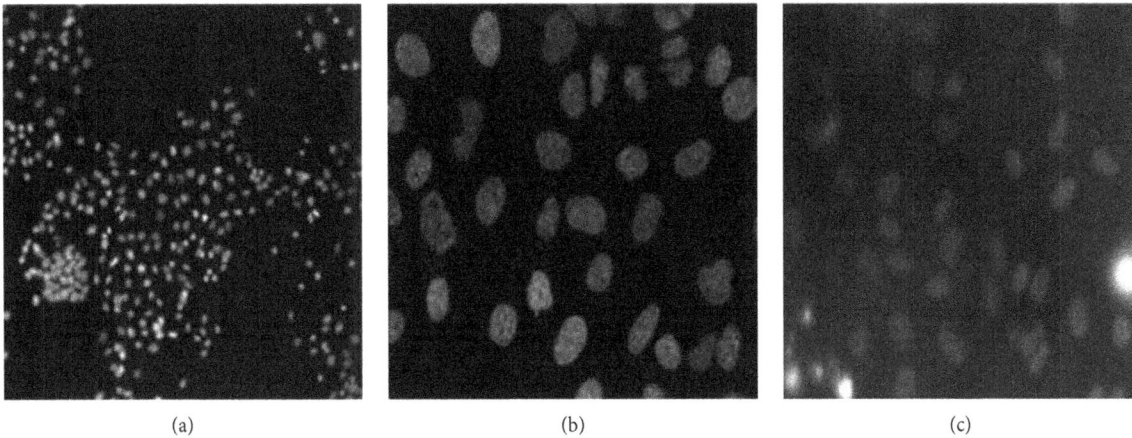

FIGURE 3: Sample dataset. (a) HT29. (b) U2OS. (c) NIH3T3.

```
(1)  Require: I grey scale image
(2)  Output: I_s segmented image
(3)  Build graph G from I
(4)  for each node a in G
(5)      λ = 20
(6)      Determine a's a–O edge weight (Figure 1) using the data term in Equation (6)
(7)      Determine a's a–B edge weight (Figure 1) using the data term in Equation (6)
(8)  end for
(9)  for each node a in G
(10)     determine a's a–b (neighbourhood) edge weight (Figure 1) using the smoothness term in Equation (6)
(11) end for
(12) Use algorithm in [21] to partition G into foreground (O) and background (B) to give I_s
```

ALGORITHM 1: Cell segmentation using Equation (6).

Figure 4 reinforces the argument, of the shrink bias, put forward. In Figure 4(b), an automatic segmentation of cells (Figure 4(f)) with adaptive λ is seen while in Figure 4(c), it is static. One can barely spot the differences in cell sizes in the two images. However, in Figures 4(d) and 4(e), there is a clear difference in cell sizes. The cells in Figure 4(d) appear bigger than that in Figure 4(e). It is obvious that cell boundaries are omitted in Figure 4(e) owing to the shrink bias of graph cut.

4.2. Statistical Significance Test of Accuracy. In order to investigate the significance of the difference in the accuracy of the interactive graph cut segmentation over the automatic graph cut model, a t-test is carried out on the F1 metric. The F1 metric is considered as it combines the precision and recall of any segmentation output. The t-test is a statistical test which indicates whether there exists a statistical significance in the segmentation accuracy of a given model over another using the F1 metric. If a p value obtained from the t-test > 0.05 [25], then there is no statistical significance in F1 metric between two models. However, if the t-test < 0.05, then there exists a statistical significance. Equation (14) gives the t-test formula:

$$t\text{-test} = \frac{M_2 - M_1}{\sqrt{(SD_2/N) - (SD_1/N)^2}}. \quad (14)$$

In Equation (14), M_2 and M_1 give the mean values of F1 score, N is the number of cell images in the considered dataset, and SD_2 and SD_1 are standard deviations of models in a considered table.

Table 7 shows the statistical significance of adapting graph cut parameter over the interactive and automatic segmentation. The interactive segmentation of cells when λ is adaptive shows statistical significance over when λ is static. Hence, the contribution of adaptive λ on interactive cell segmentation is significant in all the three datasets. However, there is no statistical significance over the automatic segmentation.

4.3. Varying Graph Cut Parameter on the Interactive and Automatic Segmentation. As observed in Figure 5(a), different segmentation accuracies are observed with different values of λ (1 to 400). This development shows that varying the graph cut parameter may influence segmentation output, confirming the claim in [21]. However, the significance of varying λ on automatic segmentation is negligible. One explanation to this is that the variability of the grey-scale intensity levels of foreground pixels is sufficiently captured

```
(1)  Require: I grey scale image
(2)  Output: I_s segmented image
(3)  Build graph G from I
(4)  for each node a in G
(5)  if (a ∈ a_E)
(6)      for edge a–O
(7)        c = 20
(8)        λ = 20 * 20 = 400 (Equation (8))
(9)        determine a's a–O edge weight (Figure 1) using the data term in Equation (7)
(10)     end for
(11)     for edge a–B
(12)       c = 0
(13)       λ = 20 * 0 = 0 (Equation (8))
(14)       determine a's a–B edge weight (Figure 1) using the data term in Equation (7)
(15)     end for
(16) else
(17)     c = 1
(18)     λ = 20 * 1 = 20 (Equation (8))
(19)     determine a's a–O edge weight (Figure 1) using the data term in Equation (7)
(20)     determine a's a–B edge weight (Figure 1) using the data term in Equation (7)
(21)  end if
(22) end for
(23) for each pixel a in G
(24)   determine a's a–b (neighbourhood) edge weight (Figure 1) using the smoothness term in Equation (7)
(25) end for
(26) Use algorithm in [21] to partition G into foreground (O) and background (B) to give I_s
```

ALGORITHM 2: Cell Segmentation using Equation (7).

TABLE 1: Interactive graph cut segmentation using the U2OS dataset.

Model	AI (%)	F1 (±std)	FN	FP	TP	TN
Interactive (λ static)	92.9	86 ± 4	92152	6779	302411	981087
Interactive (λ adaptive)	95.30	93.2 ± 2	51947	13132	340122	977925

TABLE 2: Interactive graph cut segmentation using the NIH3T3 dataset.

Model	AI (%)	F1 (±std)	FN	FP	TP	TN
Interactive (λ static)	82.9	65.5 ± 15	99621	134586	204291	937757
Interactive (λ adaptive)	85.4	73.8 ± 15	43497	156705	260414	915638

by the automatic selection of seed points. Hence, varying λ in order to add weights to graph edges may not be necessary. However, for interactive segmentation, λ may influence its segmentation output as its interactive method of seed selection may not have covered sufficiently the variability of foreground intensity levels.

4.4. Lambda (λ) Performance on Noisy Cell Images. As observed in Figure 5(b), the increase in the intensity of "salt and pepper" noise, given that λ has a constant value of 20, has a negative effect on the segmentation output on both interactive and automatic segmentation.

4.5. Receiver Operating Characteristic (ROC) Curves. Figure 6 shows the Receiver Operating Characteristic (ROC) curves for the three datasets (interactive segmentation).

Table 8 also shows the Area under Curve (AUC) for the ROC curves. The AUC close to 1 suggests good segmentation result.

Table 9 compares the best segmentation outputs from Tables 1–6 to existing segmentation models. The Otsu thresholding which is used to autoselect seed points for the automatic segmentation has segmentation outputs of 92/74/89 on U2OS, NIH3T3, and HT29 datasets, respectively. The merging algorithm has 96 % segmentation accuracy on the U2OS dataset; hence, it outperforms the best result of 95.3 % obtained from Tables 1–6.

5. Discussion

The outcome of the investigation, carried out on the three publicly available datasets, suggests that the graph cut parameter (λ) plays a significant role in improving the

TABLE 3: Interactive graph cut segmentation using the HT29 dataset.

Model	AI (%)	F1 (±std)	FN	FP	TP	TN
Interactive (λ; static)	93.5	77 ± 18	16300	735	29335	215772
Interactive (λ adaptive)	95.46	86 ± 9	10566	1331	36496	213750

TABLE 4: Automatic graph cut segmentation using the U2OS dataset.

Model	AI (%)	F1 (±std)	FN	FP	TP	TN
Automatic (λ static)	93.96	89 ± 3	75452	7584	321519	976087
Automatic (λ adaptive)	94	88.2 ± 4	75052	7601	315401	978199

TABLE 5: Automatic graph cut segmentation using the NIH3T3 dataset.

Model	AI (%)	F1 (±std)	FN	FP	TP	TN
Automatic (λ static)	85.3	70 ± 13	88923	113328	214989	959015
Automatic (λ adaptive)	85.8	70 ± 14	76778	117835	227133	954508

TABLE 6: Automatic graph cut segmentation using the HT29 dataset.

Model	AI (%)	F1 (±std)	FN	FP	TP	TN
Automatic (λ static)	96	88 ± 1	3019	7419	40043	212428
Automatic (λ adaptive)	96	88 ± 1	3019	7420	40043	212430

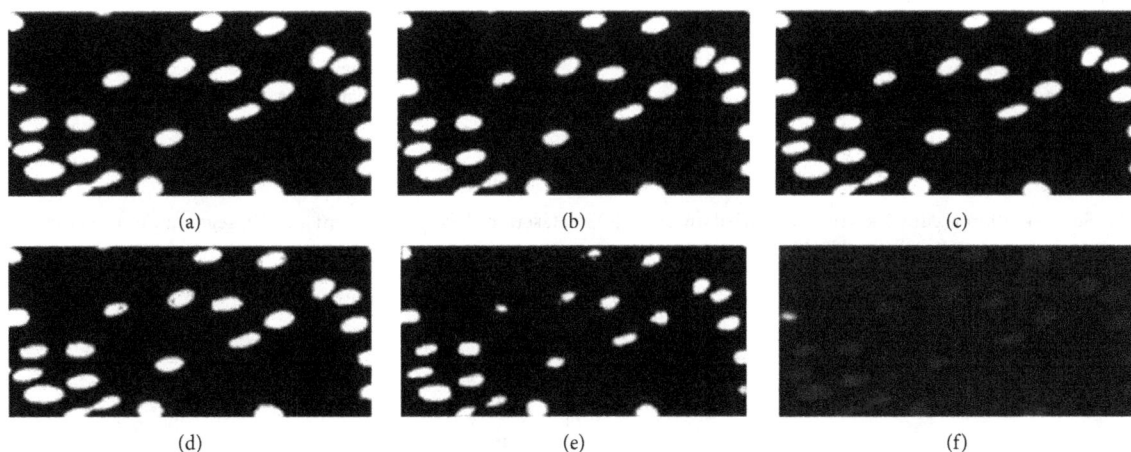

FIGURE 4: (a) Ground truth. (b) Automatic segmentation with adaptive λ. (c) Automatic segmentation with static λ. (d) Interactive segmentation with adaptive λ. (e) Interactive segmentation with static λ. (f) Original image.

segmentation accuracy and the reduction of graph cut shrink bias on interactive cell segmentation. However, its impact on automatic segmentation is negligible. Where appropriate tools have been deployed with a view to enhancing the output of automatic graph cut segmentation, the accuracy of automatic graph cut segmentation may not be significantly affected where λ is ignored. Thus, λ plays a significant role in interactive graph cut segmentation, although the performance of both (interactive and automatic segmentation) could be adversely affected by cell-image noise. Automatic graph cut segmentation is useful as it speeds up cell segmentation. However, when an area of an image is subjected to further investigation, in isolation, then the interactive

segmentation has its own advantage because it enables seed points to be selected interactively.

The automatic graph cut segmentation outperforms the interactive segmentation for one reason. As can be observed in Figures 2(b) and 2(c), the automatic segmentation captures the variability of foreground intensity levels better than the interactive segmentation.

6. Conclusion

This paper has investigated the relevance of the graph cut parameter (λ) in interactive and automatic graph cut cell segmentation strategies (using more than 5000 cells). Based

TABLE 7: Statistical significance test.

Model	T-test	p value	Statistical significance F1 score
Interactive (λ adaptive and static) U2OS	11.25	0.01	86 is statistically significant over 93.2
Automatic (λ adaptive and static) U2OS	1.11	0.2	89 is not statistically significant over 88.2
Interactive (λ adaptive and static) NIH3T3	2.7	0.01	65.5 is statistically significant over 73.8
Automatic (λ adaptive and static) NIH3T3	0	0.2	70 is not statistically significant over 70
Interactive (λ adaptive and static) HT29	2.1	0.02	77 is statistically significant over 86
Automatic (λ adaptive and static) HT29	0	0.2	88 is not statistically significant over 88

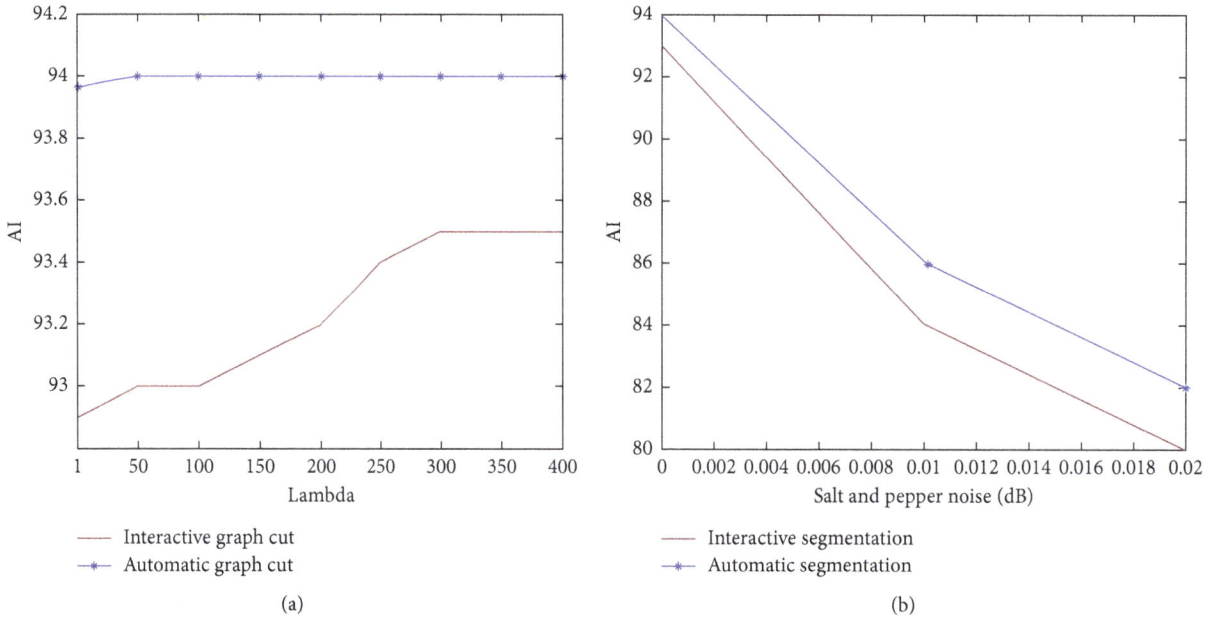

(a)

(b)

FIGURE 5: (a) Segmentation accuracies when λ is varied on the U2OS dataset. (b) Given a constant λ of 20, segmentation accuracy decreases with increase in noise intensity on the U2OS dataset.

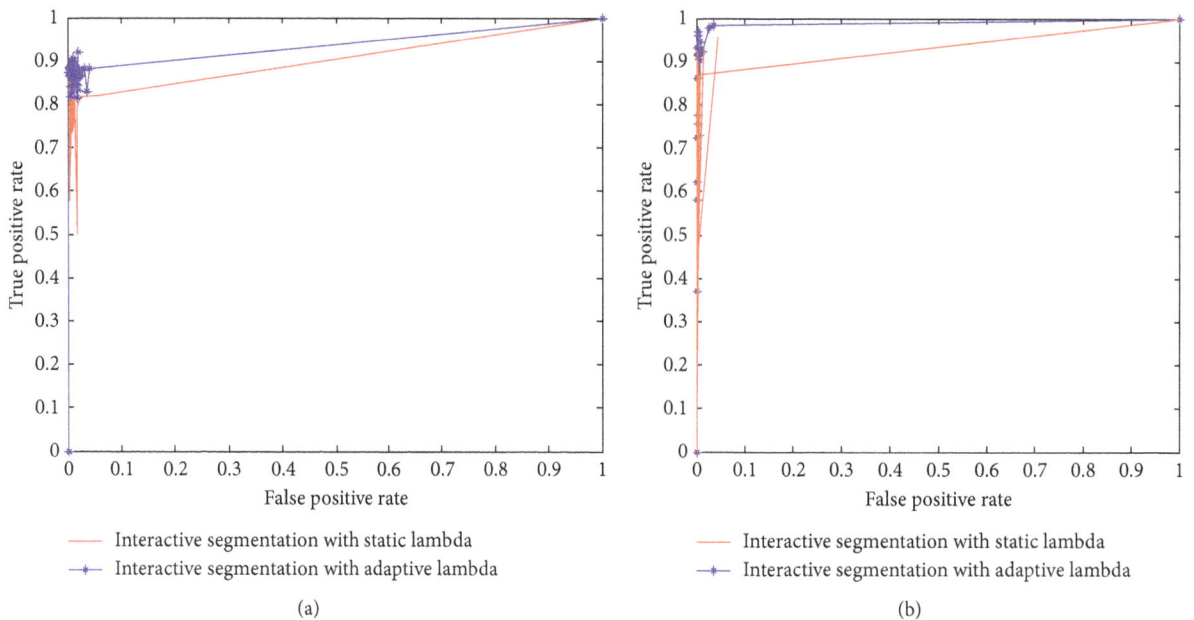

(a)

(b)

FIGURE 6: Continued.

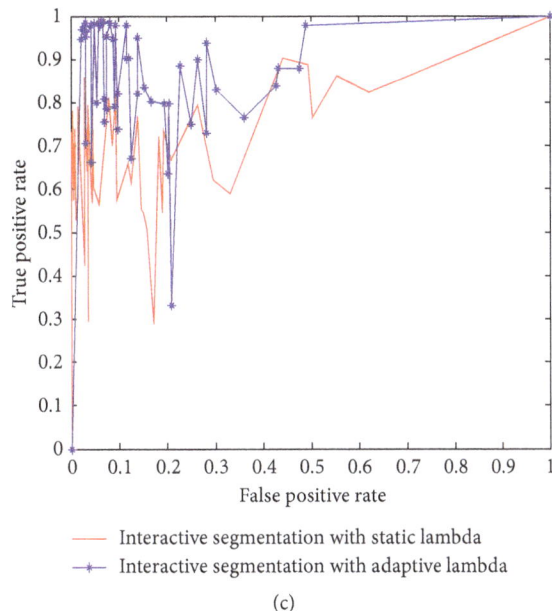

(c)

FIGURE 6: ROC curves for the interactive segmentation when λ is static and adaptive on the (a) U2OS dataset. (b) HT29 dataset. (c) NIH3T3 dataset.

TABLE 8: Automatic graph cut segmentation using the U2OS dataset.

Dataset	Area under curve
U2OS interactive (λ static)	0.95
U2OS interactive (λ adaptive)	0.96
HT29 interactive (λ static)	0.97
HT29 interactive (λ adaptive)	0.98
NIH3T3 interactive (λ static)	0.74
NIH3T3 interactive (λ adaptive)	0.84

TABLE 9: Comparison of segmentation models.

Model	AI % (U2OS/NIH3T3/HT29)
Otsu thresholding [15]	92/74/89
Watershed [15]	91/78/-
Merging algorithm [15]	**96/83/-**
K-means	92.4/83/89.3
Best results from Tables 1–6	95.3/**85.8/96**

on the investigation performed, this establishes three novel conclusions: (1) the adaptation of the graph cut parameter across various regions of the cell image minimizes the shrink bias of the interactive graph cut segmentation; (2) the adaptation of the graph cut parameter value may significantly improve segmentation performance for the interactive graph cut than the automatic graph cut; and (3) the presence of noise on cell images may reduce the performance of a chosen graph cut parameter value.

image dataset HT29 has been referenced in [23]. In addition, these datasets can be downloaded from https://data.broadinstitute.org/bbbc/BBBC008/ or from the corresponding author upon request.

Conflicts of Interest

The authors declare that they have no conflicts of interest.

Acknowledgments

This work was supported in part by the National Research Foundation of South Africa (Grant nos. 92468 and 93539).

References

[1] A. Massoudi, A. Sowmya, K. Mele, and D. Semenovich, "Employing temporal information for cell segmentation using max-flow/min-cut in phase-contrast video microscopy," in *Proceedings of International Conference of the IEEE EMBS*, pp. 5985–5988, Boston, MA, USA, August 2011.

[2] S. Dai, K. Lu, and J. Dong, "Lung segmentation with improved graph cuts on chest CT images," in *Proceedings of 3rd IAPR Asian Conference on Pattern Recognition (ACPR)*, pp. 241–245, Kuala Lumpur, Malaysia, November 2015.

[3] S. Candemir and Y. S. Akgul, "Adaptive regularization parameter for graph cut segmentation," in *Proceedings of Conference on Image Analysis and Recognition (ICIAR)*, pp. 117–126, Póvoa de Varzim, Portugal, June 2010.

[4] D. Freedman and T. Zhang, "Interactive graph cut based segmentation with shape priors," in *Proceedings of IEEE Computer Society Conference on Computer Vision and Pattern Recognition (CVPR)*, pp. 755–762, San Diego, CA, USA, June 2005.

[5] S. Vicente, V. Kolmogorov, and C. Rother, "Graph cut based image segmentation with connectivity priors," in *Proceedings of IEEE Conference on Computer Vision and Pattern Recognition (CVPR)*, pp. 1–8, Anchorage, AK, USA, June 2008.

[6] B. Peng and O. Veksler, "Parameter selection for graph cut based image segmentation," in *Proceedings of British Machine*

Vision Conference (BMVC), pp. 1–10, Leeds, UK, September 2008.

[7] D. Kirmizigul and D. Schlesinger, "Incremental learning in the energy minimisation framework for interactive segmentation," *Lecture Notes in Computer Science*, vol. 332, pp. 323–332, 2010.

[8] T. Wang, Z. Ji, Q. Sun, Q. Chen, and H. Shoudong, "Image segmentation based on weighting boundary information via graph cut," *Journal of Visual Communication and Image Representation*, vol. 33, pp. 10–19, 2015.

[9] A. Blake, C. Rother, M. Brown, P. Perez, and P. Torr, "Interactive image segmentation using an adaptive GMMRF model," *Lecture Note in Computer Science*, vol. 3021, pp. 428–441, 2004.

[10] M. Szummer, P. Kohli, and D. Hoiem, "Learning CRFs using graph cuts," *Lecture Notes in Computer Science*, vol. 5303, pp. 582–595, 2008.

[11] P. G. Nikolas and K. K. Aggelos, "Methods for choosing the regularization parameter and estimating the noise variance in image restoration and their relation," *IEEE Transactions on Image Processing*, vol. 1, no. 3, pp. 322–336, 1992.

[12] A. M. Thompson, J. C. Brown, J. W. Kay, and D. M. Titterington, "A study of methods of choosing the smoothing parameter in image restoration by regularization," *IEEE Transactions on Pattern Analysis and Machine Intelligence*, vol. 13, no. 4, pp. 326–339, 1991.

[13] D. Watzenig, B. Brandstatter, and G. Holler, "Adaptive regularization parameter adjustment for reconstruction problems," *IEEE Transactions on Magnetics*, vol. 40, no. 2, pp. 1116–1119, 2004.

[14] B. Hong, J. Koo, H. Dirks, and M. Burger, "Adaptive regularization in convex composite optimization for variational imaging problems," in *Proceedings of German Conference on Pattern Recognition*, pp. 268–280, Basel, Switzerland, September 2017.

[15] L. P. Coelho, A. Shariff, and R. Murphy, "Nuclear segmentation in microscope cell images: a hand-segmented dataset and comparison of algorithms," in *Proceedings of IEEE International Symposium on Biomedical Imaging (ISBI)*, pp. 518–521, Boston, MA, USA, June 2009.

[16] Y. Al-Kofahi, W. Lassoued, W. Lee, and B. Roysam, "Improved automatic detection and segmentation of cell nuclei in histopathology images," *IEEE Transactions on Biomedical Engineering*, vol. 57, no. 4, pp. 841–852, 2010.

[17] S. Dimopoulos, E. M. Christian, R. Y. Fabian, and S. Y. Joerg, "Accurate cell segmentation in microscopy images using membrane patterns," *Bioimage Informatics*, vol. 30, no. 18, pp. 2644–2651, 2014.

[18] R. Kechichian, H. Gong, M. Revenu, O. Lezoray, and M. Desvignes, "New data model for graph-cut segmentation: application to automatic melanoma delineation," in *Proceedings of IEEE International Conference on Image Processing (ICIP)*, pp. 892–896, Paris, France, October 2014.

[19] Y. Boykov and V. Kolmogorov, "An experimental comparison of min-cut/max flow algorithms for energy minimization in vision," *IEEE Transactions on Pattern Analysis and Machine Intelligence*, vol. 26, no. 9, pp. 1124–1137, 2004.

[20] L. Ford and D. R. Fulkerson, *Flows in Networks*, Princeton University Press, Princeton, NJ, USA, 1986.

[21] Y. Boykov and M.-P. Jolly, "Interactive graph cuts for optimal boundary and region segmentation of objects in n-d images," in *Proceedings of IEEE International Conference on Computer Vision (ICCV)*, pp. 105–112, Vancouver, Canada, July 2001.

[22] K. O. Oyebode and J. Tapamo, "Adaptive parameter selection for graph cut-based segmentation on cell images," *Image Analysis and Stereology*, vol. 35, no. 1, pp. 29–37, 2016.

[23] V. Ljosa, K. L. Sokolnicki, and A. E. Carpenter, "Annotated high-throughput microscopy image sets for validation," *Nature Methods*, vol. 10, no. 5, pp. 6–37, 2012.

[24] R. Gadde and R. Yalamanchili, *Tech Geek*, 2011, https://masterravi.wordpress.com/2011/05/24/interactive-segmentation-using-graph-cutsmatlab-code/.

[25] Table a-3., 2018, http://www.math.odu.edu/stat130/t-tables.pdf.

Permissions

List of Contributors

Hao Liu and Puming Zhang
School of Biomedical Engineering, Shanghai Jiao Tong University, Shanghai 200240, China

Jung Jun Lee, Jae-Hwan Jhong and Ja-Yong Koo
Department of Statistics, Korea University, Seoul 02841, Republic of Korea

Sung Hwan Kim
Department of Applied Statistics, Konkuk University, Seoul 05029, Republic of Korea

Mireya S. García-Vázquez
Instituto Politécnico Nacional-CITEDI, Tijuana, BC, Mexico

Jessica Beltrán
Instituto Politécnico Nacional-CITEDI, Tijuana, BC, Mexico
CONACYT, Ciudad de México, Mexico

Jenny Benois-Pineau
LaBRI, University of Bordeaux, Bordeaux, France

Luis Miguel Gutierrez-Robledo
Instituto Nacional de Geriatría, Ciudad de México, Mexico

Jean-François Dartigues
INSERM, University of Bordeaux, Bordeaux, France

Zhihua Huang
College of Mathematics and Computer Science, Fuzhou University, Fuzhou, China

Minghong Li
Department of Physiology, Yunnan University of Traditional Chinese Medicine, Kunming, China

Yuanye Ma
Kunming Institute of Zoology, CAS, Kunming, China

Hongjuan Gao
College of Information Science and Technology, Northwest University, Xi'an, China
College of Xinhua, Ningxia University, Yinchuan, China

Guohua Geng and Wen Yang
College of Information Science and Technology, Northwest University, Xi'an, China

Michael D. Vasilakakis and Dimitris K. Iakovidis
Department of Computer Science and Biomedical Informatics, University of Thessaly, Lamia, Greece

Evaggelos Spyrou
Department of Computer Science and Biomedical Informatics, University of Thessaly, Lamia, Greece
Institute of Informatics and Telecommunications, National Center for Scientific Research "Demokritos", Athens, Greece

Anastasios Koulaouzidis
Endoscopy Unit, The Royal Infirmary of Edinburgh, Edinburgh, UK

Alessandra Paffi, Francesca Camera, Chiara Carocci, Francesca Apollonio and Micaela Liberti
Sapienza University of Rome, Via Eudossiana 18, 00184 Rome, Italy

Xiaoli Zhu, Wanci Li and Wansheng Wang
Invasive Technology Department, The First Affiliated Hospital of Soochow University, No. 899, Pinghai Road, Suzhou, Jiangsu 215006, China

Zhao Ran and Xin Gao
Department of Medical Imaging, Suzhou Institute of Biomedical Engineering and Technology, Chinese Academy of Sciences, No. 88, Keling Road, Suzhou, Jiangsu 215163, China

Kangshun Zhu and Wensou Huang
Department of Minimally Invasive Interventional Radiology, The Second Affiliated Hospital of Guangzhou Medical University, No. 250, Changgang East Road, Guangzhou, Guangdong 510260, China

Ashkan Sharabiani and Houshang Darabi
Department ofMechanical and Industrial Engineering, University of Illinois at Chicago, Chicago, IL, USA

Edith A. Nutescu
Department of Pharmacy Systems Outcomes and Policy and Center for Pharmacoepidemiology and Pharmacoeconomic Research, University of Illinois at Chicago, Chicago, IL, USA

William L. Galanter
Department of Pharmacy Systems Outcomes and Policy and Center for Pharmacoepidemiology and Pharmacoeconomic Research, University of Illinois at Chicago, Chicago, IL, USA

Department of Medicine, University of Illinois at Chicago, Chicago, IL, USA

Jingming Xia, Yiming Chen and Aiyue Chen
School of Electronics and Information Engineering, NanjingUniversity of Information Science and Technology, Nanjing 210044, China

Yicai Chen
School of Mechanical Engineering, North China Electric Power University, Hebei 071000, China

Syed Muhammad Anwar
Department of Software Engineering, University of Engineering and Technology, Taxila, Pakistan

Maheen Gul and Muhammad Majid
Department of Computer Engineering, University of Engineering and Technology, Taxila, Pakistan

Majdi Alnowami
Department of Nuclear Engineering, King Abdulaziz University, Jeddah, Saudi Arabia

Francesco Montefusco
Department of Information Engineering, University of Padova, Padova, Italy

Morten Gram Pedersen
Department of Information Engineering, University of Padova, Padova, Italy
Department of Mathematics "Tullio Levi-Civita", University of Padova, Padova, Italy
Padova Neuroscience Center, University of Padova, Padova, Italy

Xinpei Wang, Chang Yan, Changchun Liu and Peng Li
School of Control Science and Engineering, Shandong University, Jinan, Shandong 250061, China

Bo Shi
Department of Medical Imaging, Bengbu Medical College, Bengbu, Anhui 233030, China

Chandan Karmakar
School of Information Technology, Deakin University, Burwood, VIC 3125, Australia

Zhennao Cai and Jianhua Gu
School of Computer Science and Engineering, Northwestern Polytechnical University, Xi'an 710072, China

Caiyun Wen
Department of Radiology, The First Affiliated Hospital of Wenzhou Medical University, Wenzhou, Zhejiang 325035, China

Dong Zhao
College of Computer Science and Technology, Changchun Normal University, Changchun 130032, China

Chunyu Huang
College of Computer Science and Technology, Changchun University of Science Technology, Changchun 130032, China

Hui Huang, Changfei Tong, Jun Li and Huiling Chen
College of Mathematics, Physics and Electronic Information Engineering, Wenzhou University, Wenzhou, Zhejiang 325035, China

Ali Ghanbarzadeh
Department of Medical Radiation Engineering, Tehran Science and Research Branch, Islamic Azad University, Tehran, Iran

Majid Pouladian
Department of Biomedical Engineering, Tehran Science and Research Branch, Islamic Azad University, Tehran, Iran

Ali Shabestani Monfared
Cancer Research Center, Medical Physics Department, Babol University of Medical Sciences, Babol, Iran

Seied Rabi Mahdavi
Radiobiology Research Center, Department of Medical Physics, Iran University of Medical Sciences, Tehran, Iran

Caroline W. Kanyiri
Department of Mathematics, Pan African University Institute of Basic Sciences, Technology and Innovation, Nairobi, Kenya

Kimathi Mark
Department of Mathematics, Machakos University, Machakos, Kenya

Livingstone Luboobi
Institute of Mathematical Sciences, Strathmore University, Nairobi, Kenya

Haihua Jiang and Bin Hu
Faculty of Information Technology, Beijing University of Technology, Beijing 100124, China

Zhenyu Liu, Xiaoyu Li and Huanyu Kang
Gansu Provincial Key Laboratory of Wearable Computing, School of Information Science and Engineering, Lanzhou University, Lanzhou 730000, China

Gang Wang
Beijing Anding Hospital of Capital Medical University, Beijing 100088, China

Lan Zhang
Lanzhou University Second Hospital, Lanzhou 730030,
China

**Francisco Gómez-Vela and Domingo S. Rodriguez-
Baena**
Division of Computer Science, Pablo de Olavide
University, 41013 Seville, Spain

José Luis Vázquez-Noguera
Carrera de Ingeniería Informática, Universidad
Americana, Asunción, Paraguay

**Rupert Faltermeier, Martin A. Proescholdt, Sylvia
Bele and Alexander Brawanski**
Department of Neurosurgery, University Hospital
Regensburg, Regensburg, Germany

Stefan Wolf
Department of Neurosurgery, University Hospital
Charite, Berlin, Germany

**Kazeem Oyeyemi Oyebode, Shengzhi Du, Barend
Jacobus van Wyk and Karim Djouani**
Department of Electrical Engineering, Tshwane
University of Technology, Pretoria, South Africa

Index

www.ingramcontent.com/pod-product-compliance
Lightning Source LLC
Chambersburg PA
CBHW080534200326
41458CB00012B/4432